CLINICAL DATA INTERPRETATION IN ANAESTHESIA AND INTENSIVE CARE

Dedication

We would like to dedicate this book to our ever optimistic wives who allowed us to work on it in the belief that it would pay for a luxurious retirement.

Commissioning Editor: Michael Parkinson
Project Development Manager: Jim Killgore
Project Manager: Nancy Arnott
Designer: Erik Bigland

CLINICAL DATA INTERPRETATION IN ANAESTHESIA AND INTENSIVE CARE

Edited by

Stephen Bonner MRCP FRCA

Consultant in Anaesthesia & Intensive Care Medicine
James Cook University Hospital
Middlesbrough, UK

Chris Dodds MRCGP FRCA

Consultant in Anaesthesia & Sleep Medicine
James Cook University Hospital
Middlesbrough, UK

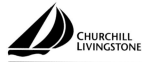
CHURCHILL
LIVINGSTONE

EDINBURGH LONDON NEW YORK PHILADELPHIA ST LOUIS SYDNEY
TORONTO 2002

CHURCHILL LIVINGSTONE
An imprint of Harcourt Publishers Limited

© Harcourt Publishers Limited 2002

◗◗ is a registered trademark of Harcourt
Publishers Limited

The right of S Bonner and C Dodds to be
identified as editors of this work has been
asserted by them in accordance with the
Copyright, Designs and Patents Act 1988

First published 2002

ISBN 0443-06453-9

British Library Cataloguing in Publication Data
A catalogue record for this book is available from
the British Library

**Library of Congress Cataloging in
Publication Data**
A catalog record for this book is available from
the Library of Congress

Note
Medical knowledge is constantly changing. As
new information becomes available, changes in
treatment, procedures, equipment and the use
of drugs become necessary. The editors,
contributors and the publishers have taken care
to ensure that the information given in this text is
accurate and up to date. However, readers are
strongly advised to confirm that the information,
especially with regard to drug usage, complies
with the latest legislation and standards of
practice.

The
publisher's
policy is to use
**paper manufactured
from sustainable forests**

Printed in China

PREFACE

The role of the anaesthetist continues to expand, beyond that of perioperative physician to acute and chronic pain specialist and critical care physician. Such an expanding role demands clinical knowledge across the breadth of hospital specialities. Anaesthetists need to rapidly interpret and judge clinical situations in intensive care or accident & emergency at all times of day and night and often in isolation, adding further pressure on decision making. This exposure is heightened by the impact of the changes in our training system. The reduction in the hours of work for trainee doctors and the shortened duration of training means that trainees have less exposure to large quantities of clinical data. In addition more consultants are finding themselves inspecting a cranial CT scan on an intubated patient at 2am, or being called to ITU to deal with an acute arrhythmia. Recent years have also seen an explosion in investigative tests, yet the benefits and pitfalls of these are rarely expounded even in current CPD journals. This book grew out of a desire to provide ongoing CPD in clinical data interpretation for both consultants as well as trainees, together with an insight into some newer methods of investigations, of relevance to Anaesthesia.

Of equal concern is that the interpretation of clinical data has often been poorly taught during anaesthesia training and has been poorly served in educational material. Yet such data is increasingly prevalent in all current clinical examinations in anaesthesia, both in the OSCEs as well as clinical vivas. The ability to rapidly interpret and act on such clinical data subsequently becomes central to clinical practice as a specialist. The topics covered in this book reflect important areas in examinations as well as providing an aid to theatre based teaching for both trainees and trainers.

The book aims to cover specific areas of current practice in anaesthesia, critical care and pain control, by providing a series of questions centred around a clinical scenario. Each clinical scenario is based around the need to interpret a piece of clinical data, followed by a series of self assessment questions meant to test your knowledge of the subject discussed. Answers and discussions are given at the end of each chapter. A table of normal values is also given. Further reading is given to encourage investigation of the area discussed in definitive texts beyond the scope of this book. The investigations used in these areas of practice are reviewed in the introduction to each chapter to highlight their utility and value as well as their limitations. However, each piece of data has been selected because of its direct applicability and usefulness in daily clinical practice in Anaesthesia or critical care as well as its appearance in the examinations. Emphasis is repeatedly placed on the need to understand the clinical picture before making judgements of any pieces of investigative data.

We would be grateful for notification of any errors or omissions in this book and hope that it provides a useful, stimulating and educational tool for consultants and trainees alike in all fields of anaesthesia and critical care.

Middlesbrough   S.B.
2002   C.D.

ACKNOWLEDGEMENTS

The editors would like to thank Richard Bore and Katie Whittam, superintendent radiographers for their help with data collection. We would also like to thank Les Maxwell, head of medical illustration and Zoe Jade Price, trainee photographer, for their help with data copying.

Stephen Bonner would like to thank Dr Andy Burns, SpR in Maxillofacial surgery for data collection of facial trauma. James De Courcy would like to thank Drs Tim Nash and Paddy Clarke for loan of images. Alistair Gascoigne would like to thank Rita Markawat, Senior Medical Technician for the pulmonary function tests and Dr DL Richardson FRCR, for his kind input on the radiology.

The systematic method of CTG interpretation described in the obstetric chapter is based on the ALSO (Advanced Life Support in Obstetrics) teaching format.

The editors would also like to thank all the patients who have given their consent for the publication of their photographs in this book.

CONTRIBUTORS

Kathryn Bell MRCP FRCA
Consultant Anaesthetist
Royal Victoria Infirmary
Newcastle upon Tyne, UK

Stephen Bonner MRCP FRCA
Consultant in Anaesthesia & Intensive
Care Medicine
James Cook University Hospital
Middlesbrough, UK

Nick Bradey FRCR
Consultant Neuroradiologist
Middlesbrough General Hospital
Middlesbrough, UK

Fiona Clarke FRCA
Consultant in Anaesthesia & Intensive
Care Medicine
James Cook University Hospital
Middlesbrough, UK

James de Courcy DCH FRCA
Consultant in Pain Management and
Anaesthesia
Cheltenham General Hospital
Cheltenham, UK

Chris Dodds MRCGP FRCA
Consultant in Anaesthesia & Sleep Medicine
James Cook University Hospital
Middlesbrough, UK

Fiona Gamlin MRCP FRCA
Consultant Anaesthetist with an interest in
vascular anaesthesia
St James University Hospital
Leeds, UK

Alistair Gascoigne BSc FRCP
Consultant in Intensive Care and
Respiratory Medicine
Royal Victoria Infirmary
Newcastle upon Tyne, UK

Richard Hartley FRCR
Consultant Radiologist
James Cook University Hospital
Middlesbrough, UK

Phil Kane FRCS
Consultant Neurosurgeon
Middlesbrough General Hospital
Middlesbrough, UK

Andy Kilner FRCA
Consultant in Anaesthesia & Intensive
Care Medicine
Freeman Hospital
Newcastle upon Tyne, UK

Moira McCarthy FRCR
Consultant Radiologist
James Cook University Hospital
Middlesbrough, UK

David Michael Ryall MB ChB FRCA
Consultant Anaesthetist
James Cook University Hospital
Middlesbrough, UK

Elizabeth Ryall MB ChB MRCOG
Consultant Obstetrician & Gynaecologist
University Hospital of North Tees
Stockton on Tees, UK

David Ryan FRCA
Consultant Clinical Physiologist
General Intensive Care Unit
Freeman Hospital
Newcastle upon Tyne, UK

Chris Snowden BMed. Sci. FRCA
Consultant & Senior Lecturer in
Anaesthesia
Freeman Hospital
Newcastle upon Tyne, UK

Mike Tremlett FRCA
Consultant Anaesthetist
James Cook University Hospital
Middlesbrough, UK

Jonathan Wyllie FRCP
Consultant Paediatrician
James Cook University Hospital
Middlesbrough, UK

CONTENTS

1

RESPIRATORY DISEASE

INTRODUCTION

The diagnosis and management of patients with respiratory disease involves the careful interpretation of a full medical history, a detailed clinical examination and the results of investigations, guided by the history and examination. In an examination setting, data interpretation should also be guided by the clinical information provided in the question. Therefore, it is vital that the question is read carefully and that data and radiographs are studied in a systematic manner.

CHEST RADIOGRAPHS

The chest X-ray (CXR) is common in the FRCA examinations and may involve laterals as well as the standard postero-anterior (PA) film. All films should be examined in a structured manner. A checklist should be employed to avoid missing important pathology, particularly when a more obvious abnormality of lesser significance may be present.

Since the CXR represents a two-dimensional image of a three-dimensional object, an understanding of basic anatomy is required to identify normal structures and the position of abnormalities. A systematic approach ensures that nothing is missed. The patient's history, in addition to name, age, gender and race, should be noted. Film projection should be noted since mobile or anteroposterior (AP) films can lead to apparent cardiomegaly as a result of magnification. Other features of AP projected films may include elevation of the clavicles, horizontal ribs and encroachment of the scapulae into the lung fields.

Appreciation of the penetration of the film is important before commenting on shadows in the lung fields. A good guide is that the intervertebral discs should just be visible through the heart in a normal exposure. The degree of rotation of the patient should also be commented on when taking into account apparent abnormalities of the mediastinum and hilar regions. The position of the patient should be noted; this is particularly important when commenting on pneumothoraces or pleural effusions on a supine film.

The next step is to examine the X-ray clinically in a sequential order. Normal PA and lateral CXRs are shown in Figure 1.1. Lateral films are taken rarely and are only required to identify structures in the lungs or behind the heart. The precise order in which a CXR is studied is debatable, depending upon the needs of the speciality and personal preference. The Advanced Trauma and Life Support (ATLS) protocol dictates 'bones, soft tissue, diaphragm, heart, mediastinum and lung fields'. Anaesthetists are used to dealing with trauma patients and this may be a suitable order. As your career progresses into Intensive Care, this may change to lung fields first, as this is where most abnormalities are found, but it remains important not to miss out any other part of the CXR. For examination purposes, it is recommended to start by saying that this is a PA CXR, well centred and penetrated etc., and then pointing out the most obvious pathology. The examiner will move you on if necessary.

Clearly, interpretation must take into account clinical information along with the data given from various investigations, but always remember that common things are common. The detection of certain abnormalities may be of great importance in anaesthesia and should not be missed. In the event of no apparent abnormality being identified, the following may have been missed by the first assessment and should be sought:

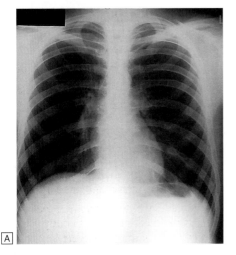

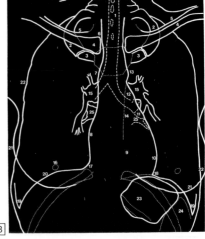

1	Air in trachea	7	Sup. vena cava	13	Aortic knuckle or knob	19	Lat. costophrenic angles
2	First rib	8	R. atrium	14	Lat. border of descending	20	R. cupola of diaphragm
3	First costal cartilage	9	R. ventricle		thoracic aorta	21	Breast shadow
4	Clavicles	10	L. ventricle	15	Pulmonary artery	22	Lat. border of throacic cage
5	Skin line over clavicles	11	L. auricle (auricular	16	R. nipple	23	Fundal air bubble
6	R. brachiocephalic v.		appendage of l. atrium)	17	Inf. vena cava	24	Spleen
	(innominate v.)	12	Pulmonary trunk (conus)	18	L. cardiophrenic angle	25	Pulmonary veins

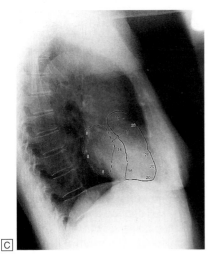

1	Trachea	6	Descending thoracic aorta	11	Site of l. atrium	16.	Vertebral body of T4
2	L. main bronchus	7	Pulmonary outflow tract	12	Site of l. ventricle	17	Vetebral body of T11
3	R. main bronchus	8	R. main pulmonary a.	13	Horizontal fissure	18	Inf. angle of scapula.
4	Ascending thoracic aorta	9	L. main pulmonary a.	14	R. oblique fissure		
5	Aortic arch	10	Site of r. ventricle	15	L. oblique fissure		

Fig. 1.1 A, B: Normal postero-anterior chest X-ray (CXR) and corresponding annotated diagram. Although the CXR is commonly viewed in clinical practice, it is still easy to miss subtle abnormalities if a system is not used. Certain areas deserve special attention, including apices, behind the heart shadow, hilae and costophrenic angles. Note that the right heart border is composed of the superior vena cava, right atrium and inferior vena cava, whilst the left heart border is formed from the aortic knuckle, pulmonary conus, left atrial appendage and left ventricle. C, D: The normal lateral CXR and corresponding annotated diagram. (Reproduced with permission from Weir J, Abraham PH 1986 *The Atlas of Radiological Anatomy*. Churchill Livingstone, Edinburgh.)

- small apical pneumothoraces
- rib fractures
- things behind the heart (is there a lateral chest X-ray?)
- correct position of lines, tubes or other foreign bodies
- hiatus hernia
- below the diaphragm
- the neck and trachea.

COMPUTED TOMOGRAPHY (CT) SCAN

The study of CT scans also requires knowledge of anatomy and interpretation in the light of the clinical details available. The image obtained is computer-generated and shows a coronal representation of a section through the chest. The main uses are in the identification of mediastinal disease, staging of carcinoma of the lung, and identification of interstitial lung disease. Scans are often performed following intravenous contrast, which enhances vascular organs as well as the major blood vessels. High-resolution scans can be performed which provide sections of the thorax down to a few millimetres in thickness, allowing for improved resolution of the interstitium and lung parenchyma. Pulmonary angiography may be combined with high-resolution CT scanning to delineate thrombi in the pulmonary arteries.

PULMONARY FUNCTION TESTS

Most tests of pulmonary function assess the expiratory phase of respiration. All pulmonary function tests can be expressed as a comparison with the mean reference value and standard deviation obtained in a healthy population, usually as a percentage of the population mean. The most commonly employed investigations are peak expiratory flow rate (PEFR), forced expiratory volume in one second (FEV_1) and forced vital capacity (FVC) obtained by performing spirometry.

PEFR can be used in assessing patients with obstructive airways disease and can be used as a simple bedside guide to the degree of reversibility with inhaled beta-agonists. A much forgotten but useful clinical tool is the forced expiratory time, which is also a reflection of obstruction to expiratory flow.

The interpretation of spirometry is one of simple pattern recognition. The patient is asked to take a maximal inspiration and then expire through the spirometer as fast and for as long as he or she is able, producing a volume–time curve. The two commonest patterns obtained at spirometry are of obstructive and restrictive defects. Various other abnormalities are sometimes detected on the spirograph, and are usually brought about by leakage around the mouth, the patient coughing or making further inspiratory effort (Fig. 1.2).

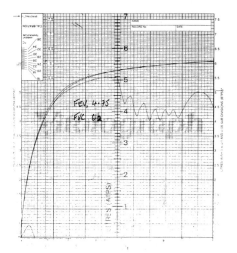

Fig. 1.2 Normal spirometry including one trace where the patient is coughing.

An obstructive defect is one where the ratio of FEV_1 to FVC is less than 75%. The curve has a characteristic nature, and in situations where the patient is able to expire for longer than the machine can move, an apparent spike is seen at the end of the curve (Fig. 1.3). A restrictive defect is seen when the FEV_1:FVC ratio is normal but there is a reduction in the absolute values compared with the normal population. A restrictive pattern will be seen following pneumonectomy, lung collapse, large pleural effusion, interstitial lung disease, mechanical deformity of the chest and neuromuscular weakness.

Patients with a condition that would usually be associated with a restrictive defect may also have obstructive spirometry if they have smoked or have asthma. Spirometry is also a useful tool in the detection of large airways obstruction, producing a straight line in the volume–time curve indicating the maximal flow that can be generated across the obstruction.

the maximal flow generated with increasing concavity of the expiratory limb as the severity of the obstruction increases (Fig. 1.5). The second pattern to recognise is that seen in large airways obstruction, where the peak expiratory flow may be reduced but is sustained throughout most

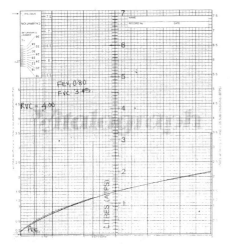

Fig. 1.3 A clearly obstructive spirogram where the patient continues to expire after the trace has finished. The true forced vital capacity is shown by the spike at the end of the trace and is therefore recorded as 3.45 L.

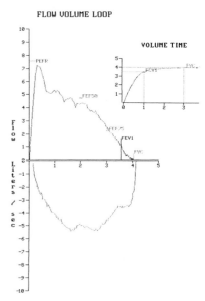

Fig. 1.4 Normal flow-volume curve.

FLOW-VOLUME CURVES

Usually, flow-volume curves are regarded with a degree of trepidation by non-respiratory physicians. However with a basic understanding of how they are generated, they are usually easy to interpret, since diagnosis is again by pattern recognition. The test involves the patient taking a maximal inspiratory effort from residual volume to total lung capacity. The patient then performs a forced expiratory manoeuvre back to residual volume. The resultant flow volume curve is then pictured on the data oscilloscope (Fig. 1.4).

The patterns described are related to both obstructive and inspiratory defects. Obstructive defects exhibit two main patterns. The first is of small airways obstruction, where there is a reduction in

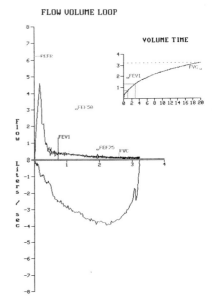

Fig. 1.5 Typical flow-volume curve seen in chronic obstructive pulmonary disease.

of expiration in a plateau manner (Fig. 1.6). This pattern is seen typically in extrathoracic obstruction. (The pattern seen in restrictive disease is characterised simply by a reduction in flow and volume as expressed against a normal population.)

Abnormalities of inspiratory flow are far less common, the main defect described being one of a late inspiratory tail seen in unilateral main stem bronchial narrowing.

DIFFUSION CAPACITY (TRANSFER FACTOR)

Tests which assess the ability of the lungs to extract oxygen usually rely on the strong affinity of carbon monoxide for haemoglobin. The precise details of the test are not required in the interpretation of the data. Two techniques are in use: single breath and steady state. Both employ the use of low-concentration carbon monoxide to assess diffusion capacity and helium to assess alveolar ventilation. The two results provided are the total lung capacity to absorb carbon monoxide (T_LCO) and the diffusion constant (KCO) which assesses the diffusion capacity per unit of lung volume. Both T_LCO and KCO can be expressed as a percentage, in comparison to a normal population taking age, gender and height into account.

Characteristically, T_LCO is reduced in circumstances where the ability of the lung to absorb oxygen is reduced. This occurs where there is loss of effective alveolar ventilation, including pulmonary oedema and pneumonia, and conditions where there is an increase in the effective distance the oxygen has to diffuse, such as interstitial fibrosis. T_LCO will also be reduced in situations where there is a total loss of lung parenchyma, such as emphysema, lobectomy and pneumonectomy. The KCO will be preserved in cases of lobectomy or pneumonectomy but not in emphysema, as in the former, the remaining lung has normal diffusion per unit volume, whereas in the latter the lung is reduced in volume and diffusion capacity.

In addition to this, there are several catches. In situations where there is effectively more haemoglobin to bind carbon monoxide, the KCO will be increased. These conditions include polycythaemia and alveolar haemorrhage. KCO may also be increased in asthma and neuromuscular weakness, as there may be increased blood per unit volume of lung.

VENTILATION–PERFUSION SCANS

Ventilation–perfusion scans may be used in both static and dynamic circumstances. The test employs the inhalation of an inert gas, such as xenon-133, followed by an intravenous injection of technetium-99m-labelled microalbumin aggregates. Both elements emit gamma radiation which can be detected easily. The initial phase is of ventilation. The patient takes several breaths of the radioactive gas, and images are taken at the time of inhalation and at equilibrium to demonstrate preferential

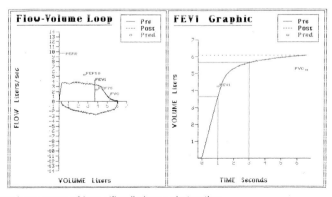

Fig. 1.6 Flow-volume curve of large 'fixed' airway obstruction.

areas of ventilation. Serial images are then obtained over time to identify delay in the washout of xenon-133, which is indicative of air trapping and thus of obstructive airways disease. During the perfusion scan, blood should flow preferentially to areas of the lung which are ventilated; the matching of ventilation and perfusion is then observed by comparing the two scans (Fig. 1.7). A chest radiograph should be taken at the same time as the scan in order to exclude pathology, as significant abnormality of the lungs may negate interpretation of the scan.

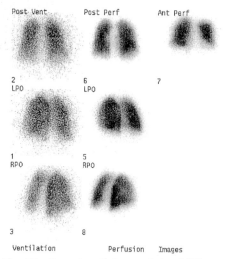

Fig. 1.7 Normal ventilation–perfusion (V/Q) scan.

Various patterns are recognisable in differing clinical states. Matched defects in both ventilation and perfusion, corresponding to a lobar or segmental distribution, are seen characteristically in lobar collapse or pneumonia. A matched defect may not correspond to an anatomical defect, such as in a pleural effusion. Multiple matched defects may be seen in patients with severe obstructive pulmonary disease identified by significant washout delay of the xenon 133 and may also be seen in interstitial lung disease and pulmonary oedema.

Ventilation–perfusion scans are characteristically used in the diagnosis of pulmonary emboli. In this situation, there will be multiple defects in perfusion with near normal ventilation (Fig. 1.8). The resulting scan is often expressed in terms of probability of pulmonary embolus, the number and size of defects being taken into consideration.

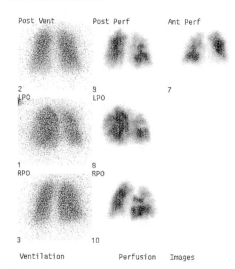

Fig. 1.8 Ventilation/perfusion (V/Q) scan showing multiple perfusion defects seen in multiple pulmonary emboli.

In situations where there is a right-to-left shunt, e.g. atrial septal or ventricular septal defects, the kidneys and liver will be highlighted on the perfusion scan owing to the aggregates passing into the systemic circulation.

Perfusion scans may also be quantitative in nature to assess the relative perfusion in patients with borderline lung function who are being considered for pneumonectomy. The correlation of relative perfusion with the pulmonary function likely to remain following surgery allows prediction of the viability of surgery in borderline cases.

FURTHER READING

Alexander RH, Proctor HJ 1997 *Advanced Trauma Life Support Student Manual*. American College of Surgeons, Chicago.

Bourke SJ, Brewis RAL 1998 *Lecture Notes on Respiratory Medicine*, 5th edn. Blackwell Science, Oxford.

Brewis RAL, Corrin B, Geddes DM, Gibson GJ 1995 *Respiratory Medicine*, 2nd edn. WB Saunders, London.

QUESTIONS

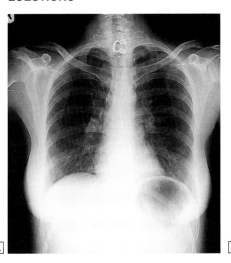
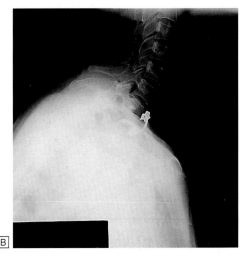

Question 1.1

You are called to A&E to see a 34-year-old woman who is in respiratory distress and complaining of a choking sensation. She says this happened shortly after the restoration of a dental crown. Her CXR is shown (A) together with lateral c. spine film (B).

a. Describe the CXR and lateral neck. What is the position of the foreign body?
b. Will a Heimlich manoeuvre help?
c. How should this be removed? What are the anaesthetic considerations?

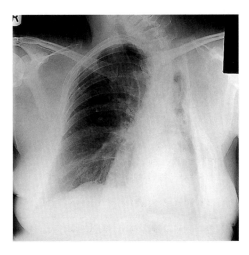

Question 1.2

You are asked to assess a patient with a previous history of tuberculosis for dental extractions under general anaesthesia. She presents with early morning confusion, somnolence and ankle swelling. Her CXR is shown.

a. Explain the radiographic abnormalities and their clinical consequences.
b. Why do you think she is confused?
c. What simple test, other than arterial blood gas analysis, may help to confirm your suspicions?

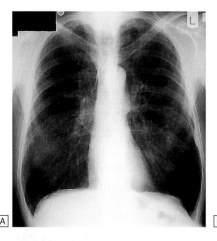 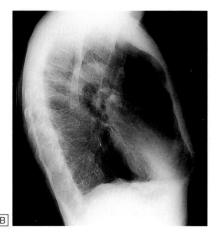

Question 1.3

A 67-year-old man is scheduled for repair of his inguinal hernia. On closer questioning he reveals a history of haemoptysis. His PA and lateral CXRs are shown in (A) and (B), respectively.

a. Describe the CXRs.
b. What are the underlying diagnoses?
c. Describe the pattern of spirometry and relative values of diffusion capacity that you would expect in this man.
d. How would you propose to anaesthetise this man?

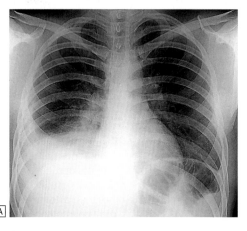 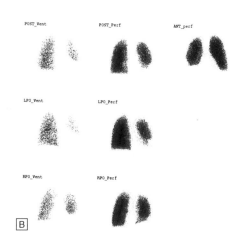

Question 1.4

A 25-year-old man is scheduled for emergency cholecystectomy. You see him on the ward and discover that he was in fact admitted 3 days ago with right-sided pleuritic chest pain. He had an ultrasound scan of his abdomen which showed gallstones and he has also had a ventilation–perfusion scan. On examination, you find an unwell-looking pyrexial man who is short of breath and his oxygen saturation is 90% on air. His CXR and V/Q scan are shown in (A) and (B), respectively.

a. What do the scan and CXR show and what further information would you request?
b. What is the probable diagnosis and what other features of the history may be pertinent?

Question 1.5

A patient is referred for complicated dental extractions requiring general anaesthesia. He is known to be on oxygen at home on an ad hoc basis. The only other thing of note is that he has complained of occasional transient loss of vision in the left eye. Clinically he is overweight and has signs of obstructive pulmonary disease. His oxygen saturation is 87% on air but there are no other abnormal findings. His lung function results are shown below:

- FEV_1 = 1.8 L (40% of predicted)
- FVC = 3.2 L (60% of predicted)
- T_LCO is 50% and KCO 125% of predicted.

a. What is the likely interpretation of the lung function tests?
b. What implications are there for anaesthesia?

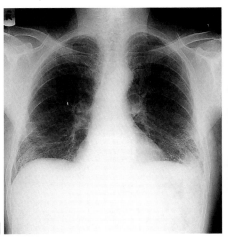
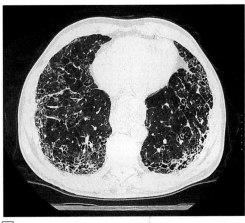

A B

Question 1.6

A 67-year-old man is referred to you for your anaesthetic opinion. He is scheduled for repair of a large non-reducible inguinal hernia. He complains of shortness of breath on going up stairs but little else. Clinically there are widespread crackles on auscultation. A CXR and CT scan of his chest are shown in (A) and (B), respectively, and his pulmonary function tests are as below:

- FEV_1 = 3.8 L (96% of predicted)
- FVC = 5.9 L (117% of predicted)
- T_LCO is 37% of predicted
- KCO is 35% of predicted.

a. What does the chest radiograph (A) show?
b. Explain the lung function tests in this context.
c. What does the CT scan (B) show?

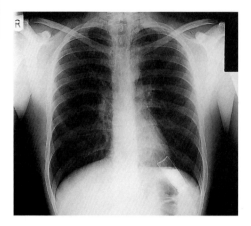

Question 1.7

You are called to A&E to see a young boy who is admitted short of breath. He has just had a prolonged bout of coughing and is complaining of crackling in his ears. His CXR is shown.

a. What are the radiological abnormalities and what are the most likely diagnoses?
b. From this, can you say what is the likely pattern of spirometry?
c. How has this happened?

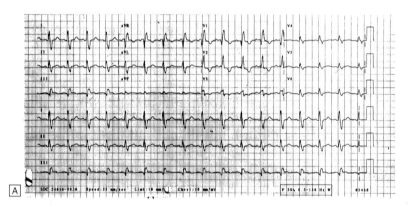

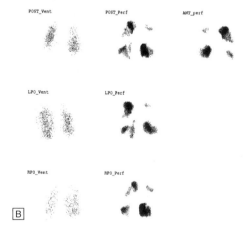

Question 1.8

You are called to a cardiac arrest on a medical ward. It is a 68-year-old lady who was confined to bed following an episode of presumed influenza 6 weeks previously and has only just been admitted to hospital. At the time of admission she was noted to be breathless and hypoxic on air but her CXR was normal. She has just collapsed and is hypotensive. She is resuscitated with fluids. An ECG (A) is performed and a V/Q scan (B) is taken on the way to ITU.

a. What does the V/Q scan show?
b. What does the ECG show?
c. How should she be managed?

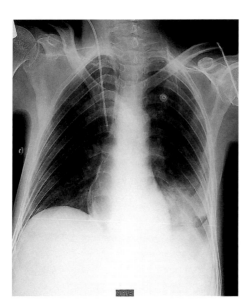

Question 1.9

This is the supine CXR of a man with ulcerative colitis who is septic and who was resuscitated on the ward prior to laparotomy. Shortly after induction, his condition deteriorated and he became difficult both to ventilate and to oxygenate.

a. What is the diagnosis on the radiograph and what is your course of action?
b. How may you confirm this?
c. What treatment will you perform?

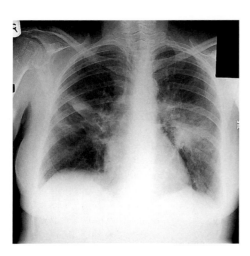

Question 1.10

An 18-year-old female presents for a diagnostic laparoscopy because of abdominal pain. In her medical history she describes increasing dyspnoea and a dry unproductive cough over a few days. There is a background of increasing malaise and reluctance to participate in sport over the preceding months and her mother added that she had noticed flecks of blood on her blouse when she had done the laundry.

Her full blood count showed a microcytic picture with a haemoglobin of 7.8 g/dL; oxygen saturation on high-flow oxygen was over 95%. Her CXR is shown. Her lung function tests are as follows:

- $FEV_1 = 2.3$ L
- FVC = 2.9 L
- T_LCO is 35% of predicted
- KCO is 114% of predicted.

a. What does the CXR show?
b. What can you conclude from the spirometry?
c. What abnormality is seen in the diffusion capacity and how do you account for the discrepancy?
d. What is a probable diagnosis?
e. What additional information is essential?

1

Q

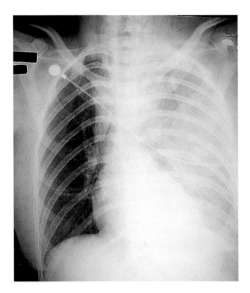

Question 1.11

The supine CXR of a 24-year-old man is shown.

a. Describe the CXR.

b. Can you work out the clinical history from it?

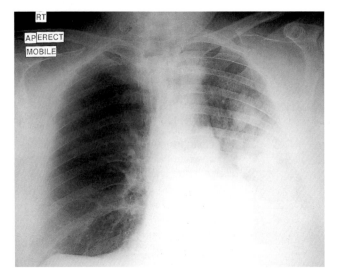

Question 1.12

This is the CXR of a 58-year-old man admitted to coronary care in respiratory failure. He was grossly obese and apyrexial. The ECG is said to have shown a non-specific T-wave abnormality. He had been found at home slumped over in a chair. His condition deteriorated rapidly, requiring emergency intubation followed by inotropic support. The only other information available is of heavy alcohol intake and progressive nocturnal dyspnoea.

a. Describe the CXR.

b. What are the possible diagnoses?

c. How will you differentiate between possible diagnoses?

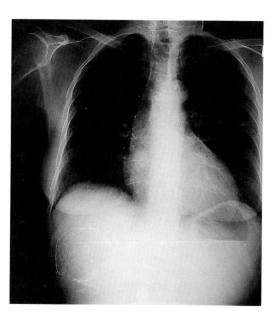

Question 1.13

This is the preoperative CXR of a 58-year-old woman who presented for a Keller's osteotomy. She was well preoperatively, complaining only of intermittent palpitations. Following induction, she developed a sinus tachycardia and became profoundly hypertensive.

a. What did you miss on the preoperative CXR?
b. What is the likely diagnosis and what will you do next?
c. After the procedure, what are you going to ask the patient and how will you advise on further investigation?

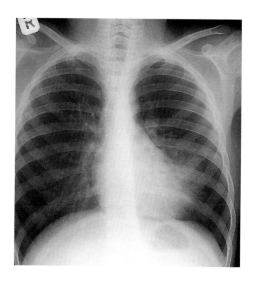

Question 1.14

This is the CXR of a child in the assessment ward awaiting routine tonsillectomy. The CXR was taken because he has a productive cough.

a. What is the diagnosis?
b. What is the treatment?

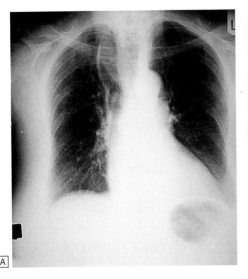 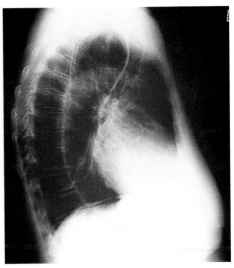

A B

Question 1.15

(A) and (B) are the PA and lateral CXRs, respectively, of a woman in her 70s who is being assessed for cataract surgery. She is apparently fit and well, but says she has had CXRs in the past and cannot remember why.

a. Describe these CXRs.
b. How would you advise her on the options for anaesthesia?

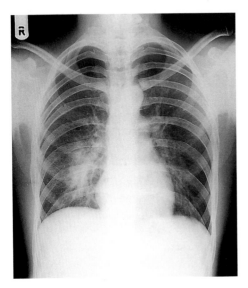

Question 1.16

This is the CXR of a 17-year-old boy who presents on your list for diagnostic laparoscopy for intermittent right hypochondrial pain over previous weeks.

a. What is the diagnosis on CXR?
b. How will you manage this condition?
c. Are you surprised by the lack of symptoms?

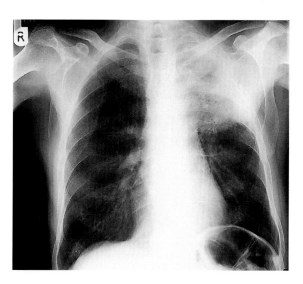

Question 1.17

You are asked to review a man in his 70s regarding his pain control, which is thought to be secondary to pneumonia. His CXR is shown.

a. Describe his CXR. What has been missed?

b. What other features may be present on questioning and examination?

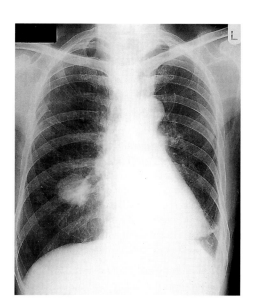

Question 1.18

This is the CXR of a 56-year-old man who has a squamous cell carcinoma. He has borderline pulmonary function and you have been asked to assess him for a right lower lobectomy.

a. Describe this CXR

b. Is this an operable tumour?

c. How would you evaluate a patient's lung function before proposed pneumonectomy?

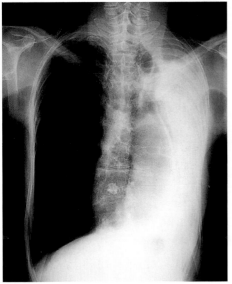
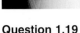
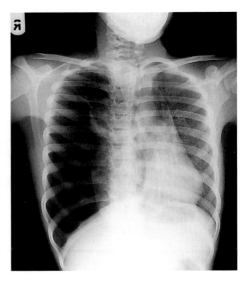

Question 1.19
You are asked to review a man on the surgical ward. He has been hypoxic since his return from theatre and is now extremely breathless. You are shown his PA CXR.

a. What is the diagnosis?
b. How should he be managed?

Question 1.20
a. What is wrong with this CXR?
b. What clinical signs would you expect to see?

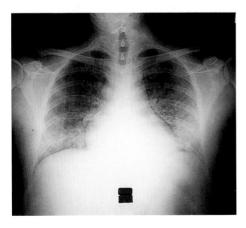

Question 1.21
This is the CXR of a 27-year-old patient who is on regular haemodialysis and is scheduled for the removal of his non-functioning renal graft. He gives a history of increasing exertional dyspnoea and dry unproductive cough. His spirometry shows a moderate restrictive defect, with 60% reduction in both T_LCO and KCO. Two weeks prior to this, the reduction had been only 20%.

a. What is the most likely diagnosis?
b. What course of action do you recommend?

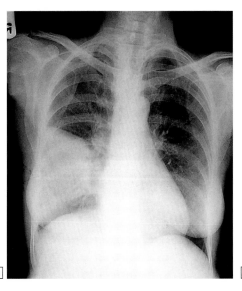

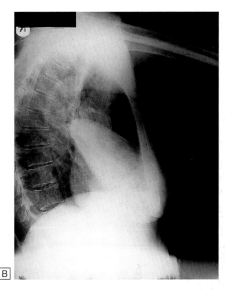

Question 1.22

These are the PA (A) and lateral (B) CXRs of a patient with a persistent cough and pyrexia following an episode of coughing at a barbecue a week previously.

a. Describe these radiographs. What is the radiological diagnosis?
b. What is the management?

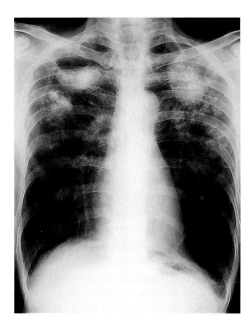

Question 1.23

This is the CXR of a 69-year-old retired coalface miner who has smoked 20 cigarettes per day since he was a teenager. He presents on your list for elective hip replacement. He says his chest is no worse than normal.

a. What does the CXR show?
b. Is he fit for anaesthesia? What assessment should be made?

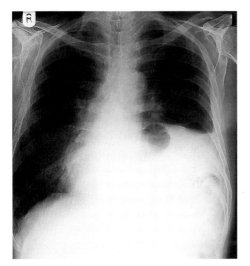

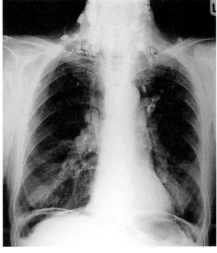

Question 1.24

This is the CXR of a man who is to undergo a laparoscopic cholecystectomy. Thirty years prior to this he was involved in a road traffic accident and as a result had to give up professional football.

a. Describe this CXR. What was the likely diagnosis 30 years ago?

b. How will this diagnosis affect your anaesthetic technique?

Question 1.25

You have been asked to assess an elderly lady on a medical ward with polymyalgia rheumatica (PMR) who is experiencing severe shoulder and neck pain. When you see her, she appears systemically unwell. Her CXR is shown.

a. What are the likely diagnoses on this CXR?

b. What needs to be done?

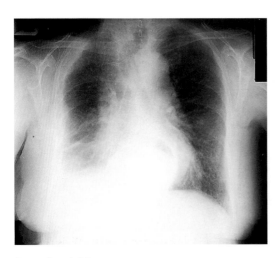

Question 1.26

A 72-year-old patient presents for a thoracoscopic pleural biopsy for possible malignancy. Her CXR is shown.

a. What else can be seen that you must be aware of and how might this affect your anaesthetic technique?

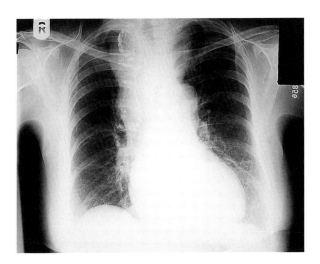

Question 1.27

This 74-year-old woman presented to A&E with a Colles' fracture requiring manipulation. She is on thyroxine replacement. She declines manipulation under local anaesthesia and is insistent on a general anaesthetic. You notice she has a slight inspiratory wheeze. This is her CXR.

a. What does it show?
b. How would you proceed?

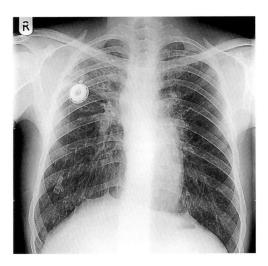

Question 1.28

This young man presents with right iliac fossa pain and an associated mass; he is unable to give a history. His relatives are not available. This is his chest radiograph. His pulmonary function shows an obstructive defect with an FEV_1 of 50%.

a. Describe the CXR.
b. What are the likely diagnoses?
c. What should be done?

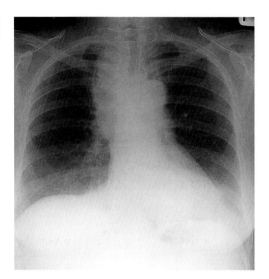

Question 1.29
You have been asked to help one of the new SHOs insert a central line in this patient on a medical ward. His face appears puffy and he is short of breath. His CXR is shown.

a. What does the CXR show?
b. What is the diagnosis and why is it difficult to insert a central line?

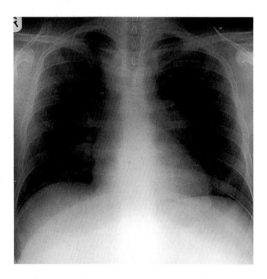

Question 1.30
This 35-year-old man presents on the trauma list for repair of a fractured tibia. He plays football in the local Sunday league. The X-ray shown was performed because he had been seen in the chest clinic of the neighbouring hospital some time ago but could not remember why.

a. What is the abnormality?
b. What impact does it have on your anaesthetic technique?

ANSWERS

Answer 1.1

a. The PA CXR is well centred and penetrated and taken on deep inspiration. The obvious abnormality is a foreign body (dental collar for crown prep) overlying the trachea. There is a notable gastric bubble (possibly from air swallowing). It is not possible to say whether it lies in the trachea, oesophagus or in another plane. Often the clinical information does not distinguish between them and a lateral is required. This shows the foreign body to be in the oesophagus.

b. Unlikely, as this is usually only of benefit for objects lodged in the trachea.

c. This will need to be removed under rigid oesophagoscopy. A full stomach should be assumed and the airway secured under a rapid sequence induction. Large objects or food boluses may distort laryngeal anatomy, but this is rare.

Muscle relaxation is usually required to perform the oesophagoscopy and reduce risk of oesophageal perforation. In small children, rigid oesophagoscopy may reduce cardiac output significantly from pressure on the great vessels in the mediastinum and this should be monitored continuously, usually with a finger on the pulse throughout surgery in addition to standard NIBP monitoring.

Answer 1.2

a. The CXR demonstrates a previous left-sided thoracoplasty and severe kyphoscoliosis. Thoracoplasty was a surgical method employed to collapse chronically either a lobe or a lung in a patient with tuberculosis and has been superseded by antituberculous chemotherapy. The long-term complication of such a restrictive defect is respiratory failure. Kyphoscoliosis may complicate thoracoplasty or occur in isolation. Respiratory and ventilatory failure in these patients may develop when their vital capacity is below 50% of that predicted.

b. The patient is confused owing to the onset of nocturnal hypoventilation, which is associated with cor pulmonale in patients with either of these mechanical defects.

c. A venous bicarbonate concentration that is raised may support the diagnosis of respiratory failure, being indicative of a compensated respiratory acidosis. This is a simple outpatient test and is a useful tool in following a patient with mechanical deformity of the thorax.

Answer 1.3

a. The plain film shows overexpansion of the chest with relatively flat hemidiaphragms. Normally, only about seven intercostal spaces should be seen. There is also calcification of the diaphragmatic pleura and a left-sided pleural plaque. The lateral film shows an increase in AP diameter with large anterior mediastinal window consistent with obstructive airways disease. Clinically the patient will be easily recognisable with a hyperinflated barrel chest.

b. The findings are consistent with overinflation typically seen in chronic obstructive pulmonary disease. The presence of pleural plaques is suggestive of previous exposure to asbestos, but the presence of haemoptysis raises the possibility of carcinoma in a smoker.

c. Spirometry would be expected to show an obstructive defect and there may be a significant reduction in both T_LCO and KCO.

d. A respiratory opinion should be obtained regarding the possibility of carcinoma, which may lead to elective surgery being delayed. Assuming the patient has no evidence of advanced malignancy and surgery goes ahead, the main anaesthetic risks are of pneumothorax as a result of positive pressure ventilation and perioperative respiratory failure. The risks of these may be minimised using a central nerve blockade, regional or local anaesthetic infiltration technique. If general

1

A

anaesthesia is required, a spontaneously breathing technique may be useful in combination with regional blockade.

Answer 1.4

a. The CXR shows a dense opacification at the right base with no visible lung markings. The V/Q scan shows a matched defect at the right base, the ventilatory defect being larger than the perfusion defect. The additional knowledge required is a full clinical history and examination.

b. The patient has a history suggestive of pneumonia and the radiograph shows a small basal effusion which is probably para-pneumonic in nature. Particular features in the history may point to the aetiology. A recent trip abroad or to the dentist or a vomiting episode may guide one to either the pathogen or the possibility of aspiration.

Answer 1.5

a. He is overweight and hypoxic at rest. His spirometry reveals obstructive pulmonary disease but this is not severe and appears out of proportion to his hypoxia. Equally, the T_LCO is reasonable at 50% of predicted. This implies that his obesity may be a significant part of the problem and he may be under-ventilating. It is likely that obstructive sleep apnoea is a contributory factor to his pulmonary hypoventilation. The transient ischaemic attacks may be secondary to polycythaemia, causing a hyperviscosity syndrome. The raised KCO would support this.

b. These patients present numerous problems for general anaesthesia. There may be significant co-morbid disease, particularly angina; maintenance of the airway and intubation may be difficult; sedative premedication should be avoided as there is a risk of airway obstruction, as there is also in the immediate postoperative period; and they should be nursed in a high-dependency or ITU setting. Regional

anaesthetic techniques may be possible.

Further reading

Isono S, Sha M, Suzukawa M et al 1998 Preoperative nocturnal desaturations as a risk factor for late postoperative nocturnal desaturations. *British Journal of Anaesthesia* 80(5): 602–605.

Johnson JT, Braun TW 1998 Preoperative, intraoperative and postoperative management of patients with obstructive sleep apnea syndrome. *Otolaryngologic Clinics of North America* 31(6):1025–1030.

Answer 1.6

a. The CXR shows interstitial shadowing, which is more marked at the bases, with some sparing of the costophrenic angles. This is consistent with pulmonary fibrosis.

b. Whilst the spirometry is normal, the diffusion capacity is severely impaired and is consistent with a diagnosis of fibrosing alveolitis obtained from the radiograph.

c. CT scan of the same patient, however, in addition to showing the characteristic changes of fibrosis in the lower lobes, also shows extensive concomitant emphysema as reflected by the apparent loss of lung parenchyma. Life is not simple and many patients may have multiple coexistent pathologies in the lung.

Answer 1.7

a. The CXR demonstrates overinflation of the chest, mediastinal emphysema and surgical emphysema in the neck. The mediastinal emphysema is shown as translucence, delineating structures in the mediastinum. An inhaler is also seen, presumably in a pocket.

b. The presence of the inhaler means that this boy is likely to have asthma and the spirometry is therefore likely to be obstructive.

c. The detection of mediastinal emphysema must be considered carefully in the context of the clinical details. It arises in circumstances where there is a sudden, massive rise in intrathoracic pressure. It is not always synonymous with pneumothorax, although once mediastinal gas is detected in a patient, a high level of suspicion must remain for the development of pneumothorax.

Answer 1.8

a. The scan shows multiple perfusion defects and near-normal ventilation, which in the context of a normal radiograph is diagnostic of pulmonary embolus.

b. The ECG shows a deep S wave in lead I, a Q wave in lead III with T-wave inversion in lead III. The chest leads show a dominant R wave and evidence of right ventricular strain.

c. Additional oxygen should be supplied along with intravascular volume loading to provide increased cardiac filling pressures, thus improving cardiac output. Opiate analgesia may be required for anxiety or pain. Ventilatory support may be required if she tires clinically. The current management of catastrophic pulmonary embolus would be to use an intravenous thrombolytic agent such as streptokinase or alteplase (rtPA, tissue-type plasminogen activator), followed by subcutaneous low-molecular-weight heparin and warfarin. Direct pulmonary artery thrombectomy on cardiopulmonary bypass is associated with a high mortality, but may need to be considered in catastrophic embolic events, particularly if the patient cannot be given thrombolytic agents, e.g. in the perioperative period. Further emboli may be treated with a temporary venocaval filter.

Answer 1.9

a. The radiograph shows a subtle anterior pneumothorax in the right hemithorax. The lungs are relatively radiolucent in comparison to the left. The right heart border is particularly distinct in comparison to the left heart border due

to the interface with air. The more obvious abnormality is the left-sided consolidation which focuses the attention.

b. If ventilation is difficult then a chest drain should be inserted. If the patient is stable, well oxygenated and the diagnosis is far from being clear-cut, then an erect film may be performed and, if still uncertain, a CT scan may confirm the presence of an anterior (occult) pneumothorax. His erect CXR is shown below and illustrates the need to take radiographs in the erect position when checking the position of intravenous catheters and attempting to exclude pneumothoraces.

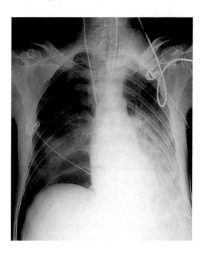

c. The subsequent radiograph demonstrates the progression of the pneumothorax and the need for the insertion of an intercostal underwater seal chest drain. Occult pneumothoraces are more common than has been recognised previously, being diagnosed by CT scan alone in 39% of trauma cases in one series. Controversy remains over the treatment of occult pneumothoraces that remain occult on CXR, but if the patient is ventilated, a chest drain is usually recommended. If treated conservatively, the patient must be followed up rigorously, both clinically and radiologically.

Further reading

Hill SL, Edmisten T, Holtzman G, Wright A 1999 The occult pneumothorax: an increasing diagnostic entity in trauma. *American Surgeon* 65: 254–258.

Answer 1.10

a. The CXR shows widespread air space shadowing. The differential diagnoses are pulmonary oedema, pneumonia and alveolar haemorrhage.
b. The spirometry shows a normal ratio of FEV_1 to FVC; however, without predicted values it is not possible to pass further comment.
c. The diffusion capacity shows a reduction in T_LCO, implying a low total diffusion capacity of the lung and yet the KCO is supranormal. In the presence of a low haemoglobin, alveolar haemorrhage should be considered.
d. The probable diagnosis is Goodpasture's syndrome.
e. Obviously this patient is not fit for elective surgery. Renal function should be assessed and either a lung or renal biopsy may be required to confirm the diagnosis of Goodpasture's syndrome.

Answer 1.11

a. The CXR shows opacification of the left hemithorax. To those who have not studied the film carefully, the answer may have been given as consolidation, but note the lack of air bronchogram. This appearance is typical of a large left pleural effusion taken in the supine position. Note the slight shift of the mediastinum to the right, away from the massive effusion. In addition, there is evidence of swelling in the neck along with surgical emphysema.
b. This patient has probably been stabbed. The combination of a massive effusion (haemothorax) and surgical emphysema means a penetrating injury is the likely mode of injury. Obviously this could also have been caused by blunt thoracic trauma, but the absence of rib fractures makes this less likely.

Answer 1.12

a. This is a mobile, AP CXR. The obvious abnormality is unilateral left-sided air space shadowing with total loss of the left hemidiaphragm.
b. Possible diagnoses include pneumonia, aspiration pneumonia (particularly if found lying on the left-hand side) and unilateral pulmonary oedema.
c. The history leads you away from the diagnosis of pneumonia as the patient is apyrexial. Fibreoptic bronchoscopy will help to identify the presence of gastric secretion or purulent sputum in the lungs, and transoesophageal echocardiography or a pulmonary artery flotation catheter will help to identify pulmonary oedema. This is a cautionary tale as the diagnosis in this case was pulmonary oedema and a dilated cardiomyopathy possibly related to alcohol. Unilateral pulmonary oedema does occur, since pulmonary oedema, or fluid of any other origin, will always be more marked in dependent areas.

Answer 1.13

a. The CXR at first glance appears normal. However, on closer inspection, a calcified mass is evident under the right hemidiaphragm. Calcification is seen running alongside the ribs under the diaphragm.
b. The differential diagnosis of a tachycardic hypertensive response post-induction includes light anaesthesia, thyrotoxic crisis, malignant hyperthermia and a phaeochromocytoma. Given the calcification on the CXR, this is likely to be due to the release of catecholamines from a phaeochromocytoma. These events should herald the termination of the procedure and treatment with beta-blockers and alpha-blockers.
c. Following recovery, a full history should be taken to elucidate any history of panic or anxiety attacks, sweats, headache etc. A family history should be taken as phaeochromocytomas can be familial, e.g. multiple endocrine adenoma syndromes, as well as Von

Recklinghausen's disease, and the patient should be referred to an endocrinologist for further investigation.

The CT scan below demonstrates a massive calcified mass arising in the right adrenal gland. Whilst the diagnosis may be slightly aesthetic, this question highlights the need to look at the whole film as the pathology may have been easily missed. Phaeochromocytomas are rare, but like malignant hyperthermia, they occur commonly in the examination setting.

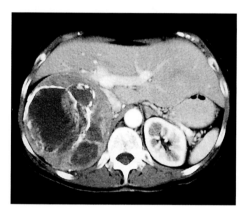

Further reading
Desmonts JM, Marty J 1984 Anaesthetic management of patients with phaeochromocytoma. *British Journal of Anaesthesia* 56: 781–789.
Sellevold OF, Raeder J, Stenseth R 1985 Undiagnosed phaeochromocytoma in the perioperative period: Case reports. *Acta Anaesthesiologica Scandinavica* 29: 474–479.

Answer 1.14

a. There is loss of definition of the left heart border, with consolidation. The left hemidiaphragm is clear. This represents a lingula pneumonia.
b. The child should be assessed fully, antibiotics administered accordingly and the procedure postponed.

Answer 1.15

a. The PA CXR shows a large linear opacity in the right hemithorax and mediastinum, the impression being of an air-filled cavity. The lateral film confirms the diagnosis of a mega-oesophagus.
b. The patient should be asked about symptoms of reflux or aspiration. If she is able to lie flat without symptoms, then local anaesthesia would be a good option. If general anaesthesia is to be administered, a rapid-sequence induction should be performed.

Answer 1.16

a. There is a small right pneumothorax in addition to the more obvious right midzone shadowing, which may be collapse or consolidation.
b. This may be the cause for the right-sided hypochondrial pain and the need for surgery should be reviewed. If surgery is not performed as this is a young fit man with a relatively small, asymptomatic pneumothorax, then this may be observed with repeat CXRs. If it enlarges (halfway towards the mediastinum) then it requires simple aspiration. If it becomes recurrent after aspiration or if the patient needs surgery (and therefore artificial ventilation), an intercostal underwater seal chest drain should be inserted.
c. Not at all. Spontaneous pneumothoraces are not uncommon (particularly in young, thin, fit men) and often present with minimal symptoms.

Further reading
Miller AC, Harvey JE 1993 Guidelines for the management of spontaneous pneumothorax. Standards of Care Committee, British Thoracic Society. *British Medical Journal* 307: 114–116.

Answer 1.17

a. There is a left upper lobe pneumonia. There is also a pleural cap and loss of the second rib, which is most likely to be secondary to a bronchial neoplasm.
b. The patient may complain of systemic symptoms in addition to cough and haemoptysis. Clinically the patient may have a left-sided Horner's syndrome (anhydrosis, meiosis, ptosis and

enophthalmos). The patient may complain of pain in the distribution of T1 and T2, along with wasting of the small muscles of the hand.

This question highlights the need to look at the bones very closely. An easier way to look at the ribs is to turn the film through 90° and then look at eye level.

Answer 1.18

a. This is a PA erect CXR which is slightly off-centre and underpenetrated. There is a large opacification in the lower zone of the right lung which is well circumscribed and likely to be a bronchocarcinoma. In addition, there are multiple metastases in the right lung (seen as small circular opacifications in the periphery of the lung) and there is also destruction of the posterior portion of the fifth rib.

b. This is not an operable tumour as there is extensive evidence of metastatic disease.

c. The ability of a patient to withstand lung resection is complex and depends upon the functional contribution of the lung to be resected and therefore, by definition, the function of the remaining lung tissue. In general terms, Olsen's criteria remain true: he proposed a maximum ventilatory capacity > 50% of predicted, FEV_1 > 2 L and 50% of FVC, predicted postoperative FEV_1 > 800 mL, balloon occlusion P_aO_2 > 6 kPa (45 mmHg) and mean pulmonary artery pressure < 4.5 kPa (35 mmHg) as being acceptable. If any of these criteria are not met, more sophisticated testing of split lung function is required. These may include inhaled xenon radiospirometry to assess ventilation combined with a technetium scan to assess perfusion; this will predict postoperative lung function. If the predicted postoperative FEV_1 is below 800 mL, the risk of pulmonary insufficiency postoperatively is high and further invasive techniques to assess function of the remaining lung should be performed. The pulmonary artery of the lung to be removed may be occluded using a pulmonary artery flotation catheter. If significant pulmonary hypertension (> 35 mmHg) or hypoxaemia (P_aO_2 < 6 kPa) do not occur, then the remaining lung may be considered to be able to take the entire cardiac output. It has been suggested that preoperative studies of exercise capacity may give a more accurate guide to predicting postoperative status than these invasive tests. This measurement is attractive because it is non-invasive and may more accurately reflect physiological reserve. In particular, the patient's capacity for maximal oxygen uptake ($Vo_{2\,max}$) of > 20 mL/kg/min is associated with few postoperative pulmonary complications.

Further reading

Gal TJ 1996 Anaesthesia for the patient with lung disease. In: Pearl RG, ed. *Baillière's Clinical Anaesthesiology; The Lung in Anaesthesia and Intensive Care*. Baillière Tindall, London.

Olsen CN, Block AJ, Swensen EW 1975 Pulmonary function evaluation of the lung resection candidate. *American Review of Respiratory Disease* 111: 379–387.

Answer 1.19

a. The patient has total collapse of the left lung with deviation of the trachea to the left and overinflation of the right lung. There are lung markings all the way out to the periphery on the right and therefore this should not be confused with a tension pneumothorax. A hidden clue would be that it is a PA film and therefore departmental. A patient with a tension pneumothorax could not stand! It is most likely that the lung collapsed owing to a missed endobronchial intubation.

b. He requires high-flow oxygen and urgent physiotherapy and possibly facial continuous positive airways pressure (CPAP). Fibreoptic bronchoscopy and removal of secretions may be required, as well as artificial ventilation if he tires clinically. His post re-inflation CXR (below) shows the left lung to be smaller than the right as a result of previous tuberculosis. The right lung remains overinflated, suggesting obstructive pulmonary disease.

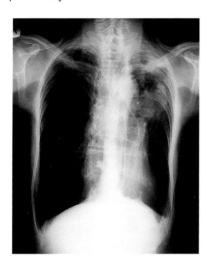

Answer 1.20

a. This CXR should never have been taken since it is of a right-sided tension pneumothorax. This should have been obvious clinically and since this is a life-threatening emergency, it should have been treated on clinical grounds with an intercostal chest drain and underwater seal.

b. Clinical signs of a tension pneumothorax include respiratory distress, tracheal deviation to the opposite side, tachycardia followed by cardiovascular collapse, distended neck veins and hyperresonance with decreased air entry on the affected side.

Answer 1.21

a. The CXR shows the so-called 'reversed bat's wings' sign, which in this context is most likely to represent *Pneumocystis carinii* pneumonia (PCP). The cardiac outline appears enlarged, which may be due to the AP projection.

b. PCP does not usually present with an acute deterioration but more often with a slow decline over a week or so prior

to presentation. The surgery should be postponed. The patient should be started on high-dose intravenous co-trimoxazole, and steroids are indicated if the patient is hypoxic. He should be referred for consideration of bronchoscopy with bronchoalveolar lavage, although 60% of cases may be picked up on an induced sputum sample.

Answer 1.22

a. The PA CXR shows right middle lobe consolidation, the superior limits being marked by the horizontal fissure. The right heart border is obscured, confirming that the middle lobe is involved and the diaphragm is spared, which would normally be involved in a lower lobe pneumonia. The position and borders of the right middle lobe are well shown on an area of consolidation on the lateral film.

b. The patient requires a rigid bronchoscopy to diagnose and remove the probable foreign body, which may have been aspirated at the barbecue.

Answer 1.23

a. This is a PA CXR which is well centred and penetrated. The lungs are overinflated, suggesting airways obstruction, and there are the characteristic changes of progressive massive fibrosis (PMF).

b. The patient should have spirometry with an attempt to assess reversibility to inhaled beta-agonists. If there is a significant obstructive defect, a steroid trial should be given. Emphysema is likely as well, in view of his history of cigarette smoking and the overinflation on the X-ray. This will reduce the diffusion capacity. PMF usually occurs in miners with a long history of smoking. Although changes on CXR in PMF look alarming, they may remain unchanged for years and fitness for anaesthesia is on clinical grounds, particularly exercise tolerance and spirometry.

Answer 1.24

a. This PA CXR shows opacification at the left lower zone with gas-containing spaces within it. This is the result of a ruptured central tendon of the diaphragm with stomach herniating into the chest. The barium swallow (below) confirms the presence of the stomach herniating through into the chest.

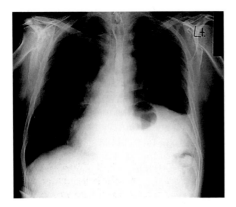

b. The assessment should involve lying and standing spirometry to assess lung function. If there is significant loss of diaphragmatic function on the left, the supine spirometry will be reduced significantly. The patient will require a rapid-sequence induction.

Answer 1.25

a. This is a well-centred and penetrated CXR. There is extensive calcification in the neck and, to a lesser extent, in the chest. This represents old TB and is merely a distraction. The worrying abnormality is the free gas under both hemidiaphragms. The patient has polymyalgia and has most likely perforated an abdominal viscus. The presence of abdominal signs may be masked by steroids. This information was not given in the history but was implied by the diagnosis of PMR.

b. She needs an urgent laparotomy for perforated abdominal viscus.

Answer 1.26

a. There is an obvious interstitial shadowing, particularly marked at the right base, which is likely to be neoplastic and draws your attention. However, there is also an air–fluid level seen behind the heart. This is likely to represent a hiatus hernia and will need to be assessed clinically; it may require appropriate premedication and consideration for rapid-sequence induction. The trachea is tortuous; this may be an incidental finding and may detract from other more significant abnormalities.

Answer 1.27

a. There is a mass in the superior mediastinum with associated calcification. The most likely diagnosis is of previous haemorrhage into a retrosternal goitre.

b. The main concern with the presence of possible stridor is the possibility of a compromised airway. The CT scan of the thoracic inlet (next page) shows the calcification in the retrosternal goitre on the right and a degree of tracheal compression. Spirometry should be the first investigation of choice. Whilst flow volume curves may yield more information, they are not universally available and are less familiar. Under any circumstances, general anaesthesia is hazardous in this lady and it should be emphasised that local anaesthetic techniques will be safer. In cases of mid-tracheal obstruction, intubation is rarely a problem but clinical obstruction is common. The fibreoptic or rigid bronchoscope may be useful for the placement of an endotracheal tube (ETT) distal to the level of the goitre. The degree and level of compression should be assessed by CT scan and plans made accordingly. An emergency tracheostomy in case of loss of the airway is not an option as it is unlikely to pass the obstruction. Most narrowings will allow placement of a 7.0 armoured ETT.

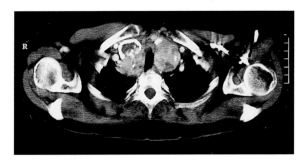

Further reading

Mason RA, Fielder CP 1999 The obstructed airway in head and neck surgery. Editorial. *Anaesthesia* 54: 625–628.

Answer 1.28

a. This PA CXR shows bilateral loss of volume of the upper lobes, as indicated by the drawing upwards of the hilar structures and tenting of the diaphragms. In addition, there is patchy fibrosis, air space shadowing and the suggestion of cysts. There is also an indwelling intravenous line and port.

b. The CXR diagnosis is cystic fibrosis. The abdominal pain is most likely due to intestinal obstruction.

c. A surgical opinion should be sought for the possible intestinal obstruction, although it should respond to conservative management. Specialist help should be sought for the management of cystic fibrosis.

Answer 1.29

a. The CXR shows a large right-sided mediastinal mass. This is likely to be neoplastic and is most likely causing superior vena cava obstruction (SVCO).

b. SVCO presents acutely with swelling of the arms, neck and face as well as lacrimation. The great veins are distended. As the situation becomes chronic, venous collaterals develop over the chest wall. Central access for pressure monitoring will remain difficult, if not impossible, since although the neck veins may be distended, the SVC is compressed and lines rarely thread properly.

Answer 1.30

a. The abnormality is one of bilateral hilar adenopathy. The differential diagnosis includes sarcoidosis, lymphoma and metastatic disease, and may be confused with bilateral pulmonary enlargement as seen in pulmonary hypertension. This man is otherwise well and the diagnosis is most likely to be sarcoidosis.

b. This is a disease of unknown aetiology characterised by granulomatous inflammation. To all intents and purposes, it bears little relevance to anaesthesia in the acute form unless there is associated hypercalcaemia and this should be checked. In the chronic form, there is loss of pulmonary function which will be evident from the clinical history and these patients will need lung function tests preoperatively. Rarer complications are covered by the rule 'If you don't know, ask'.

2

CARDIOLOGY

The most commonly encountered investigations of cardiac structure or function in clinical practice are the electrocardiogram (ECG) and the chest X-ray (CXR). They are also those most likely to be encountered in the FRCA examinations. Other investigations, however, frequently provide the clinical anaesthetist with valuable information, and may reasonably be expected in an examination. Therefore an understanding of echocardiography, angiography and isotope studies is important.

ELECTROCARDIOGRAPHY

Interpretation of an ECG depends upon an understanding of how it is generated. The resting potential across a myocardial cell membrane of −90 mV is maintained by the relative impermeability of the membrane to sodium ions (Na^+), and high permeability to potassium ions (K^+). Sodium and potassium are exchanged across the cell membrane by Na/K-ATPase in order to maintain Na^+ as the principal extracellular cation and K^+ as the principal intracellular cation. K^+ moves out of the cell down its concentration gradient, resulting in a negative interior charge. During muscle activation, Na^+ channels open briefly, allowing sodium ion influx, equalising and slightly overshooting zero potential (Fig. 2.1). The positive plateau potential is then maintained by a slow influx of calcium ions, and finally repolarisation is achieved by the restoration of membrane potassium permeability.

As this charge passes from cell to cell, a wave of depolarisation can be detected at skin surface electrodes and converted into an electrocardiographic trace (ECG). In the normal heart, this depolarisation is initiated in the sinoatrial node in the right atrium, spreads across the atria to the atrioventricular node and from there is rapidly passed down the conduction tissue of the bundle of His, via the two left and single right bundles and the subendocardial Purkinje tissue to the muscle fibres (Fig. 2.2).

At each time point, waves of depolarisation will be progressing in different directions. These can be regarded as vectors, some of which will be of equal magnitude travelling in opposite directions and will therefore cancel each other out. When the magnitude and direction of each

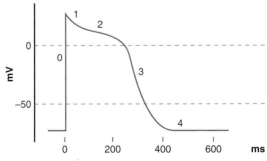

Fig. 2.1 Diagrammatic representation of a myocardial cell action potential. Phase 0, sodium influx via fast, voltage-dependent sodium channels; phase 1, potassium efflux; phase 2, calcium influx via slow voltage-dependent calcium channels; phase 3, potassium efflux along the concentration gradient, and restoration of Na/K-ATPase activity; phase 4, continued slow leak of potassium along the concentration gradient.

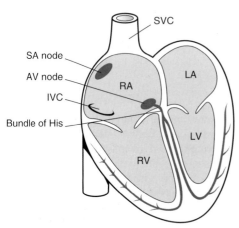

Fig. 2.2 Cross-section of the myocardium and conducting system. Depolarisation is initiated in the sinoatrial node (SAN), spreads across the right atrium (RA) to the atrioventricular node (AVN), and then via the bundle of His and bundle branches to both ventricles.

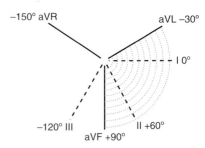

Fig. 2.3 Diagrammatic representation of the angle of interrogation in the vertical plane for each of the standard limb leads. The hatched area represents the normal range for the axis, or principal vector.

vector at any single time-point is taken into account, the result is a single overall vector which is recorded on the ECG. If this vector is directed towards the exploring electrode, the deflection on the ECG will be positive; if away, the deflection will be negative. The size of the deflection depends on the mass of tissue being depolarised, and so atrial depolarisation causes a small deflection, whereas ventricular depolarisation results in a large deflection. Therefore the normal wave of depolarisation produces a characteristic pattern in each of the ECG leads. An understanding of the normal pathway and the view of each lead of the ECG aids interpretation.

The standard limb leads (I, II, III) and the unipolar limb leads (aVR, aVL, aVF) interrogate the heart in the vertical plane (Fig. 2.3). The chest leads progress across the anterior chest wall from V1 (right ventricle) to V5/6 (left ventricle).

Interpreting the ECG
Developing a systematic approach to examining the ECG helps in the detection of any abnormalities. A simplified representation of the ECG is shown in Figure 2.4. The morphology of these

deflections will vary depending on the lead being examined, but some features will be constant throughout all leads, i.e. those relating to timing. Usually an ECG will be recorded at a rate of 25 mm/s, and therefore each small square on the tracing represents 0.04 s and each large square 0.2 s. Each ECG recording should specify the speed at which it was recorded, and also show a calibration deflection to confirm that 1 mV corresponds to 10 mm on the y axis.

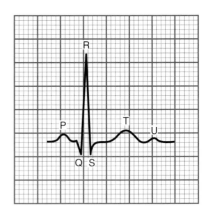

Fig. 2.4 An idealised electrocardiographic trace of a single depolarisation.

Rate
A systematic approach to reading an ECG generally starts with rate. This is most easily calculated by counting the number of large squares between consecutive R

waves and dividing this number into 300. If the rate is not regular then counting the number of R waves in a 15 cm strip and multiplying by 10 gives a more accurate figure.

Rhythm

First decide which area of the heart is acting as pacemaker, e.g. sinus node, atria, atrioventricular node or ventricle, and whether the rhythm is regular. If irregular, is there any repetitive pattern (regularly irregular) or no discernible pattern (irregularly irregular)? Supraventricular and ventricular extrasystoles may be present in a normal tracing.

P wave

The P wave relates to atrial depolarisation which normally spreads from the SA node in the right atrium. The wave of depolarisation is therefore predominantly right to left and so the P wave is positive in the left-sided leads. It is usually negative in aVR and may be so in leads III, V1 and aVL. A single P should precede each QRS, not exceed 2–3 mm in height and be no longer than two to three small squares (0.1 s).

PR interval

This is the time taken for the depolarisation initiated in the SA node to reach the ventricular muscle and is measured from the beginning of the P wave to the beginning of the QRS complex. The normal interval is 0.12–0.2 s, i.e. three to five small squares. A longer interval would signify a delay in conduction somewhere along the normal route, for example at the AV node. A shorter interval suggests accelerated depolarisation from either an abnormal pacemaker or aberrant conduction pathways.

The QRS complex

The QRS corresponds to the depolarisation of the ventricular muscle mass. As the left ventricle is the largest mass, this exerts the greatest influence over the morphology of the complex in each lead. Therefore leads interrogating the right surface of the heart will be predominantly negative with large S waves, and those on the left will be predominantly positive with large R waves. This results in a gradual shift from predominantly negative complexes in right-sided chest leads to predominantly positive complexes in left-sided leads, i.e. R wave progression (see Fig. 2.5).

The initial depolarisation in the ventricles is across the septum from left to right. Therefore there may be a small Q wave in the left-sided leads (I, aVL, aVF, V5, V6). These should be no more than 1 mm wide

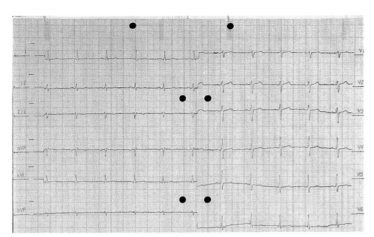

Fig. 2.5   The normal ECG. Note the normal progression in r wave height across the anterior chest leads.

and 2–3 mm deep, and the entire QRS complex should be less than 2 mm wide (0.06–0.08 s).

The voltage criteria for ventricular hypertrophy is generally a deflection of the R or S wave greater than 25 mm; however, this may be a normal variant in young, thin, fit individuals.

Axis

The axis refers to the direction in which the principal wave of depolarisation travels through the ventricles, the principal vector, and is calculated by looking at the QRS complexes in the limb leads (see Fig. 2.3). The lead with the tallest R wave will be closest to the axis, whilst the lead with the deepest S will be closest to 180° from the axis. Any lead in which the R and S waves are approximately equal will be at 90° to the axis. An axis between −30° and +90° (110° according to some references) is considered normal. The axis will be shifted if the normal route of depolarisation is altered, such as a bundle branch block, or if an increased muscle mass shifts the principal vector, as in ventricular hypertrophy.

ST segment

The ST segment corresponds to phase 2 of the action potential during which there is no change in polarity; therefore the ST segment should be isoelectric. It may curve upwards towards the T wave, and may also be slightly elevated, particularly in young, healthy males, but by no more than 1–2 mm. Any depression of greater than 0.5 mm is abnormal.

T wave

A normal T wave is in the same direction as the principal deflection of the QRS and corresponds to ventricular repolarisation. It may therefore be inverted in III, V1 and V2. Inversion in other leads, flattening or exaggeration of the T wave is abnormal.

U wave

U waves may be associated with hypokalaemia, but they are generally normal when associated with normal T waves.

QT interval

The QT interval is measured from the beginning of the QRS to the end of the T wave, and represents the total time for ventricular depolarisation and repolarisation. The normal time varies with heart rate and sex, and tables of normal values are available; however, for general purposes, at normal heart rates the interval should be less than 0.44 s (11 small squares).

RADIOLOGY

Evaluation of the normal CXR is covered in detail in Chapter 1. Particular areas of interest for the cardiovascular system include the mediastinum, cardiac outline and the appearance of the pulmonary vasculature. Other important clues include features such as rib notching in coarctation of the aorta or artificial heart valves or vascular clips in patients following cardiac surgery. When assessing the dimensions of the anterior mediastinum, in particular the cardiac outline, the PA view is the most accurate. This is because, in this view, the structures are closest to the film and so are less subject to magnification by the X-ray beam as it spreads out from the source (Fig. 2.6).

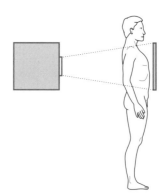

Fig. 2.6 Orientation and positioning of patient and X-ray source for a PA chest film. This minimises the magnification of the anterior mediastinal organs.

As with the ECG, the CXR should be reviewed systematically (see Ch. 1). It is important to note projection, rotation, exposure, degree of inspiration and whether the patient was erect or supine, particularly when looking for vascular signs or effusions.

The mediastinum itself is generally examined from the top down, tracing the left and right borders to detect any abnormality of outline, such as a double outline, suggesting free air in the mediastinum, or prominence of the aorta, main pulmonary artery or left atrium. Then look at the upper mediastinum for any widening, suggesting aortic aneurysm or dissection. Moving down, check the hilae for prominence and position; the left is slightly higher than the right due to the position of the left atrium. Assess the heart shadow itself for size and position. In an appropriately positioned film without excessive rotation, two-thirds of the heart shadow should be to the left of the spinous processes, and one-third to the right. The widest part of the heart should not be greater than half of the total width of the thorax measured from the internal border of the ribs. When examining the rest of the chest film, look in particular at the vascularity of the lung fields, checking for hyper- or hypoperfusion. In a normal erect film, pulmonary vessels in the upper zone are smaller than the same generation of vessels in the lower zone because of the gravitational effect. Upper zone vessels of a similar or larger diameter suggest pulmonary venous hypertension. Check also for evidence of extravascular fluid such as peribronchial cuffing, Kerley's B lines, collection in the fissures, and blunting of the costophrenic angle suggesting pleural effusions. Most of these changes occur when left atrial pressures exceed 22 mmHg.

ECHOCARDIOGRAPHY

Ultrasonic waves directed through a tissue will be absorbed, reflected or pass though the tissue, depending on characteristics such as density and interface with other tissues. Echocardiography detects the reflected energy and converts it into a visual image. The image is constructed from the time it takes the signal to return to the transducer, i.e. the distance between the structure and the transducer. Different modes of echocardiography give different information.

M-mode
A single beam is directed through a tissue and reflected from the various structures along its length. The linear image is plotted against time, so the y axis represents the distance of the structure from the transducer, and the x axis time. M-mode can be used to examine moving structures such as the mitral valve, assessing valve opening (Fig. 2.7).

Two-dimensional echocardiography
A sequence of signal beams is used to construct a two-dimensional image of the area under examination (Fig. 2.8). This mode is useful for examining both structure and function of the heart. The image can be frozen and measurements taken, e.g. the cross-sectional area of the aortic valve or ventricular dimensions. Real-time images can assess valve and ventricular function, and can visualise abnormal structures such as septal defects or vegetations.

Doppler echocardiography
The Doppler effect is used to calculate the velocity and direction of blood movement in the heart by detecting the frequency shift in sound waves returning to the transducer. In pulsed-wave (PW) Doppler, a single transducer sends and receives sound waves. It is therefore able to time 'gate' the received signal, and so precisely sample the area under examination. Unfortunately, it cannot detect high-velocity flow. Continuous-wave (CW) Doppler has separate transducers for sending and receiving, and therefore can detect high velocity flow, but cannot be gated to sample at a particular depth. Both PW and CW Doppler can be used in conjunction with two-dimensional imaging to direct the probe accurately (Duplex scan). CW Doppler can be directed across a valve, and an instantaneous pressure gradient calculated from the Bernoulli equation.

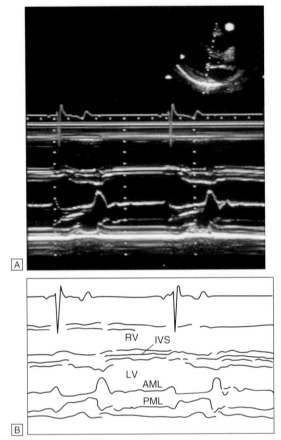

Fig. 2.7 M-mode image (A) and associated line drawing (B) of the mitral valve. RV, right ventricle; IVS, intraventricular septum; LV, left ventricle; AML, anterior mitral valve leaflet; PML, posterior mitral valve leaflet.

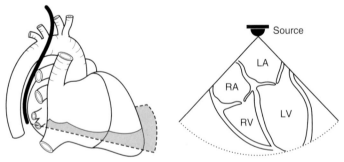

Fig. 2.8 Diagrammatic representation of two-dimensional acquisition via a transoesophageal probe. The diagram on the right shows a simplified long axis two-dimensional image. RA, right atrium; LA, left atrium; RV, right ventricle; LV, left ventricle.

Colour flow mapping

Multiple PW Doppler samples are collected and superimposed onto a two-dimensional image. Each sample is coded according to direction of flow in relation to the transducer (BART – blue away, red towards). Regurgitant flow and flow across abnormalities such as atrial septal defects (ASDs) can be easily detected (Fig. 2.9).

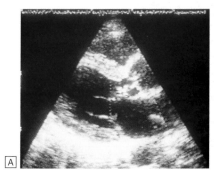

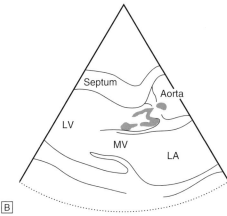

Fig. 2.9 A: Colour flow mapping showing regurgitant flow across the aortic valve during diastole. The flow is away from the probe and therefore appears blue. B: Line drawing of (A). LV, left ventricle; LA, left atrium; MV, mitral valve. The hatched area represents the regurgitant flow across the aortic valve.

Transthoracic versus transoesophageal echocardiography

Transthoracic echocardiography is non-invasive and easy to perform, but can be difficult in some subjects, such as the obese and patients with lung disease in whom air between the heart and the transducer causes distortion of the image. It is also more difficult to obtain good information on posterior structures such as the mitral valve and the descending aorta.

Transoesophageal echocardiography often gives better quality images because of the proximity of the probe to the heart, and is more accurate at examining mitral valve function and atrial structures. Sedation is required to pass the probe

down the oesophagus. There is also a risk of local damage, including arytenoid dislocation and oesophageal tears. The procedure is contraindicated in the presence of varices or oesophageal stricture.

Stress echocardiography

A two-dimensional transthoracic examination of the left ventricle is made before and after physical or pharmacological stress is induced. Changes in wall motion or thickness suggest ischaemia. The inotrope dobutamine and vasodilator dipyridamole are the most commonly used pharmacological agents, and the technique is particularly valuable in patients unable to exercise for non-cardiac reasons.

ISOTOPE STUDIES

Myocardial perfusion is assessed by injecting radioisotopes such as thallium or technetium-99m intravenously. They distribute according to blood flow, ischaemic areas showing up as 'cold' spots on a gamma camera image. Tomographic imaging gives three-dimensional representations, and stress testing can be incorporated to detect reversible ischaemia. In gated ventriculography, radiolabelled blood cells are injected and the heart is imaged to detect the blood in the ventricles. Repeated imaging throughout the cardiac cycle, 'gated' against the ECG, allows estimation of ventricular volumes and ejection fraction.

MAGNETIC RESONANCE IMAGING (MRI)

Cardiac MRI gives high-resolution images of cardiac and aortic structure, and cinematic MR angiography can give information on blood flow, e.g. in coronary grafts. Blood flowing at a rate of greater than 3 cm/s gives no signal, so a signal void in the image indicates patency. Further development of cinematic cardiac MRI stress testing is being carried out and it is considered suitable for patients unable to exercise and in whom echocardiographic image resolution is inadequate, particularly those with respiratory disease and the obese, although there is some limitation as to the size of patients able to undergo MRI.

CARDIAC CATHETERISATION

Although catheterisation remains the gold standard in cardiac investigation, it is being superseded in many conditions by non-invasive techniques. Much of the information to be gained from cardiac catheterisation, such as data on myocardial and valve function, detection of anatomical defects and shunts, an estimate of cardiac output and measurement of intracardiac pressures (Table 1), can be provided by increasingly sophisticated echocardiography and MR techniques. Echocardiography and MRI are replacing angiography as the primary investigation in aortic disease. The main indication for cardiac catheterisation is therefore coronary angiography, although this is the group with the highest mortality, in the order of 0.1%. Figure 2.10 demonstrates the normal coronary anatomy.

Table 1 Intracardiac pressures measured during cardiac catheterization

Chamber	Upper limit of pressure (mmHg)
Right atrium	6
Right ventricle	30/5
Pulmonary artery	30/15
Left atrium (PAWP)	12
Left ventricle	150/12
Aorta	150/90

PAWP, pulmonary artery wedge pressure.

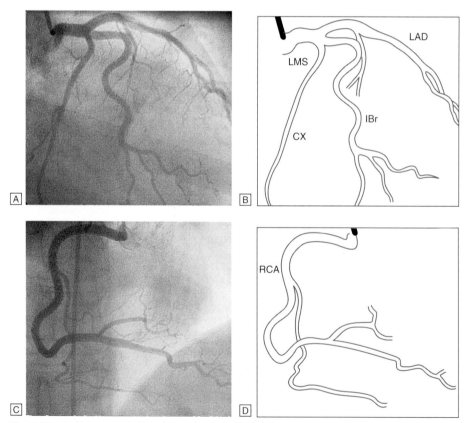

Fig. 2.10 Angiograms (A, C) and line drawings (B, D) of normal coronary anatomy. RCA, right coronary artery; LMS, left main stem artery; LAD, left anterior descending artery; CX, circumflex artery (this vessel traverses the atrioventricular groove, giving it the straight appearance clearly seen in this example); IBr, intermediate branch (this is a normal variant and is unusually large in this example).

QUESTIONS

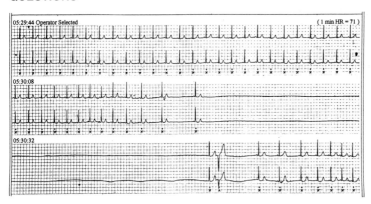

Question 2.1

This is the 24-h Holter monitor of a 68-year-old woman presenting for cholecystectomy. She was referred for this investigation from the preoperative screening clinic having complained of intermittent palpitations and shortness of breath.

a. What is the diagnosis?
b. What specific perioperative precaution is required?
c. What are the other indications for such intervention?

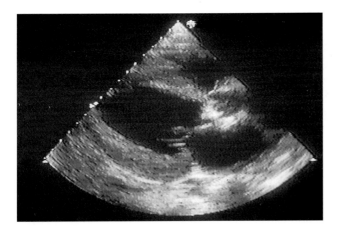

Question 2.2

A 36-year-old primigravida complains of excessive tiredness and shortness of breath at 37 weeks gestation. On examination, a murmur is noted and an echocardiogram performed.

a. What is the diagnosis and the most likely underlying cause?
b. Outline the initial management.
c. Outline perioperative problems and anaesthetic management.

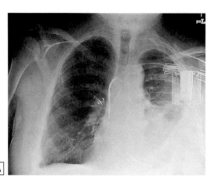

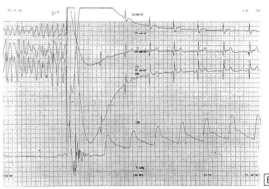

A | B

Question 2.3

(A) is the CXR of a 78-year-old man who has been admitted with a chest infection. You are asked to review him for possible ITU admission, but there are no cardiology notes available. The ECG trace (B) was found in his notes and was recorded with the intra-arterial pressure trace shown during a previous anaesthetic.

a. What do the CXR and ECG trace show?
b. What is the device shown on the CXR?
c. What are the implications for anaesthesia?

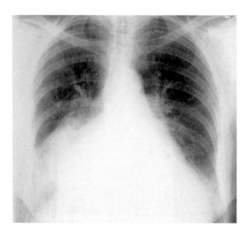

Question 2.4

A 76-year-old woman is listed for a dynamic hip screw for a fractured neck of femur. She is mildly confused and unable to give a history. She is found to be in atrial fibrillation with a rate of 120. Her CXR is shown.

a. What abnormalities are present and what is the diagnosis?
b. How would you confirm the diagnosis?
c. Describe your anaesthetic management.

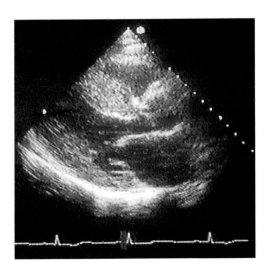

Question 2.5

A 19-year-old is admitted for knee surgery following a football injury. He has recently taken up the sport to improve his level of fitness and reports that on occasions he has felt light-headed and short of breath during the games.

a. What is this image and what does it show?
b. What are the symptoms of this abnormality?
c. What are the implications for anaesthesia?

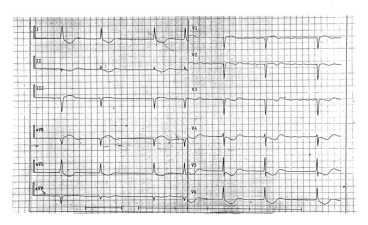

Question 2.6

An 80-year-old woman is admitted for sigmoid colectomy following a diagnosis of malignant disease. She has been on digoxin for several years, and her GP has recently started her on a new 'heart tablet', the name of which she cannot remember. Her preoperative ECG is shown.

a. What abnormalities are present?
b. What are the possible causes?
c. How would you manage this patient?

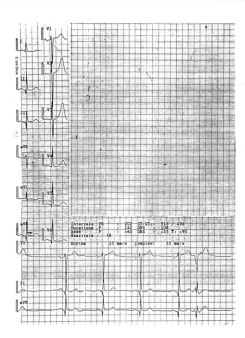

Question 2.7

A 65-year-old man is admitted for elective cholecystectomy. He is a regular smoker and takes a β-blocker for hypertension but is otherwise well. He had a full health insurance medical 2 months ago, including an ECG which was reported as satisfactory. His admission ECG is shown.

a. What abnormalities are present on the ECG?

b. What are the implications for surgery?

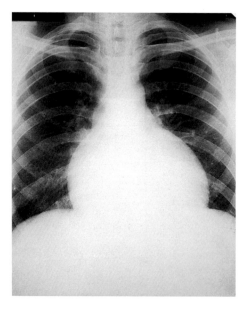

Question 2.8

An obese 68-year-old man is brought by ambulance to the A&E department. He has apparently been unwell and generally tired for several months, but hasn't seen his GP. Over the last few days his condition has deteriorated and his admission was precipitated by a collapse at home. On examination, level of consciousness is depressed, he has cold peripheries, is hypotensive with a blood pressure recorded as 80/40 mmHg, and is tachypnoeic. His CXR is shown.

a. What abnormalities are present, what is the diagnosis and what are the possible causes?

b. What physical signs would help to confirm the diagnosis?

c. What further investigations may be indicated?

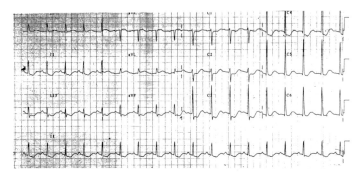

Question 2.9

A 48-year-old woman with insulin-dependent diabetes since childhood is admitted with right calf rest pain. She has been dialysis-dependent for 2 years and is under regular follow-up for severe diabetic retinopathy. She has no cardiac symptoms. On examination she has severe ischaemia of her feet and a gangrenous toe.

a. What abnormalities are present on the ECG?
b. What is the significance of the lack of symptoms?
c. Discuss the preoperative preparation of this patient.

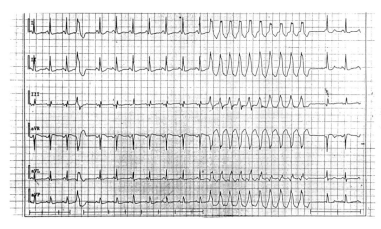

Question 2.10

A 46-year-old woman presents to A&E complaining of palpitations. This is her ECG.

a. What is the differential diagnosis?
b. What feature may help to confirm a diagnosis?
c. Outline the management of this patient?

2
Q

Question 2.11

These are the results of cardiac catheterisation in a 64-year-old man 1 week post-myocardial infarction:

Chamber	Blood oxygen saturation
RA	72%
RV	88%
PA	86%
LA	97%
LV	97%

a. What is the diagnosis?
b. How could you assess the severity?
c. What clinical features may be present and what other investigations could have confirmed the diagnosis?

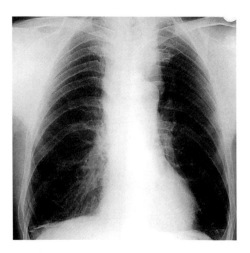

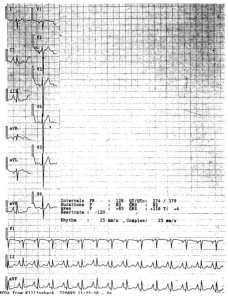

Question 2.12

A previously well 41-year-old male presents for open reduction and internal fixation of a fractured ankle sustained in a road traffic accident. Clinical examination is unremarkable except for a blood pressure of 190/80 mmHg. His CXR is shown.

a. What abnormalities are present and what is the diagnosis?
b. What clinical signs may be elicited?
c. What are the important considerations for anaesthesia?

Question 2.13

This is the ECG of a 170 cm, 120 kg man presenting for a Roux-en-Y procedure.

a. What is the likely diagnosis?
b. What tests or features would support the diagnosis?
c. What else may cause this ECG abnormality?

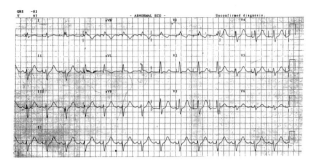

Question 2.14

A 74-year-old man is admitted for transurethral resection of prostatic enlargement. This ECG was recorded as part of his preoperative screen.

a. What does the ECG show?
b. What intervention is required prior to surgery?
c. Describe the perioperative management of this patient.

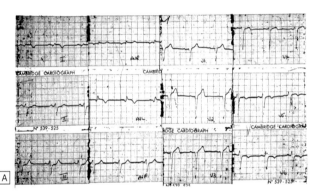

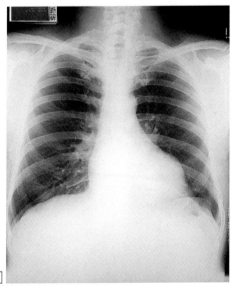

Question 2.15

A 53-year-old man with known ischaemic heart disease and a history of myocardial infarction 2 years previously presents for inguinal hernia repair. His ECG (A) and preoperative chest film (B) are shown.

a. What abnormality is present on the chest film?
b. What features of the ECG may support the diagnosis?
c. What further investigation is indicated?

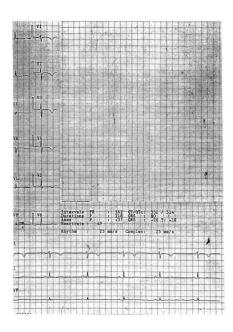

Question 2.16

A 69-year-old man requires AP resection for rectal carcinoma. He underwent coronary artery bypass grafting 4 years ago and has been well since, although he remembers that in the days immediately following his operation there were some problems with his heart rhythm and he remains on medication for this. His ECG is shown.

a. What are the abnormalities?
b. What are the possible causes?
c. What risks are associated with this abnormality?
d. What is the management?

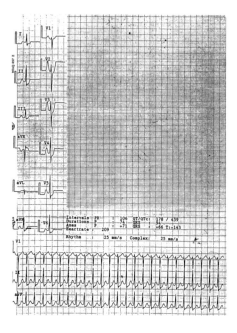

Question 2.17

A 23-year-old woman attends a day-case unit for extraction of wisdom teeth under general anaesthesia. She has no past history of note except occasional 'panic attacks'. In the anaesthetic room she complains of dizziness, and a 12-lead ECG is recorded, as shown.

a. What is the diagnosis?
b. What is the underlying cause?
c. How would you treat this dysrhythmia?

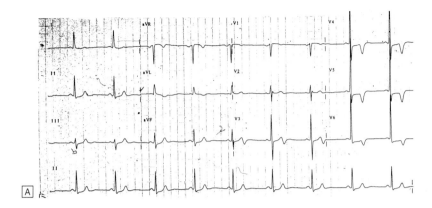

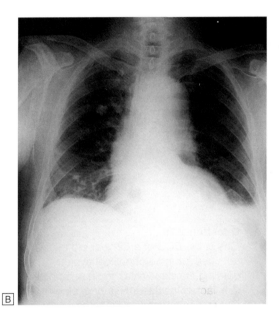

Question 2.18

A 67-year-old man is admitted to the A&E department complaining of severe chest pain. His ECG and CXR are shown in (A) and (B), respectively.

a. What abnormalities are present and what is the diagnosis?
b. What clinical features may be present and which further investigations are indicated?
c. Describe your initial management.

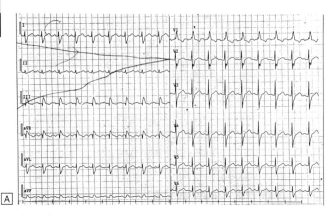

A

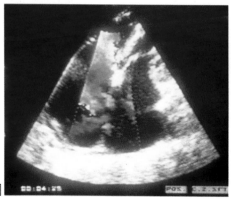

B

Question 2.19

This is the ECG (A) and two-dimensional echocardiogram (B) of a 24-year-old woman presenting for cardiac surgery.

a. What are the abnormalities?
b. Classify the cardiac abnormality.
c. What other investigations may be indicated?

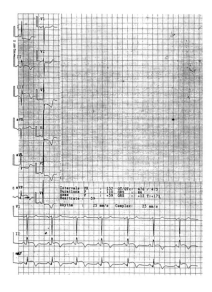

Question 2.20

This is the ECG of a 62-year-old man admitted for femoropopliteal bypass grafting. He claudicates at 50 m, and his risk factors include a history of smoking, non-insulin-dependent diabetes with poor control, and a body mass index of 31. He complains of feeling unwell for several days, and now has chest discomfort worse on lying down. His medication includes aspirin, gliclazide and bendrofluazide.

a. What is the diagnosis?
b. What are the possible causes of the current pain?
c. Outline initial investigations and early management.

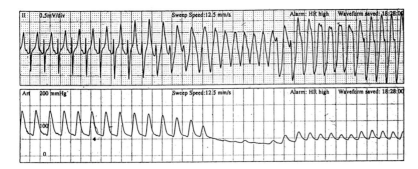

Question 2.21

A young male is brought to hospital following a road traffic accident in which he was hit from the side. He requires a chest drain for pneumothorax, has fractures of his pelvis and right femur, and peritoneal lavage is heavily bloodstained. He is transferred to theatre for laparotomy, and during the subsequent orthopaedic procedure this ECG and arterial pressure trace is recorded.

a. What are the abnormalities and likely cause?
b. What factors may have contributed to this situation?
c. How would you correct the abnormality?

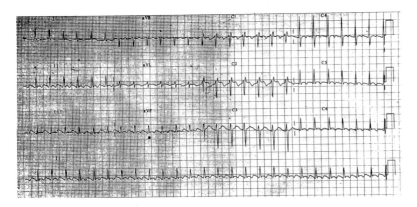

Question 2.22

A 50-year-old 46 kg woman is brought to the A&E department complaining of shortness of breath and palpitations. Her ECG is recorded as shown.

a. What abnormalities are present and what is the rhythm?
b. What procedures could confirm the diagnosis?
c. What are the possible causes of the rhythm?
d. How would you manage this patient?

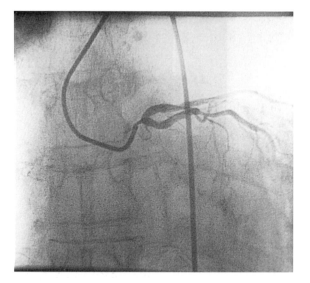

Question 2.23

This is the coronary angiogram of a 57-year-old man who has been admitted for coronary artery bypass grafting.

a. What lesion is shown?
b. What are the implications for anaesthesia?

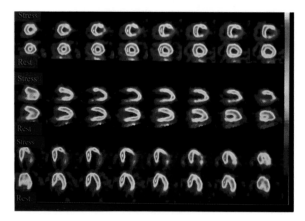

Question 2.24

A 67-year-old male presents for investigation 4 weeks after suffering a myocardial infarction for which he received thrombolysis. He is a lifelong smoker and complains of calf pain after walking 200 yards.

a. What is the investigation shown and what does it indicate?
b. What further investigation is indicated?
c. Which vessel is involved?

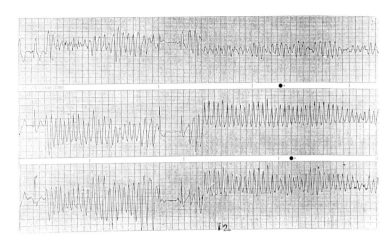

Question 2.25

The ECG shown was recorded from a 62-year-old man 48 h following coronary artery bypass grafting. He was sedated, intubated and ventilated and required inotropic support and pharmacological control of recurrent tachydysrhythmias.

a. What does the ECG show?
b. What are the possible causes?
c. What is the management of this dysrhythmia?

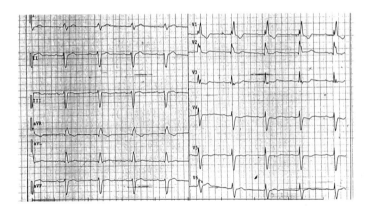

Question 2.26

A 59-year-old male smoker with no past history of note is admitted for repair of a left inguinal hernia. He reports shortness of breath on moderate exercise, which he attributes to his smoking and to being a little overweight. His routine ECG is shown.

a. What abnormalities are present on the ECG?
b. What is the significance of these abnormalities?
c. What specific management, if any, is required?

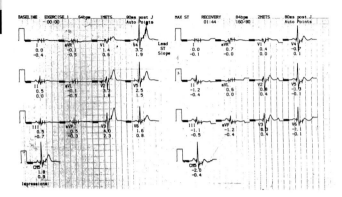

Question 2.27

This is the summary of the exercise ECG of a 65-year-old male smoker referred for investigation of atypical chest pain. He achieved an exercise time of 5 min and 8 s of a Bruce protocol test, a maximum heart rate of 112 beats/min, and a workload of 7 METS. The test was terminated when the patient complained of shortness of breath and tired legs.

a. Is the test positive or negative, and why?
b. What other features may indicate a positive test?
c. What does the term METS mean?
d. During peak exercise this man's blood pressure fell from 170/90 to 120/60 mmHg. What is the significance of this?

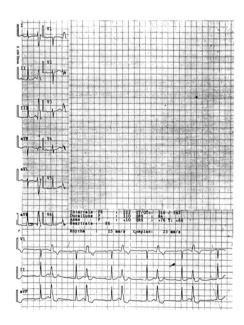

Question 2.28

This ECG was recorded from a 76-year-old patient listed for urgent transurethral resection of prostate (TURP) following admission for acute urinary retention.

a. Describe the abnormalities.
b. What are the possible causes?
c. What interventions, if any, are required?

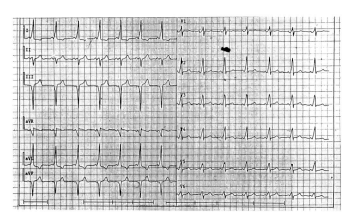

Question 2.29

This is the ECG of a 44-year-old woman who has been admitted for a total abdominal hysterectomy.

a. What abnormalities are present?
b. What is the diagnosis?
c. Describe any appropriate anaesthetic considerations.

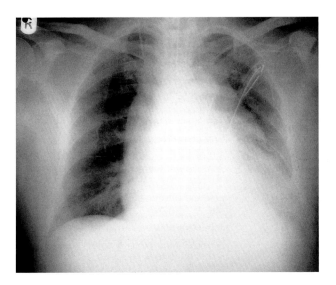

Question 2.30

This is the CXR of a woman aged 65 years. She is a long-term smoker with a history of hypertension. The X-ray was taken 4 h after admission to ICU following coronary artery bypass grafting (CABG). She was initially stable, but after sedation was stopped she became agitated. She then rapidly deteriorated, becoming tachycardic and hypotensive.

a. What is the diagnosis and what are the possible causes?
b. What other signs may be present?
c. Outline the appropriate management.

2

A

ANSWERS

Answer 2.1

a. The tape shows a background of sinus rhythm with periods of sinus bradycardia and sinus arrest. There is no evidence of tachydysrhythmia, but the history is suggestive. The diagnosis is sick sinus syndrome.

b. Temporary pacing. Sinus node disease is generally accepted as an indication for perioperative pacing. This is particularly important in procedures such as laparoscopic surgery which may cause vagal stimulation and prolong any sinus pauses. In the case of this symptomatic patient, permanent pacing is indicated, in combination with pharmacological control of any tachydysrhythmias.

c. Indications for perioperative pacing include:

   (i)   Mobitz II type second-degree heart block
   (ii) complete heart block
   (iii) symptomatic bifascicular block
   (iv) bifascicular block with prolonged PR interval (trifascicular block).

Patients with a first-degree heart block, Wenkebach type second-degree heart block or bundle branch block do not require pacing as they rarely proceed to complete heart block. In addition, patients in groups (iii) and (iv) above uncommonly develop a complete heart block, their poor outcome being principally due to the underlying cardiac disease. The advent of alternative pacing techniques, such as non-invasive transcutaneous pacing (NTP), means that emergency pacing can be readily available without requiring invasive procedures. Patients with symptomatic trifascicular block will probably require a permanent pacing system, and a temporary wire may be inserted if surgery is urgent.

Further reading

Amar D, Gross JN 1993 Patients with pacemakers. In: Simpson JI, ed. *Anaesthesia and the Patient with Co-existing Heart Disease*. Little, Brown & Co., Boston.

Answer 2.2

a. The two-dimensional echocardiogram shows a uniformly or concentrically thickened left ventricular wall, suggesting an increase in afterload. The aortic valve appears bright, indicating the presence of calcification. The diagnosis is aortic stenosis. The echocardiography report will include a measured gradient across the aortic valve. A gradient of 50 or more indicates severe stenosis, and in general the valve area in these patients is reduced to less than 0.7 cm^2 (normal $2.6–3.5 \text{ cm}^2$). The most likely cause is a congenitally stenotic valve, usually bicuspid. Stenosis may develop in early adult life, but calcification is rare before the age of 30. Rheumatic disease accounts for less than 3% of cases.

b. This is a severe stenotic lesion and the patient has symptoms suggestive of the development of left ventricular failure. She requires admission, rest, regular cardiovascular monitoring, cardiological referral and preparation for urgent caesarean section.

c. The presence of a severely stenotic valve results in a fixed stroke volume. The increased afterload causes concentric hypertrophy to develop, with a resulting reduction in left ventricular compliance. Left ventricular end-diastolic pressure rises and ventricular function becomes dependent on elevated end-diastolic volume. The patient is therefore at risk of myocardial ischaemia, particularly if tachycardia develops and diastolic coronary perfusion time is reduced, and of haemodynamic instability if either systemic vascular resistance or left ventricular preload fall. Full invasive monitoring, including a pulmonary artery catheter to monitor left ventricular preload, is indicated. Although there is controversy over whether carefully conducted regional anaesthesia is appropriate in mild-to-moderate aortic stenosis, in severe lesions general anaesthesia is recommended. Careful patient positioning is particularly relevant for patients with aortic stenosis. A high-dose narcotic technique may also be necessary. In particular, it is important to avoid tachycardia, bradycardia, a reduction in systemic vascular resistance or excessive fluid shifts. Treatment of hypotension should be directed to fluid therapy, titrated against left ventricular preload, and pure vasoconstrictors such as phenylephrine. V5 ECG monitoring is helpful in detecting any myocardial ischaemia. In cases of severe stenosis, the procedure should take place where facilities for cardiopulmonary bypass are available for urgent valve replacement. It is also important to pay close attention to fetal monitoring and resuscitation, particularly when high-dose opioid techniques are utilised.

Further reading

Pittard A, Vucevic M 1998 Regional anaesthesia with a sub-arachnoid microcatheter for Caesarean section in a parturient with aortic stenosis. *Anaesthesia* 53: 169–191.
Wlody D 1993 The pregnant patient with cardiac disease. In: Simpson JI, ed. *Anaesthesia and the Patient with Co-existing Heart Disease.* Little, Brown and Co., Boston.

Answer 2.3

a. The CXR shows signs of a left lower lobe pneumonia. In addition, there is a device implanted in the left chest wall. The ECG trace shows a period of ventricular fibrillation with no output shown on the intra-arterial trace, followed by a shock with restoration of sinus rhythm and cardiac output.
b. This is an implanted cardioverter defibrillator device (ICD), consisting of a transvenous intraventricular lead connected to a control unit. Modern devices are able to differentiate between ventricular tachycardia and fibrillation. Overpacing is triggered to overcome tachycardia. If this is unsuccessful or if fibrillation occurs, a DC shock is initiated. The control unit has sensed ventricular fibrillation and delivered a

shock directly to the ventricle, restoring sinus rhythm. Devices also have a pacing function if required. Older devices comprised an epicardial pad which required thoracotomy to position, and a control unit placed in the abdominal wall.
c. The implications for anaesthesia depend not only on the device but also on associated patient factors. Regarding the device itself, the use of perioperative equipment, particularly electrocautery, may be misinterpreted by the ICD as a dysrhythmia and result in either a DC shock or the device attempting overpacing. The device should therefore be deactivated prior to surgery and external cardiac monitoring substituted.

The patient requiring an ICD is likely to have significant cardiac disease, with continuing ischaemia and cardiac failure, and may be taking a variety of medications. In addition, the patient is known to be at risk of cardiac dysrhythmias, and therefore external defibrillation equipment should be immediately available. If required, the defibrillator paddles should be placed as far away from the device as possible.

Further reading

Amar D, Gross JN 1993 Patients with pacemakers. In: Simpson JI, ed. *Anaesthesia and the Patient with Co-existing Heart Disease.* Little, Brown and Co., Boston.
Gaba DM, Wyner J, Fish KJ 1985 Anaesthesia and the automatic implantable cardioverter/defibrillator. *Anesthesiology* 62: 786–792.

Answer 2.4

a. There is marked cardiomegaly. The left atrium is grossly enlarged, suggesting either mitral stenosis or regurgitation, which would be consistent with atrial fibrillation. There is perihilar pulmonary oedema and septal lines are present. The right costophrenic angle is blunted, probably secondary to a pleural effusion. Pulmonary oedema occurs more frequently with stenosis and, if present with a regurgitant valve, suggests the development of left

2

A

ventricular dysfunction. In this case there is pulmonary congestion with left ventricular enlargement, suggesting a diagnosis of mitral regurgitation or mixed mitral valvular disease.

b. Physical examination may reveal the characteristic plethoric 'mitral facies' of mitral valve disease. If mitral stenosis is predominant, there may be a tapping apex beat, loud first heart sound, an opening snap, a mid-diastolic murmur, and if the patient is in sinus rhythm a presystolic accentuation of the murmur may also be heard. Signs of mitral regurgitation include a displaced apex beat, pansystolic murmur of regurgitation, soft diastolic murmur of ventricular filling, and a third heart sound.

The investigation of choice is echocardiography, with transoesophageal examination providing most accurate information on the mitral valve. The diagnosis may be confirmed and the severity of the lesion assessed. The gradient across the valve and orifice area can be calculated, and other associated abnormalities such as mural thrombus can be detected.

c. The problems of mitral stenosis include a relatively fixed cardiac output depending heavily on left atrial filling and the duration of diastole. In addition, this patient also has marked pulmonary oedema. Pulmonary hypertension and right ventricular strain are probably also present. Preoperative stabilisation includes control of heart rate with digoxin, correction of any electrolyte abnormality, if possible, and diuretic therapy for pulmonary oedema.

In contrast, the problems of mitral regurgitation are mainly those of left ventricular overload. Systemic vasodilatation improves forward flow and a faster heart rate reduces ventricular size.

Anaesthetic considerations include careful monitoring of left and right filling pressures, optimisation of left ventricular filling and avoidance of tachycardia if stenosis is predominant, although a mild

tachycardia is often beneficial if regurgitation is predominant. Factors known to exacerbate pulmonary hypertension such as acidosis or hypoxia should be avoided. A low-dose volatile and opioid technique is probably the most appropriate, although careful fully monitored epidural may be considered.

Answer 2.5

a. The image is a two-dimensional transthoracic echocardiogram. The left atrium, mitral valve and left ventricle can be clearly seen. The right ventricle can also be seen at the top of the image, and the abnormality is a thickened ventricular septum especially in the basal area (see figure below). The diagnosis is hypertrophic cardiomyopathy (HCM). In most cases of HCM the thickening of the ventricular wall is asymmetric, preferentially involving the interventricular septum. Lesions with basal involvement cause outflow obstruction due to both a sphincter effect of the thickened muscle and a Venturi effect which draws the mitral valve into the outflow tract, coincidentally causing mitral regurgitation.

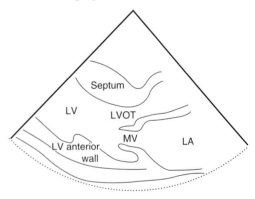

b. Individuals with HCM may be asymptomatic, however some dyspnoea is common secondary to reduced diastolic function. Angina may occur because of reduced coronary flow and increased myocardial oxygen demand. Dysrhythmias are common, and syncope can result either from rhythm disturbance or from an inability to increase cardiac output during exercise. Sudden death is a risk, particularly in children and young adults.

c. Patients with known obstructive HCM may already be on medical treatment with β-blockers, calcium channel blockers or amiodarone. These medications should be continued throughout the perioperative period as far as possible. The principal aim is to avoid increasing the gradient across the outflow tract. Increasing cardiac contractility exacerbates the obstruction, and therefore sympathetic stimulation or sympathomimetic drugs should be avoided. Similarly, hypovolaemia or drugs or manoeuvres which reduce the afterload also increase the gradient. Tachycardia is detrimental for the same reasons as in aortic stenosis. Moderately cardiodepressant agents such as volatile anaesthetics can actually improve ventricular dynamics. Monitoring should include V5 ECG to detect ischaemia. Invasive arterial pressure monitoring is useful but CVP monitoring gives no valuable information on left ventricular loading. Pulmonary artery flotation catheter may help, but perioperative transoesophageal echocardiography gives the best information on left ventricular function and filling. Arrhythmias are common and need to be treated aggressively. Cardioversion should be immediately available, and agents such as short-acting β-blockers may be valuable in supraventricular tachycardias.

Further reading

Casthely PA, Lee SY, Komer CA 1993 Cardiomyopathies. In: Simpson JI, ed. *Anaesthesia and the Patient with Co-existing Heart Disease.* Little, Brown & Co., Boston.

Julian DG, Campbell CJ, McLenachan JM 1998 Diseases of the pericardium and myocardium. In: *Cardiology* 7th edn. WB Saunders & Co., London.

Answer 2.6

a. The rhythm is atrial fibrillation with a slow ventricular response. Other abnormalities present include inferior Q waves, poor R wave progression in the anterior chest leads and widespread downsloping ST depression. The first complex in the standard leads has a broad QRS and is probably ventricular in origin.

b. Causes of atrial fibrillation include mitral valve disease, thyrotoxicosis, alcohol, ischaemic heart disease, pericarditis and recent cardiac surgery. In this case there is evidence of ischaemic heart disease. The widespread downsloping ST-segment depression, the so-called reverse tick, suggests digoxin toxicity. Many dysrhythmias may complicate digoxin toxicity, including atrial tachycardias, atrioventricular block and complete heart block, junctional rhythm, and ventricular dysrhythmias such as ectopics, VT and VF. In this case the development of digoxin toxicity on a background of long-term problem-free administration indicates that there has been a change in plasma protein binding, renal clearance or sensitivity to digoxin. Several cardiac drugs affect one or more of these factors, including verapamil, amiodarone and nifedipine. The most likely explanation is that the new tablet is a diuretic and a fall in plasma potassium has increased the patient's sensitivity to digoxin. Hypocalcaemia, hypomagnesaemia and hypothyroidism can have similar effects.

c. The plasma digoxin level should be checked. In the presence of hypokalaemia, the first step would be to normalise plasma potassium. In situations of severe toxicity, digoxin antibodies (Digibind) may be administered to reduce plasma levels acutely. Digoxin is not removed by dialysis. Cardioversion should not be used in digoxin toxicity as it may result in malignant ventricular dysrhythmias or asystole. Complete heart block may require temporary pacing, and other dysrhythmias should be treated pharmacologically if necessary.

2
A

Answer 2.7

a. The rhythm is sinus with a rate of 48 consistent with β-blockade. Pathological Q waves in leads II, III and aVF indicate a previous full-thickness inferior myocardial infarction. There are also voltage criteria to suggest LVH consistent with long-term hypertension. As the MI was asymptomatic and Q waves are permanent, it is normally impossible to give any indication as to when it occurred. However, in this case, the patient presumably had a normal ECG at his medical 2 months earlier, dating the event to within that period.

b. The most important consideration is the timing of the surgery. Most risk indices for patients undergoing non-cardiac surgery (e.g. Goldman et al, Detsky et al, below) include myocardial infarction (MI) within 6 months as a major contributor to increased risk of perioperative MI. The risk of re-infarction within 1 week of MI is as high as 40%, whilst by 6 months most texts report the risk to be reduced to 5–6%. Although more recent work has suggested that there is no relationship between timing and re-infarction (Shah et al, below), the improvement probably reflects the increased use of invasive monitoring and intensive care facilities. The incidence of silent perioperative ischaemia has also been shown to correlate with outcome (Mangano et al, below). As this procedure is elective and the mortality from perioperative MI is high (up to 70%), it would be appropriate to delay surgery. In addition, the patient would benefit from cardiological referral for exercise testing and treatment optimisation in addition to his current β-blockade, such as adding aspirin and lipid-lowering agents if required.

Further reading

Detsky AS, Abrams HB, McLaughlin JR et al 1986 Predicting cardiac complications in patients undergoing non-cardiac surgery. *Journal of General Internal Medicine* 1: 211–219.

Goldman L, Caldera DL, Nussbaum SR et al 1978 Multifactorial index of cardiac risk in non-cardiac surgical procedures. *Medicine* 57: 357–370.

Mangano DT, Browner WS, Hollenberg M et al 1990 Association of perioperative MI with cardiac morbidity and mortality in men undergoing non-cardiac surgery. The Study of Perioperative Ischaemia Research Group. *New England Journal of Medicine* 323: 1781–1788.

Shah KB, Kleinman BS, Sami H et al 1990 Re-evaluation of perioperative MI in patients with prior MI undergoing non-cardiac operations. *Anesthesia and Analgesia* 71: 231–235.

Answer 2.8

a. The CXR shows a generalised increase in heart size not suggestive of any particular chamber enlargement. The lack of signs of pulmonary congestion suggests that the cause is not cardiomegaly and myocardial failure. The patient is shocked, with a reduced level of consciousness suggesting poor cardiac output, and cold peripheries confirming peripheral vasoconstriction. The diagnosis is pericardial effusion with cardiac tamponade.

   The possible causes of pericardial effusion include neoplastic disease, infection such as tuberculosis, heart failure, myxoedema, and generalised disorders such as uraemia, rheumatoid arthritis and systemic lupus erythematosus.

b. Signs of the effusion itself include difficulty palpating the apex beat, quiet heart sounds and occasionally a friction rub. Signs of tamponade are an elevated JVP (which rises on inspiration), tachycardia, hypotension and pulsus paradoxus.

c. An ECG may show low-voltage complexes across all leads, and possibly flattened or inverted T waves. The most useful investigation is transthoracic echocardiography to confirm the presence of pericardial fluid and elicit signs of cardiac tamponade, i.e. right ventricular and atrial diastolic collapse. In severe cases the left atrium may also collapse in late diastole. Echocardiography will also aid in emergency pericardiocentesis if indicated.

Further reading
Cheitlin MD, Sokolow M, McIlroy MB 1993 Pericarditis. In: *Clinical Cardiology*. 6th edn. Appleton and Lange, Connecticut.

Answer 2.9

a. There is a sinus tachycardia of approximately 100. The axis is within the normal range, but there are tall R waves in leads V3–V5 suggestive of left ventricular hypertrophy. There is extensive downsloping ST depression and T wave flattening in the inferior leads and throughout the chest leads.

b. This patient has evidence of multiple end-organ disease associated with her diabetes. This includes diabetic nephropathy, retinopathy, peripheral vascular disease and coronary artery disease. In addition, the lack of symptoms from her myocardial ischaemia and presumably ischaemic toes, coupled with the elevated resting heart rate, may indicate diabetic neuropathy.

c. Diabetes is regarded as an independent risk factor in indices such as Eagle; however, this may be due to end organ disease rather than the diabetes itself. This is a situation of limb salvage, and therefore investigation should be directed at defining risk factors and addressing those which may be improved in the short term. The severity of the end organ disease may indicate poor diabetic control. Close monitoring of blood glucose and tighter control by increased frequency of either subcutaneous or intravenous infusion of insulin should improve wound healing and reduce postoperative infection. Renal failure is established, but the anaesthetist should establish the dialysis schedule, ideal weight and daily fluid allowance of the patient. Urea and electrolytes should be monitored prior to surgery.

Most importantly, this patient has evidence of silent myocardial ischaemia. CXR is required to assess heart size and any evidence of failure. Transthoracic echocardiography may be indicated to assess left ventricular function, detect diabetic cardiomyopathy and detect regional wall motion abnormalities indicative of ischaemia/infarction. Although stress testing to assess the need for coronary angiography is probably unrealistic in this urgent setting, cardiological involvement in pharmacological optimisation is desirable.

Further reading
Roizen M 2000 Anaesthetic implications of concurrent disease. In: Miller RD, ed. *Anaesthesia*, 5th edn. Churchill Livingstone, Philadelphia.

Answer 2.10

a. The ECG shows an intermittent broad complex tachycardia. The differential diagnosis is:

- ventricular tachycardia (VT)
- supraventricular tachycardia (SVT) with aberrant conduction, either pre-existing or as a result of the tachycardia
- Wolf–Parkinson–White syndrome with retrograde atrioventricular node conduction, and antegrade accessory pathway conduction.

b. Broad complex tachycardias are generally considered VT unless there is evidence to the contrary, e.g. known paroxysmal SVT. Certain ECG features may be present and help to differentiate between VT and SVT. VT – a QRS wider than 3.5 small squares; dissociated P waves; fusion beats; capture beats; left axis deviation; SVT – similar morphology during tachycardia and sinus rhythm.

In this trace, the complexes during the tachycardia are more than 3.5 small squares wide and are of variable morphology suggesting ventricular tachycardia. The other confirmatory features are not present in this case but an earlier premature beat without a preceding P wave is of a similar morphology to the tachycardia. The rhythm is therefore intermittent ventricular tachycardia. Clinical features may also help, e.g. the presence of cannon waves in the JVP indicates VT.

c. In a haemodynamically compromised patient the first step should be urgent cardioversion. In more stable situations, if the diagnosis is uncertain, carotid sinus massage or adenosine may abolish an SVT but leave VT unaffected.

If the rhythm is established as VT then lignocaine, flecainide or amiodarone may be considered in a stable patient. VT is generally a result of serious heart disease, and therefore further investigation of the underlying cause, e.g. MI, is required once sinus rhythm is re-established.

Further reading
Chou TC 1996 Differential diagnosis of tachycardia. In: *Electrocardiography in Clinical Practice*. WB Saunders, Philadelphia.

Answer 2.11

a. There is a step up in oxygenation from the right atrium to the right ventricle, indicating a left-to-right shunt at the level of the ventricle. The most likely diagnosis is a post-myocardial infarction ventricular septal defect. These occur in approximately 1% of patients after anterior or inferior myocardial infarction.

b. The pulmonary:systemic flow ratio can be calculated using the formula:

$$\frac{Q_p}{Q_s} = \frac{\text{Saturation in aorta} - \text{saturation in right atrium}}{\text{Saturation in aorta} - \text{saturation in pulmonary artery}}$$

A ratio of > 2:1 is haemodynamically significant.

c. This complication of myocardial infarction usually results in rapid development of severe cardiac failure. A pansystolic murmur at the left sternal edge may be confused with that of papillary muscle rupture and severe mitral regurgitation. Transthoracic echocardiography provides the most rapid reliable diagnosis, with colour Doppler clearly illustrating flow across a ventricular defect. Shunt can be calculated by estimating cardiac output in the pulmonary artery and the aorta. In most cases the treatment of choice is urgent surgical correction.

Answer 2.12

a. The left subclavian artery is prominent giving rise to the '3' sign, and there is notching of the inferior borders of the ribs. The diagnosis is coarctation of the aorta distal to the origin of the left subclavian artery.

b. The clinical signs are left ventricular hypertrophy giving rise to an apical heave, radiofemoral delay of the pulse, higher measured blood pressure in the upper limbs compared with the lower limbs and potentially two different types of murmur. A late systolic murmur from the coarctation itself may be heard between the scapulae and a continuous murmur from the collaterals over the ribs.

c. Left ventricular hypertrophy develops, predisposing to subendocardial ischaemia, especially if afterload is excessive. Anaesthesia should therefore be tailored to prevent surges in blood pressure. Infective endarteritis is a risk and therefore antibiotic prophylaxis is indicated.

Surgery to the thorax or abdomen may be complicated by excessive bleeding from the very large collateral vessels. In addition, in major surgery the possibility of reduced blood flow to the lower half of the body, particularly in terms of renal perfusion, needs consideration and appropriate monitoring.

Answer 2.13

a. There is evidence of right ventricular hypertrophy (RVH), with right axis deviation, and deep S waves in the lateral chest leads. Although not present in this example, other features of RVH would include a dominant R in V1 and evidence of right ventricular strain in leads V1–V3. In addition, there is an abnormally peaked P wave, especially in lead II, indicating right atrial hypertrophy. A possible cause in this case is pulmonary hypertension secondary to hypoxia associated with obstructive sleep apnoea and obesity.

b. A careful history may elicit suggestive symptoms such as loud snoring, morning headache, daytime somnolence and difficulty concentrating. A CXR may show right ventricular enlargement and prominent pulmonary arteries, and blood gas analysis may reveal elevated bicarbonate. On clinical examination there may be a right ventricular heave and the JVP may be elevated with a prominent 'a' wave. Formal sleep studies can confirm the diagnosis.

c. Any cause of right ventricular overload such as cor pulmonale, pulmonary stenosis, recurrent pulmonary emboli or Eisenmenger's syndrome.

Answer 2.14

a. There is a pacing spike with no constant relationship to either the P wave or QRS complex. The underlying rhythm is sinus with a normal PR interval. The mean QRS axis is shifted leftwards and the morphology in lead V1 is of RBBB (right bundle branch block). The ECG therefore shows bifascicular block and a pacemaker which is neither sensing nor capturing.

b. As bifascicular block is not in itself an indication for permanent pacing; this patient was presumably symptomatic. This would suggest that his cardiac function is significantly compromised, and therefore cardiological referral to re-establish pacemaker capture prior to surgery is required.

c. General perioperative and anaesthetic care will need to be tailored to the patient's compromised cardiovascular status. Specific attention needs to be paid to patients with pacemakers (see Bourke 1996, below). Firstly it is important to know the classification of the pacemaker. Each patient should have a pacemaker record card detailing the make, model and mode of the pacemaker. This is recorded as a string of up to five letters:

Position I   Chamber paced
Position II   Chamber sensed
Position III   Response
Position IV   Programmability
Position V   Anti-tachycardia function

Often only the first three letters are designated, e.g.:

VVI   Ventricular sensing and pacing; response to sensing is inhibition of pacing

DDD   Dual (atrial and ventricular) sensing and pacing; response may either be inhibition or triggering

Modern pacemakers all have some programmable features. An R at position IV indicates rate responsiveness. This provides an increase in heart rate in response to various stimuli such as increased respiratory rate, increased blood temperature or increased muscle activity, which would indicate an increase in exercise. This may cause problems in the operating theatre with artificial ventilation or change in body temperature and is therefore disabled prior to surgery. Battery and function check of the pacemaker should be carried out preoperatively if not done recently.

Chest X-ray will demonstrate the number and position of leads, and special views can be sought to demonstrate any suspected lead fracture.

Urine and electrolytes (U&E) need to be checked, particularly with regard to serum potassium, as imbalance may cause problems with capture.

Intraoperative problems are mostly related to electromagnetic (EM) interference in the operating theatre. Modern devices are well shielded and so this is less of a problem; however, monopolar electrocautery may still temporarily inhibit pacemaker function. Earth plates should therefore be as far from the pulse generator as practicable, electrocautery kept to short bursts, or bipolar used if possible. Formerly, it was recommended that magnets should be available during surgery. A magnet placed over a pulse generator usually reverts the function to fixed rate. However, in the new programmable models, it may initiate a threshold self-test in the unit, and if in place during EM interference may even result in haphazard reprogramming of the unit.

Microshock transmitted down the leads to the myocardium is also a theoretical risk. This is most likely during DC cardioversion, especially with external (temporary) pacemaker leads. In order to minimise this risk, and the risk of damage to the pulse generator itself, defibrillation pads should be placed at right angles to the pacing leads away from the generator box.

Further reading
Bourke ME 1996 The patient with a pacemaker or related device. *Canadian Journal of Anaesthesia* 43(5): R24–32.

Answer 2.15

a. Tracing the left heart border, there is an abnormal bulge above the apex. This is consistent with a left ventricular aneurysm developing as a complication of myocardial infarction.
b. The ECG features of ventricular aneurysm are deep QS waves and persistent ST elevation over the affected area. In this patient there are extensive QS waves across the anteroseptal leads and ST elevation in leads V2 and V3. The axis is shifted to the left, suggesting left anterior hemi-block, and there are non-specific ST and T wave changes in the lateral leads.
c. The ECG changes suggest extensive aneurysm. Transthoracic echocardiography is non-invasive and relatively simple to arrange

preoperatively. It will clarify the area of the lesion, quantify ventricular function and allow identification of any associated problem such as mural thrombus formation or papillary muscle dysfunction.

Answer 2.16

a. There is a sinus bradycardia with a rate of 50 beats/min and widespread T wave inversion across the anteroseptal chest leads. In addition, the QT interval is prolonged, even when corrected for heart rate (Bazett's formula: $QT_c = QT/PR$). An interval greater than 0.44 s (11 small squares) is generally regarded as prolonged.

b. The T wave inversion may indicate ongoing anteroseptal ischaemia, a recent non-Q wave MI, or may be persistent following an old MI. There is no evidence of right ventricular hypertrophy to suggest that it represents a 'strain' pattern. There are various causes of a prolonged QT interval:

- *Inherited*: Romano–Ward syndrome
- *Metabolic*: hypocalcaemia – may also cause T wave inversion
- *Drug-induced*:
  Class IA antiarrhythmics
  —Disopyramide
  —Quinidine
  —Procainamide
  Class III antiarrhythmics
  —Sotalol
  —Amiodarone
  Tricyclic antidepressants
  Terfenadine (with ketoconazole or erythromycin)
- *Other causes*:
  Ischaemic heart disease
  Hypothermia
  Myxoedema
  Intracranial haemorrhage.

c. The long QT interval predisposes to R on T phenomena, increasing the risk of ventricular dysrhythmias, usually torsade de pointes, and sudden death.

d. The management of long QT involves treatment of the underlying cause if possible. In this case the patient may well be on antiarrhythmic agents following his stormy postoperative course. This may also explain his bradycardia. The need for the drugs could be reviewed and, if necessary, the dosage or drug altered. The bradycardia may, however, also be related to his underlying cardiac disease.

Answer 2.17

a. There is a narrow complex tachycardia with a rate of approximately 200. The diagnosis is paroxysmal supraventricular tachycardia (SVT). SVT generally has a rate of 140–220 with normal morphology of the QRS complex, although there can be aberrant conduction causing a broad complex tachycardia which may be confused with VT (see Question 2.11).
b. The cause of SVT is a re-entrant circuit between the atria and the ventricles, either via the AV node itself or via an accessory pathway (Kent bundle) as in Wolf–Parkinson–White syndrome.
c. Most episodes of SVT are self-terminating. Mechanisms to slow or temporarily block AV node conduction, such as carotid sinus massage, Valsalva manoeuvre or intravenous adenosine, may terminate the re-entrant rhythm.

Answer 2.18

a. Abnormal signs on the CXR are a widened upper mediastinum, a left pleural effusion, displaced trachea and downward displacement of the left main bronchus. The ECG exhibits voltage criteria for the left ventricular hypertrophy and anterolateral ischaemic changes indicative of a left ventricular hypertrophy with strain pattern.

The diagnosis is aortic dissection in a patient with evidence of long-standing hypertension. The ischaemia on the ECG may represent pre-existing coronary disease or involvement of the coronary arteries in the dissection process.

Aortic dissection is most commonly associated with elderly hypertensive men, but may also occur in conditions causing disease of the aortic media, e.g. Marfan's disease, hypothyroidism or pregnancy. Classification has been simplified into type A dissections involving the ascending aorta, which may also extend to the descending aorta, and type B in which only the descending aorta is involved.
b. The patient often appears shocked with pallor, sweating and tachycardia. The blood pressure may appear normal, but it should be remembered that these patients are usually hypertensive. Hypotension may result if the true lumen of the aorta becomes occluded.

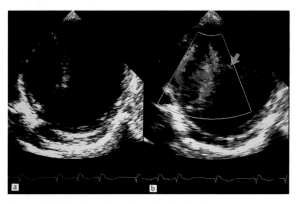

Echocardiographic views of aortic dissection.

Involvement of major vessels leads to loss of pulses in the affected limb, or to symptoms such as abdominal pain or decreased level of consciousness. If the aortic root is involved, severe aortic incompetence and left ventricular failure can lead to rapid deterioration.

Further investigations will depend on the degree of suspicion and the status of the patient. Formerly, the investigation of choice was an arch aortogram. Aortography may still be required to assess the extent of dissection accurately, but transoesophageal echocardiography provides a rapid diagnosis allowing early transfer to theatre if appropriate. A cross-sectional echocardiographic view of an aortic dissection is shown in the figure on page 63. The arrow indicates flow through the tear seen when colour flow Doppler is applied. CT and MRI are also highly sensitive but more time-consuming.

c. Initial management is aimed at preventing propagation of the dissection, essentially by controlling blood pressure. The alpha- and beta-blocking effects of labetalol are useful, with vasodilators such as sodium nitroprusside providing additional control.

Further management depends upon the type of dissection. In type A, the mortality is extremely high (up to 90%) unless urgent surgical repair is undertaken. In type B, however, the mortality rate is very similar for medical or surgical management. Surgery is therefore usually reserved for cases in which there are complications, such as continued propagation of the dissection or occlusion of major vessels.

Further reading
Oliver WC, Nuttall G, Murray MJ 1999 Thoracic aortic disease. In: Kaplan JA, ed. *Cardiac Anaesthesia*, 4th edn. WB Saunders, Philadelphia.

bundle branch block (RBBB). The mean frontal axis is deviated to the right. The echocardiogram shows a view of the atria with a large defect of the intra-atrial septum. Colour flow Doppler highlights the flow across the atrial septal defect.

b. Atrial septal defects can be classified as:

- *patent foramen ovale* – in which the septum primum and septum secondum fail to fuse
- *primum defects* – in which the defect is adjacent to the atrioventricular valves and may be associated with valvular abnormalities
- *secundum defects* – which do not encroach on the valve area. These are the commonest, and the type shown in this example. Unlike primum defects, which present early in life, secundum defects may be asymptomatic until the third decade in life.

c. ASD secundum defects may be surgically corrected in young adults to prevent the development of pulmonary vascular disease, right ventricular failure and paradoxical emboli. A cardiac catheterisation may be required to assess the shunt across the defect and to assess pulmonary hypertension, although this information can also be derived from echocardiographic Doppler and contrast examination. If no pulmonary hypertension is present, surgery is more strongly indicated in young women, as pregnancy can precipitate rapidly progressive pulmonary vascular disease. Chest radiography may show an increased cardiothoracic ratio and enlarged pulmonary arteries.

Further reading
Redington A, Shore D, Aldershaw P, 1994 *Congenital Heart Disease in Adults; a practical guide.* WB Saunders, London.

Answer 2.19

a. The ECG shows an RSR' pattern in the anterior chest leads, indicating right

Answer 2.20

a. This patient has multiple risk factors for ischaemic heart disease. There are Q waves and T wave inversion in leads II, III and aVF, indicating an inferior infarction. Whilst the presence of inferior Q waves suggests an old infarction, the ST elevation suggests a more recent re-infarction. T waves may take several weeks to return to normal, or remain permanently inverted. In addition, the R waves in the lateral chest leads fulfil the voltage criteria for left ventricular hypertrophy, and there are widespread ST and T wave ischaemic changes across the chest leads.

b. There may be ongoing ischaemia/infarction causing further pain, or pericarditis may have developed. This diagnosis is supported by the exacerbation of the pain on lying down. Pericarditis of other aetiology may cause concave ST elevation, which may be confused with MI. Such changes are usually more generalised and Q waves would not occur.

c. In addition to a full clinical examination, chest X-ray and baseline biochemistry, cardiac enzyme measurement may confirm the diagnosis. Further ECGs should be recorded if there is any suggestion of ongoing ischaemia. Urgent angiography may be necessary if there is ischaemia to assess whether angioplasty or surgery is indicated.

Management includes early transfer to a cardiology unit. As the infarct is greater than 12 h old, thrombolysis is not appropriate. The patient is already taking aspirin, but the addition of β-blockers both in the acute phase and for long-term prevention has been shown to reduce mortality (ISIS-1, Norwegian Timolol Trial). ACE inhibitors also reduce short- and long-term mortality after MI, especially if cardiac failure is present (ISIS-4, AIRE trials).

Further reading

First International Study of Infarct Survival Collaborative Group 1986 Randomised trial of intravenous atenolol among 16 027 cases of suspected acute myocardial infarction: ISIS-1. *Lancet* 2(8498): 57–66.

ISIS-4 (Fourth International Study of Infarct Survival) Collaborative Group 1995 ISIS-4: a randomised factorial trial assessing early oral captopril, oral mononitrate, and intravenous magnesium sulphate in 58,050 patients with suspected acute myocardial infarction. *Lancet* 345(8951): 669–685.

The Acute Infarction Ramipril Efficacy (AIRE) Study Investigators 1993 Effect of ramipril on mortality and morbidity of survivors of acute myocardial infarction with clinical evidence of heart failure. *Lancet* 342(8875): 821–828.

The Norwegian Multicenter Study Group. Timolol-induced reduction in motality and reinfarction in patients surviving acute myocardial infarction. *New England Journal of Medicine* 304:801–7.

Answer 2.21

a. The ECG shows a tachycardia and tall, peaked T waves. The initial QRS complexes are narrow but rapidly widen and degenerate to a broad complex tachycardia associated with a sudden loss of cardiac output. The diagnosis is ventricular tachycardia secondary to hyperkalaemia. T wave changes may occur when serum potassium exceeds 5.5 mEq/L. The loss of P waves may precede QRS widening and ultimately asystole or ventricular fibrillation may occur.

b. Hyperkalaemia may result from renal failure, acidosis, drugs such as potassium-sparing diuretics, adrenal insufficiency and administration of potassium. This patient has suffered major trauma and will have received a large volume of blood. The serum potassium of stored blood may be as high as 16 mEq/L and rapid transfusion of unwashed blood can cause rapid rises in a patient's serum potassium. In addition, the patient is likely to be acidotic, not only as a result of blood transfusion, but also secondary to poor peripheral circulation and tissue hypoxia.

c. Urgent DC cardioversion is required followed by correction of the metabolic abnormality. Calcium salts stabilise the myocardium and will also correct any transfusion-related hypocalcaemia. Dextrose and insulin infusion will control the hyperkalaemia, and acidosis may need correcting with bicarbonate. If ongoing bleeding is a problem, the use of a cell saver to recycle lost blood and wash transfused blood will help to prevent further hyperkalaemia.

Answer 2.22

a. There is a regular tachycardia with a rate of 150. The complexes are narrow, suggesting a supraventricular origin for the tachyarrhythmia. The rate of 150 is strongly suggestive of atrial flutter with 2 to 1 atrioventricular block, as atria characteristically flutter with a rate of around 300. At this rate, the flutter waves tend to be difficult to distinguish from the P and T waves of a sinus tachycardia. In addition, there is an RSR' pattern in the right-sided chest leads without widening of the QRS, indicating a partial right bundle branch block. This partial block may be a temporary phenomenon related to the tachycardia.

b. Any method of slowing down AV conduction will reduce the ventricular response rate. Valsalva, carotid sinus massage or pharmacological intervention such as adenosine or β-blockade will reveal the flutter waves more clearly (see below).

c. Atrial flutter is associated with ischaemic heart disease, rheumatic heart disease, myocarditis and thyrotoxicosis. In this patient, although we do not know her height, her weight of only 46 kg may be further evidence of elevated T4 levels.

d. In this patient, the tachycardia is of recent onset and appears to be associated with symptoms of cardiac failure; therefore low-energy DC cardioversion under general anaesthesia is likely to revert the patient to sinus rhythm and improve cardiac function. If the arrhythmia is persistent or paroxysmal then digoxin may help to control the rate. Amiodarone or sotalol may revert the rhythm to sinus. Any underlying cause such as hyperthyroidism needs to be corrected if possible. If the cause is a localised atrial re-entry circuit, ablation may be curative.

Answer 2.23

a. The principal lesion shown is a tight stenosis of the left main stem.

b. A tight stenosis of the left main coronary artery severely restricts oxygen supply to a large mass of left ventricular myocardium. Therefore, anaesthesia needs to be directed at minimising the myocardial oxygen requirement whilst maintaining myocardial oxygen delivery. In practice, this means avoiding stresses such as increased heart rate, contractility, afterload or preload. Although premedication should be sufficiently sedative to prevent anxiety, there may be significant left ventricular dysfunction, in which case the dosage may need to be altered to avoid hypotension and reduced coronary blood flow. Similar considerations are important during the conduct of anaesthesia, in that drugs need to be tailored to obtund responses to stimulation such as intubation and sternotomy, whilst maintaining diastolic

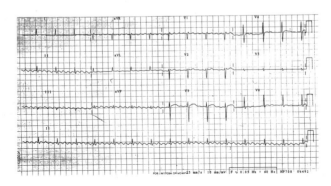

blood pressure and hence coronary perfusion. This may be achieved with a high-dose opioid induction and maintenance technique with or without the addition of low-dose volatile. Close monitoring for ischaemia by continual five-lead ECG is required. Transoesophageal echocardiography will allow detection of new ischaemia-induced regional wall motion abnormalities.

Answer 2.24

a. This is a radioisotope myocardial perfusion scan during rest and under stress. In this case, the radioisotope is technetium-99m which produces a better image than thallium-201. Nuclear cardiological stress testing can be useful in patients with an abnormal ECG in whom interpretation of conventional exercise testing is more difficult. Presumably pharmacological stress has been necessary in this case, as the patient's claudication is severely limiting. The views shown are short axis, vertical long axis and horizontal long axis. There is a clear deficit in perfusion during the stress phase not present in the resting phase, indicating an area of reversible ischaemia. The area of reduced perfusion corresponds to the posterolateral wall of the left ventricle.

b. The lack of a significant cold spot on the resting scan indicates that the thrombolytic treatment of this patient was successful. He still has a physiologically significant lesion, however, for which angiography is indicated to assess severity of disease and suitability for angioplasty or surgery.

c. Broadly speaking, the area of reduced perfusion is in the territory of the circumflex artery.

Answer 2.25

a. There are occasional narrow QRS complexes with preceding P waves. The majority of the tracing shows a broad complex tachycardia. The morphology of the tachycardia varies in that the voltage appears to increase and decrease cyclically. The rhythm is torsade de pointes VT. In addition, the initial complexes of the dysrhythmia are unlike either the pre-existing complexes or the complexes of the dysrhythmia itself, and are probably fusion beats, i.e. a combination of the normally paced beat and of the ventricular beat.

b. Torsade de pointes VT is associated with long QT syndromes either inherited or acquired (see Question 2.16). The physiological abnormality is a depression of myocardial ion channels, particularly potassium channels, causing delayed repolarisation. In this patient, the most likely cause is metabolic or drug-induced. Hypokalaemia increases the risk for drug-induced torsades de pointes.

c. The management of torsades de pointes differs from that of non-polymorphic VT. DC cardioversion is indicated if there is haemodynamic instability, but antiarrhythmic agents should be avoided as they may exacerbate the problem. This is particularly relevant to class 1a drugs such as procainamide which prolong the action potential duration. Intravenous magnesium may be effective, as hypomagnesaemia may trigger the dysrhythmia. Serum potassium levels should be checked and maintained at 4.5–5.5 mmol/L. Overpacing may also be effective in preventing recurrences whilst the underlying cause is corrected.

Further reading

Viskin S 1999 Long QT syndromes and torsade de pointes. *Lancet* 354(9190): 1625–1633.

Answer 2.26

a. The rhythm is sinus. The PR interval is prolonged (> 5 small squares), indicating a first-degree atrioventricular (AV) block. The mean frontal axis is shifted to the left. The positive and negative deflections in lead I are approximately equal, indicating that the

2

A

axis is approaching 90° away from lead I. As lead II is predominately negative, the axis is to the left of lead I, i.e. left axis deviation. The QRS complex is widened in all leads (> 3 small squares), indicating intraventricular block. The RSR pattern in V1–V3 indicates a right bundle branch block (RBBB). RBBB does not itself cause a shift in axis. The individual fascicles of the left bundle may be damaged independently. Left anterior fascicular block causes a left axis deviation, whereas left posterior hemiblock causes right axis deviation. The ECG therefore shows trifascicular block, i.e. bifascicular block and first-degree AV block.

b. Although the patient is asymptomatic, the ECG changes are associated with significant ischaemic heart disease. In addition, he has risk factors for ischaemic heart disease, in that he is male, middle-aged, overweight and a smoker.

c. If the surgery is not urgent, the patient would benefit from further investigation of his cardiac disease. Exercise ECG stress testing would be difficult to interpret due to his abnormal resting ECG, but stress echocardiography or radioisotope studies would allow assessment of the severity of his disease. Regarding anaesthesia, the presence of trifascicular block has been considered an indication for perioperative temporary pacing, as there is a risk of developing complete heart block (see Question 2.1). In asymptomatic patients with chronic bifascicular block, there is a high incidence of perioperative bradydysrhythmias and hypotension. These are usually responsive to pharmacological intervention, and even in conjunction with a prolonged PR interval, progression to complete heart block is rare. Therefore, ensuring availability of appropriate drugs and perhaps non-invasive transcutaneous pacing is probably appropriate rather than transluminal pacing.

Further reading

Gauss A, Hubner C, Radermacher P et al 1998 Perioperative risk of bradyarrhythmias in patients with asymptomatic chronic bifascicular block or left bundle branch block. Does an additional 1st degree atrioventricular block make any difference? *Anesthesiology* 88(3): 679–687.

Answer 2.27

a. The second set of complexes refers to the recovery period, and exhibits ST depression in leads II, III, aVF and V4–V6. In these leads, the depression is either down-sloping or planar, and therefore is more reliable as an indicator of ischaemia than up-sloping depression would be. The sensitivity and specificity of exercise ECG are not particularly high, but are improved by taking into account other factors which influence the probability of the test being positive or negative, e.g. symptoms, age and sex, as well as the degree of ST depression. Therefore, in this case, there is a high probability that the patient has significant coronary heart disease.

b. ST elevation may indicate severe ischaemia. Arrhythmias, such as an increase in ventricular ectopic activity, may occur in the presence of ischaemia or left ventricular dysfunction.

c. The term METS relates work to oxygen uptake (Vo_2). At rest, or 1 MET, the Vo_2 is approximately 3.5 mL/kg per min. A normal, not particularly fit, individual should be able to exercise to around 10 METS. Although Vo_2 is not actually measured during exercise testing, approximate equivalents have been calculated so that different exercise protocols can be compared. Therefore, for the Bruce protocol, stage 1 approximates to 3 METS, and stage 3 to 10 METS.

d. Heart rate and blood pressure normally rise during exercise. The rise in heart rate can be affected by medication such as β-blockers. Blood pressure can also be affected by β-blockers, especially in combination with other drugs such as calcium antagonists; however, the most likely reason for such a fall in blood pressure is ischaemia-related left ventricular dysfunction.

Answer 2.28

a. Each sinus beat with a narrow QRS complex is coupled to a broad complex ventricular premature beat (VPB). The rhythm is ventricular bigemini. There is a compensatory pause after each VPB caused by retrograde depolarisation of the SA node. The VPBs are unifocal in origin. In addition, the PR interval is prolonged, indicating a degree of AV blockade.

b. VPBs may be associated with ischaemic heart disease or cardiomyopathies, and in such cases may indicate a worse prognosis. They may also be related to electrolyte disturbance, ventricular escape in association with bradycardia, or drug toxicity such as digoxin toxicity. Further history is required to suggest a cause in this patient. The ECG itself does not indicate any ischaemia or ventricular enlargement. The combination of AV block and bigemini could indicate digoxin toxicity. Renal impairment secondary to obstructive uropathy may have resulted in elevated plasma digoxin levels if the patient was previously digitalised.

c. Any precipitating factor such as electrolyte disturbance should be corrected. If digoxin toxicity is suspected, levels need to be checked and managed as outlined in Question 2.6. Features of VPBs thought to pose a greater risk of degeneration to VT or VF include multifocal ectopics, bigemini and R-on-T phenomena. Pharmacological treatment is generally limited to situations in which there is haemodynamic instability, as the treatment itself may lead to adverse outcome. Drugs which may be used include lignocaine, procainamide and β-blockers.

Further reading

Atlee JL 1997 Perioperative cardiac dysrhythmias. *Anesthesiology* 86: 1397–1424.

Answer 2.29

a. The features are a short PR interval, a slurred upstroke on the R wave (delta wave), and a broad QRS complex. The delta wave represents premature activation of the myocardium via an accessory pathway.

b. The diagnosis is Wolf–Parkinson–White (WPW) syndrome. During episodes of tachycardia where the forward conduction is via the AV node, the delta wave disappears as the accessory pathway is conducting retrogradely. If the circuit is reversed and the forward conduction is via the accessory pathway, a broad complex tachycardia would result.

c. The aim of anaesthetic management is to avoid any drugs or manoeuvres which would tend to precipitate tachycardia. Therefore, adequate sedative premedication and perioperative analgesia are required. Atropine and other tachycardia-inducing drugs should be avoided, and if neuromuscular blockade is needed, short-acting agents reduce the requirement for reversal. If tachycardias occur, they may be treated with vagal stimulation, β-blockers or DC cardioversion if necessary.

Drugs that may be used for longer-term control of WPW include flecainide, disopyramide, β-blockers and amiodarone. Verapamil may also be used but only if there is no atrial fibrillation, as it can enhance conduction in the accessory pathway and lead to ventricular fibrillation. Radiofrequency ablation of the accessory pathway is the long-term treatment of choice for symptomatic WPW.

Answer 2.30

a. The cardiac silhouette is grossly enlarged, and in the post-CABG situation the most likely cause is bleeding. The speed of the deterioration would suggest significant surgical bleeding, probably arterial, perhaps related to a period of hypertension during emergence. Post-cardiopulmonary bypass coagulopathy secondary to heparin, haemodilution, platelet depletion or fibrinolysis may also be implicated.

b. There may be increased drainage from the mediastinal drain, and significant blood loss will lead to hypotension and tachycardia. Frequently, however, the drain may be unable to cope with rapid haemorrhage, or may be obstructed by clot leading to tamponade. Signs of tamponade, such as elevated CVP, may be masked by hypovolaemia.

c. Fluid resuscitation should be started and arrangements made for urgent chest reopening to evacuate clot and identify the source of the bleeding. If the patient is very unstable from excessive losses or tamponade, it may be necessary to proceed on the ward rather than transfer to theatre. Re-anaesthesia using a cardiostable technique, such as opioid-based anaesthesia, is indicated. Coagulation tests should be sent to guide appropriate use of blood products such as fresh frozen plasma, cryoprecipitate and platelet infusions. Antifibrinolytic agents may be a useful adjunct to improve haemostasis.

3

NEUROSURGERY

Recent advances in neuroimaging have increased diagnostic ability and safety since the days when the highly invasive tests of pneumoencephalography, ventriculography, cerebral angiography and myelography were the only tools avaliable. CT scanning has been avaliable since the early 1970s and MRI since the early 1980s. In addition, isotope imaging has developed its potential with the evolution of SPECT (single photon emission computed tomography) and PET (positron emission tomography) scanning. These latter two techniques exploit the ability of nuclear medicine to provide functional (as opposed to anatomical) information, whereas MRI can provide both. This chapter will include examples of CT, MRI and angiography, the techniques commonly encountered in anaesthetic practice. The results of this imaging are not to be viewed in isolation. Correlation of the neuroimaging with the clinical picture and the results of monitoring are essential. Continuous monitoring of intracranial pressure and jugular bulb oxygenation using invasive transducers is now commonplace in neurosurgical intensive care units alongside non-invasive techniques such as transcranial Doppler ultrasound.

PLAIN FILMS

Despite advances in imaging technology, plain X-rays remain an important investigation. They have high spatial resolution and can provide an essential overview of spinal problems. Although one should not delay CT scanning in head-injured patients in order to perform skull X-rays, some non-displaced skull fractures may only be convincingly demonstrated on plain films. They may also demonstrate the presence of

cerebral tumours by raised intracerebral pressure changes, tumour calcification or erosion of the skull vault. Signs of raised intracerebral pressure include suture diastasis in children or erosion of the dorsum sella in adults. Occasionally, lateral displacement of a calcified pineal gland may indicate the presence of a tumour in one hemisphere.

CEREBRAL ANGIOGRAPHY

Although cerebral angiography has been practised for decades, it still retains a central role in neuroimaging. It is the prime diagnostic tool for the investigation of subarachnoid haemorrhage and thromboembolic cerebrovascular disease. Although MRI may provide angiographic data sets useful for screening in subarachnoid haemorrhage, the exact relationship of the aneurysm neck to the parent vessel prior to embolisation or open craniotomy may only be identified by angiography. The same applies to arteriovenous malformations (AVMs).

NUCLEAR MEDICINE

SPECT and PET scanning provide functional rather than anatomical information. The use of PET scanning is limited by the need for a cyclotron to produce the short-lived isotropes; however, SPECT scanning only requires a gamma camera. SPECT has become more widely used with the avaliability of technetium-based compounds such as HMPAO (hexamethyl amine penta-acetic acid). Technetium-99m decays with a half-life of 6 h and generates photons of 140 keV, close to ideal for detection by the gamma camera. HMPAO is lipophilic, and therefore cerebral take-up is flow-dependent, thus making it useful as a marker of perfusion. Its main uses are in stroke, epilepsy and psychiatry. Unlike PET, SPECT is only semi-quantatitive. A further role for SPECT involves the use of thallium-201-labelled thallous chloride in the assessment of tumour grade, the differentiation between radio necrosis and recurrent tumour, and between lymphoma and toxoplasmosis in the AIDS patient. The interpretation of such cases by anaesthetists is unlikely, and therefore will not be discussed further.

COMPUTED TOMOGRAPHY

CT scanning was introduced into clinical practice in 1972 and revolutionised neuroradiology. This is due to its high-contrast resolution, enabling good soft tissue discrimination so that haemorrhage, air, fat, calcium and oedema could all be differentiated from normal brain. In addition, white matter could be distinguished from grey matter. CT, like plain films, depends on differential absorption of X-rays by tissue. Contrast resolution is dependent on different electron densities between tissues. Resolution and speed of operation have increased greatly with the advent of rapid helical/spiral scanning. The basic principles

of operation are, however, unchanged. The patient slides through a circular gantry made up of multiple fine X-ray detectors that detect a tightly collimated beam of X-rays. The X-ray densities are converted into the final image by a series of algorithms that make assumptions about the patient and the spatial distribution of the data.

CT scanning provides good detection of fresh blood, is quick to perform, convenient for patient monitoring and is widely available (Fig. 3.1). These factors make it the first line of investigation for the acutely head-injured patient. It is, however, limited in the planes available for scanning. Acutely ill patients are scanned in the transverse (axial) plane. Movement of the patient is needed for direct coronal scanning. Clearly this is a drawback in a restless or intubated patient.

MAGNETIC RESONANCE IMAGING

Magnetic resonance image scanning depends on the phenomenon of nuclear magnetic resonance (in essence nuclei with unpaired electrons, usually hydrogen, behave like magnets). When nuclei are placed in an external magnetic field, they rotate, aligning themselves in the direction of the applied field. When a second

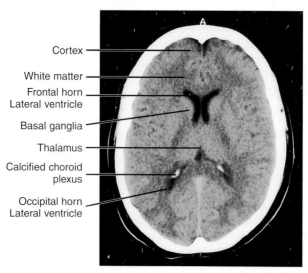

Cortex
White matter
Frontal horn
Lateral ventricle
Basal ganglia
Thalamus
Calcified choroid plexus
Occipital horn
Lateral ventricle

Fig. 3.1 A normal CT scan—axial section at the level of the thalamus.

(transverse) magnetic field is applied briefly at right angles to the first (static and constant), the nuclei are tipped in the direction of the second field. When the second field is turned off, the nuclei return to their original position in alignment with the static (longitudinal) field and at the same time release the energy absorbed as a radiosignal which is picked up by detectors. The signal produced therefore depends on the proton (water) content of the tissue. The rate of return of the nuclei depends on the element involved, the strength of the applied fields and the local chemical and magnetic environment of the nuclei (see Fig. 3.2).

Magnetic resonance imaging has many advantages: ionising radiation is not used, it can scan in any direction without moving the patient and has better contrast resolution than CT. In CT images, the contrast is dependent on electron density. In MRI there are other influences such as TI and T2 relaxation times, proton density, blood flow, diffusion and perfusion and chemical shift phenomena. Currently MRI remains a more time-consuming process than CT and has attendant monitoring problems. Not only is the patient less visible in the middle of the large-bore magnet, but access to intravenous infusions is difficult and access to the

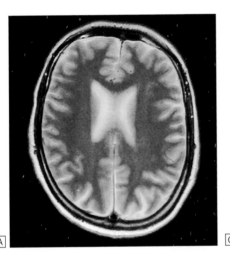

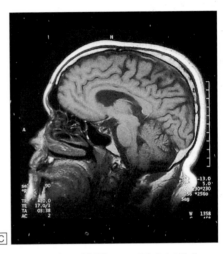

Fig. 3.2 A normal MRI scan. (A) Axial T_2 image at the level of lateral ventricles; (B) axial T_1 image at the level of the circle of Willis; (C) sagittal T_1 image in midline.

Globe

Optic nerve

Middle cerebral artery

Cerebral peduncle

Aqueduct

Cortex

White matter

3

endotracheal tube is impossible without bringing the patient out of the magnetic field. All anaesthetic equipment must be non-ferromagnetic. Technology in this field is rapidly evolving and some problems inherent with MRI may be overcome using low field resistive (permanent) magnets.

MRI scanning shows most congenital, neoplastic and inflammatory lesions of the brain better than CT and can clearly delineate many vascular lesions. MRI angiography gives results that approach direct cerebral angiography and may one day supersede it. MRI is also superior to CT for imaging the posterior fossa and spinal cord and for differentiating grey and white matter in the brain.

Interventional neuroradiology is an exciting and rapidly evolving field where many vascular lesions inaccessible to open surgery may be embolised. Venous thrombosis may also be amenable to treatment by indwelling catheter-delivered thrombolytics. In many clinical circumstances, several modalities are necessary in neuroradiology to obtain the full picture. Increasingly, treatment of vascular lesions may be carried out using interventional radiological techniques.

SELECTION OF IMAGING TECHNIQUE

In the situation of acute cerebral trauma or a deteriorating patient on ITU, CT scan is the investigation of first choice because MRI may be misleading in the context of hyperacute haemorrhage and acute cerebral oedema, but it may reveal diffuse axonal shearing injuries and small petechiae in diffuse head injuries that are missed on CT. These are of important prognostic significance. MRI is also the technique of choice in the diagnosis of sinus thrombosis. This is shown non-invasively and directly by MRI due to its flow sensitivity, whereas CT can only provide indirect evidence. Angiography has limitations due to contrast dilution by non-opacified blood.

QUESTIONS

Question 3.1

You are contacted by a junior doctor in the A&E department regarding the management of a young adult male patient with a head injury who needs a CT scan of the brain. The patient was a pedestrian in a road traffic accident and was hit by a car travelling at approximately 40 mph. The doctor informs you that the patient is unconscious and has a Glasgow Coma Score (GCS) of 2. The patient does not make any sounds or open his eyes to painful stimuli but does extend his left arm. The right arm does not make any movement in response to the painful stimulus. The patient is tolerating an oral airway. You are asked to escort the patient to the CT scanner.

a. Is the patient's Glasgow Coma Score 2?
b. What advice do you give regarding airway management?

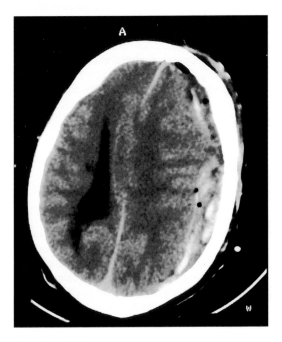

Question 3.2

A 52-year-old woman presents to the A&E having been hit by a car. She has a large laceration over the left side of her head and a GCS of 11. She has no other injuries on primary or secondary survey. Her CT scan is shown.

a. What does her CT scan show?
b. What is her prognosis?
c. Outline treatment priorities for this patient's head injury.

3

Q

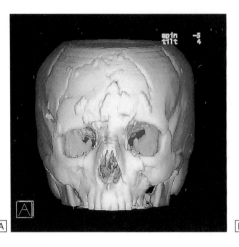

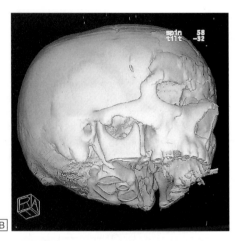

Question 3.3

An 18-year-old girl is admitted to casualty after being kicked by her horse. On arrival in A&E she was noted to have a severe head injury with superficial abrasions over the frontal area and a GCS of 5. She was cardiovascularly stable and had no other injuries. After intubation and ventilation, she was transferred to the ITU following a CT scan.

a. Describe the CT images in A and B.
b. Outline her immediate treatment.

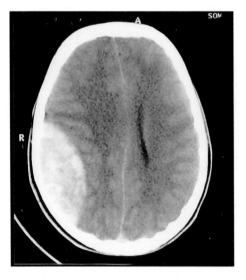

Question 3.4

A 23-year-old patient presents to A&E in an unconscious state. He was the passenger in a car involved in a high-speed accident and was found unconcious by the paramedics, having been ejected from the car. He has extensive contusions over the right temporoparietal scalp area, with a fixed and dilated right pupil. He groans and withdraws his limbs from painful stimuli on the right, but does not move his left side. He will not open his eyes. His CT scan is shown.

a. What is his Glasgow Coma Score?
b. What does the CT scan show?
c. What are the associations, treatment and prognosis of this type of injury?
d. Is the mode of presentation usual for this type of injury?
e. Outline your treatment plan in A&E as the anaesthetist preparing this man for theatre.

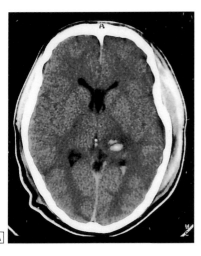 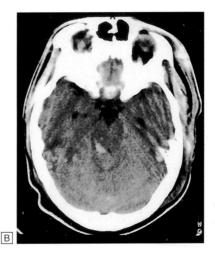

A | B

Question 3.5

An 18-year-old man was the passenger in a car involved in a high-speed road traffic accident. On arrival at A&E, his Glasgow Coma Score is 7/15 and he has a right hemiparesis. He is intubated and ventilated and a CT scan is performed, following which he is transferred to the ITU.

a. Describe the appearances of his CT scans (A, B).
b. What is the underlying mechanism of injury in this case?
c. Why does he have a hemiparesis?
d. His parents ask you if he will be 'all right'. What can you say about his neurological recovery?

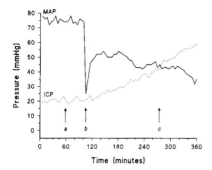

Question 3.6

A 22-year-old male pedestrian is admitted to the intensive care unit after a high-velocity road traffic accident. He has a severe diffuse brain injury and a cardiac contusion. An intracranial pressure monitor is inserted. The recordings for the 6-hour period following admission are shown. He experiences a cardiac event at point 'b' and inotrope support is indicated.

a. How is cerebral perfusion pressure calculated?
b. What is the cerebral perfusion pressure at 'a' and 'b'?
c. What options are available for controlling the ICP?
d. What has occurred at point 'c'?

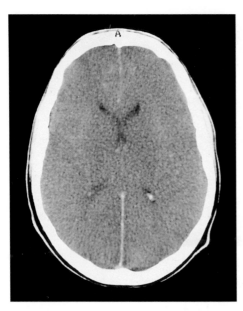

Question 3.7

A 21-year-old man is brought to A&E by the paramedics. He was discovered unconscious at home. The paramedics tell you that he was in electromechanical dissociation with a severe bradycardia when they first assessed him. They intubated him at the scene, gave him adrenaline and brought him to A&E. They were told that he had taken intravenous heroin. This is his CT scan later that day.

a. Describe his CT scan.
b. What is the underlying diagnosis on CT findings?
c. What are the neurological implications based on this scan?

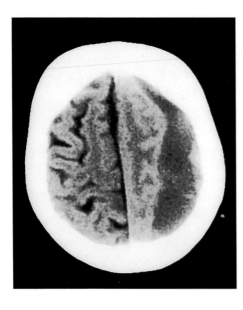

Question 3.8

A 74-year-old lady is admitted to the neurosurgical ward with a history of a fall 6 weeks previously, whilst shopping, that resulted in a Colles' fracture of her left wrist. This was reduced under an uneventful Bier's block. At the time she was fully lucid and orientated, and was discharged back to her nursing home. Since then she has become confused and unsteady on her feet. When you see her, she appears to have a mild right hemiparesis. This is one image from her CT scan.

a. What does the image show?
b. What is the most appropriate treatment?
c. Describe the anaesthetic and postoperative problems that may be encountered.

Question 3.9

You are asked to assist a senior neurosurgeon in the assessment of a 22-year-old male patient for the determination of brain stem death. The patient was admitted to the intensive care unit 4 days previously after sustaining a severe head injury in a witnessed fall of 40 feet. He has been unconscious from the outset and was intubated by the paramedic team at the scene of the accident because of respiratory irregularity. He has been ventilated since arrival at hospital. The CT scan shows extensive brain contusion affecting both frontal and temporal lobes. All sedating and paralysing agents and analgesics have been discontinued for > 24 h and the nursing staff have not noted any respiratory effort or pupillary response.

a. Does the patient fulfil the criteria for consideration of brain stem death? Are there any other questions you may ask?
b. Subsequently, the tests of brain stem reflexes are performed. No response is elicited. You are asked to supervise the performance of apnoea testing. How do you test for apnoea?

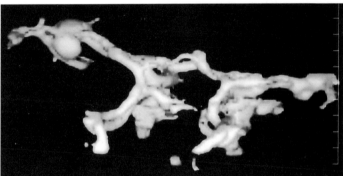

Right   Left

Question 3.10

A 23-year-old lady presents having collapsed at work. Her Glasgow Coma Score is 6/15 at presentation to A&E. She is intubated, ventilated and transferred to ITU. A CT shows blood in the right sylvian fissure consistent with a subarachnoid haemorrhage. Subsequently, a CT angiogram is performed as shown.

a. Describe the appearance of the angiogram image.
b. Describe the immediate management plan in the ITU.
c. What options exist for definitive treatment and when might this be considered?
d. What are the main anaesthetic problems to be considered if this lady presents for definitive treatment of this lesion?

3
Q

Question 3.11

A 43-year-old man is scheduled for clipping of an anterior communicating artery aneurysm. He had a subarachnoid haemorrhage 3 days ago and has been mildly confused since then. Before this, he was entirely healthy. Following are some of his biochemical laboratory results: sodium, 121 mmol/L; potassium, 4.6 mmol/L; chloride, 101 mmol/L; bicarbonate, 26 mmol/L; urea, 5.3 mmol/L; creatinine, 56 mmol/L; Hb, 10.4 g/dL; WCC, 18.9×10^9/L; platelets, 380×10^9/L.

a. What biochemical abnormality is present?
b. What other investigations would you order?
c. What is the likely cause for this disturbance?
d. What treatment would you recommend?

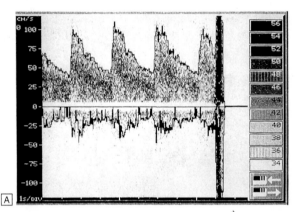

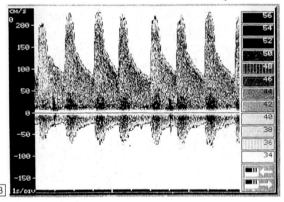

Question 3.12

A 37-year-old woman is admitted with a 3-day history of headache. The onset of the headache was consistent with a non-coma-producing subarachnoid haemorrhage and the diagnosis is confirmed on CT scan. The patient has no abnormal neurological signs on admission and is designated 'grade 1' by the neurosurgical team. The morning after admission you assess the patient with a view to cerebral angiography and note that she has weakness of her left arm and drooping of the left side of her face. (A) and (B) show transcranial Doppler ultrasound recordings taken on admission and just prior to your assessment.

a. What does the designation 'grade 1' subarachnoid haemorrhage mean?
b. What does transcranial Doppler measure?
c. What diagnosis do the transcranial Doppler readings suggest?

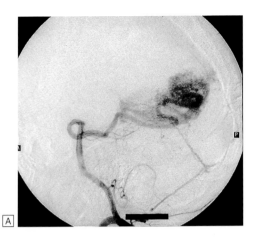
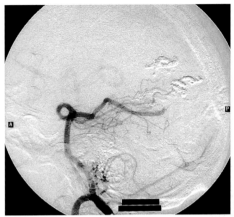

Question 3.13

A 42-year-old woman presents to the neurosurgical team with a history of headache and visual changes. These have become much more pronounced over the last few weeks and she now has nausea, especially on lying down or moving. She has had a CT of her head that identified a large arteriovenous malformation (AVM) in the left occipital lobe. The images shown are part of a sequence from her cerebral angiography of the vertebral artery.

a. What is the cause of the 'blush' in (A)?
b. What can be seen to have been achieved in (B)?
c. Describe the anaesthetic requirements for this procedure on this patient.

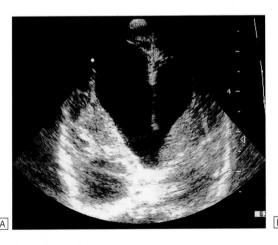
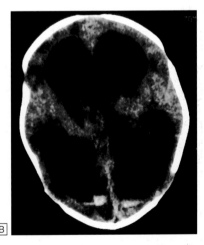

Question 3.14

You are the resident doctor on the neonatal intensive care unit. The nursing staff ask you to assess a premature baby boy (born at 34 weeks' gestation) who is feeding poorly and is sleepy. A colleague who saw the child earlier has arranged an ultrasound (A) and a CT scan (B). You find that the child has a bulging, but not tense, fontanelle.

a. What does the radiological investigation show?
b. What action do you take?
c. Are there problems if the CSF drainage is too effective?

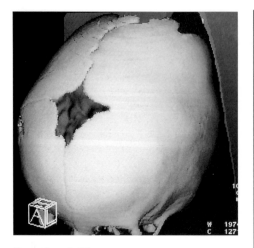

Question 3.15

a. What is this investigation and what abnormality does it show?

b. With which syndrome is this most commonly associated?

c. This child presents for surgery to have the defect corrected. What are the problems facing the anaesthetist during the operation?

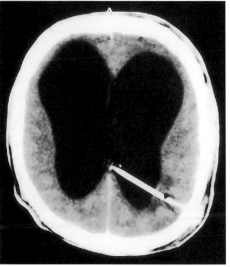

Question 3.16

You are urgently called to A&E to assess a 14-year-old youth who has been found collapsed at home. He is somnolent and has been vomiting.

a. What does his CT scan show?

b. During your assessment he abruptly deteriorates with loss of consciousness and respiratory arrest. What are your priorities in management?

Question 3.17

A 32-year-old man presents with increasing weakness of his arms of several years' duration. On examination he has ataxia of the upper limbs with wasting of the small muscles of his hands and loss of sensation to pain. This is his MRI scan.

a. What does his MRI scan show?

b. What is this condition and by which eponymous name is it known?

c. How does this condition present?

d. Surgical treatment is proposed. What is the nature of the surgery and what are the anaesthetic considerations of this procedure?

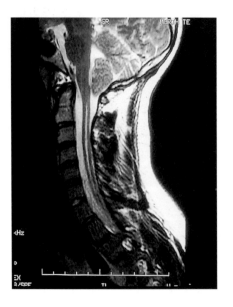

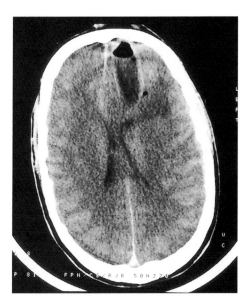

Question 3.18

You are asked to take over the anaesthetic management of a patient in the emergency department. The patient is a male vagrant of unknown identity. He was witnessed to have a grand mal seizure, and on arrival in the emergency room had a depressed conscious level and an apparent weakness of his right arm and leg. He had a further seizure in the department and has been intubated and ventilated as part of his management. The casualty consultant has requested a CT scan, which is shown, and has asked you to escort the patient to the scanner.

a. What preparations/precautions do you take prior to transfer?
b. What does the CT scan show?
c. The neurosurgical registrar indicates that the patient needs an operation. What further precautions/actions do you take prior to surgery?

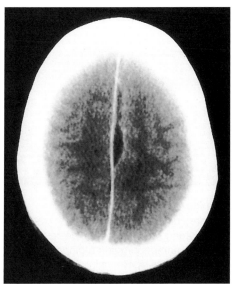

Right   Left

Question 3.19

You are called to the acute medical admissions unit to assist in the management of a 42-year-old woman who has been brought to the hospital in status epilepticus. The patient's family report that she had experienced increasing headache over the previous 48 h and that prior to the onset of her seizures she had appeared 'unwell' and confused. The seizures have persisted despite administration of intravenous benzodiazepines and an appropriate loading dose of intravenous phenytoin. Past medical history is unremarkable. The patient had an upper respiratory tract infection 10 days previously, which had responded to simple remedies.

a. What is your immediate management?
b. The patient subsequently undergoes a CT scan of brain. What does the scan show?
c. What additional treatment can you initiate?
d. You are the most senior doctor present and are asked to talk to the patient's family. What advice will you give them?

3
Q

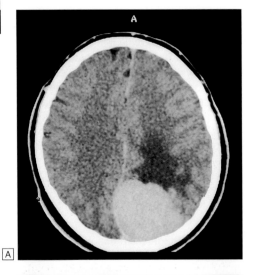

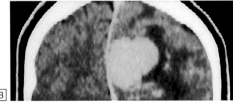

Question 3.20

A 59-year-old man presents with a 12-month history of increasing headache and, more recently, visual disturbance. Over recent weeks he has been falling frequently and has a mild right-sided weakness on clinical examination. (A) and (B) are CT scans of his head (pre-contrast axial and coronal reformation of a contrast enhanced examination, respectively).

a. Describe the scan. What is the probable diagnosis?
b. What is the particular relevance for the anaesthetist of a post-contrast examination?
c. Why has it taken so long for this patient to present?
d. This patient presents for surgical excision of this lesion. What are the potential problems for the anaesthetist?

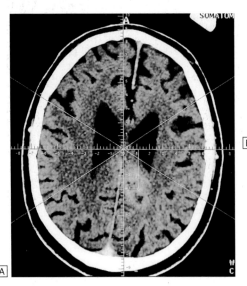

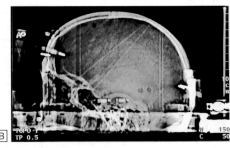

Question 3.21

You are called to theatre to assist with administering general anaesthesia to a 57-year-old man undergoing a biopsy of an intracranial lesion. He initially consented to undergo biopsy under local anaesthesia but is now distressed and requests a general anaesthetic.

a. What do his CT scans (A, B) show?
b. What difficulties may be encountered with administering a general anaesthetic in this situation?

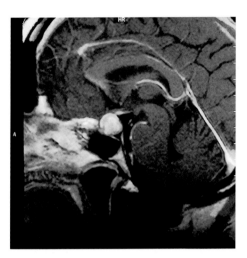

Question 3.22

You are asked to see a 43-year-old man for preoperative assessment. The patient has presented with visual failure. A representative section of his coronal MRI scan images is shown. The table below shows some of his preoperative blood results.

a. What does his scan show?
b. What is the characteristic field defect associated with this lesion and why does it occur?
c. What is your interpretation of the results of the blood tests?
d. What further investigations would you request? Give reasons.

Random cortisol	330 nmol/L (resting = 190–720 nmol/L, midnight < 220 nmol/L)
Luteinising hormone (LH)/follicle-stimulating hormone (FSH)	LH = 0.9 IU/L, FSH = 1.2 IU/L (LH 1.8–8.3 IU/L; FSH 1.6–11 IU/L)
Prolactin	520 mIU/L (57–357 mIU/L)
Thyroid function	TSH = 1.6 mIU/L (0.27–4.2 mIU/L) Free T$_4$ = 17 pmol/L (12–23 pmol/L)
Random growth hormone	95 mIU/L
Testosterone	3.1 nmol/L (9.1–55.2 nmol/L)

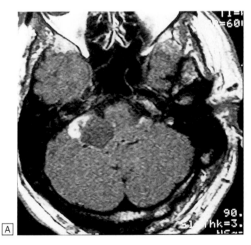

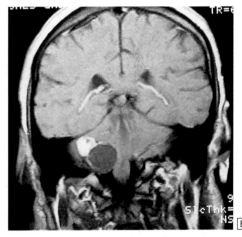

Question 3.23

A 62-year-old man presents with unilateral deafness of several years' duration. He is seen by an ear, nose and throat surgeon and an MRI scan performed. He is then referred to a neurosurgeon. This is his post-contrast MRI scan at the level of the petrous bones (A) and cerebellopontine angle (B).

a. Describe the appearances on MRI scan.
b. What is the diagnosis?
c. What are the treatment and prognosis?
d. What are the anaesthetic challenges of definitive surgical treatment?

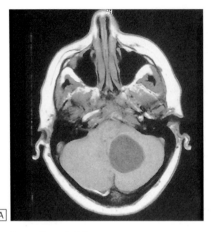 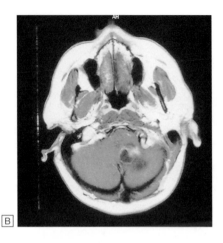

A   B

Question 3.24

You are asked to carry out a preoperative assessment on a 42-year-old man prior to surgery for a cerebellar lesion. During your assessment you note that he is tachycardic at rest, and review of the nursing charts show this to have been an intermittent problem since admission. (A) shows his pre-contrast MRI scan, (B) is his gadolinium-enhanced MRI scan.

a. What do the MRI scans show? What is the most likely diagnosis?
b. Is his tachycardia relevant?
c. What questions do you consider asking?
d. What recommendations do you make?

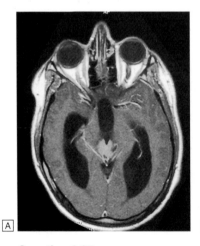 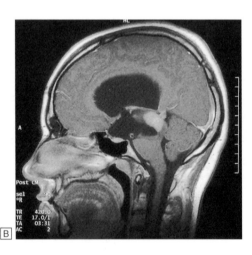

A   B

Question 3.25

A 20-year-old woman presents with a 6-week history of headache and blurred vision. (A) and (B) are gadolinium-enhanced sagittal T1-weighted and axial MRI scans of her brain, respectively.

a. What do the scans show?
b. The neurosurgeon caring for the patient decides he is going to operate on the lesion and wishes to use the supracerebellar approach with the patient in the sitting position if possible. Outline the specific concerns of anaesthesia in the sitting position and an approach to dealing with them.

ANSWERS

Answer 3.1

a. The patient's Glasgow Coma Score (GCS) is 4. The Glasgow Coma Scale is a simple, reliable and reproducible method of defining the level of consciousness by observing and scoring the patient's best response as follows:

Speech	Oriented	5
	Confused	4
	Inappropriate words	3
	Incomprehensible sounds	2
	None	1
Eye opening	Spontaneously	4
	To speech	3
	To pain	2
	None	1
Motor	Obeys commands	6
	Localises pain	5
	Normal flexion to pain	4
	Abnormal flexion to pain	3
	Extension	2
	None	1

It should be noted that the score can never be less than 3.

Practical difficulties can be encountered in describing normal and abnormal flexion in telephone communications. Response to central pain (e.g. supraorbital ridge pressure) is preferred. It may be better to ask for a description of the responses rather than accepting a score over the phone.

The scale was devised for use in adults, and difficulties can arise in the assessment of verbal response in very young children. There is no widely accepted variant of the scale for use in children.

b. The patient is unconscious. Coma is defined as a GCS of 8 or less. The patient will require a definitive airway as part of his management. It is inappropriate to transfer the patient to a potentially unsafe environment such as the CT scanner without adequate airway control.

Answer 3.2

a. There is a rim of high-density material extending from the left frontal to the occipital area consistent with a severe acute subdural haematoma. There is midline shift to the right with compression of the lateral ventricles and evidence of loss of grey/white differentiation. Air can be seen within the haematoma, indicating an open head injury, most likely a base of skull fracture.

b. Subdural haematomas usually arise from rupture of bridging veins between the cortex and dura, but may also arise from lacerations of the brain or cortical arteries. They are more common than extradural haematomas (30% of severe head injuries) and carry a poorer prognosis than extradural haematoma because of underlying severe primary brain injury. The mortality remains high at 60%.

c. Treatment is aimed at preventing secondary brain injury, initiating measures to reduce intracranial pressure (ICP) and the preparation for craniotomy. Intubation and ventilation are not required at the moment, as the GCS is 11, but if this fluctuates or falls, she should be intubated without delay to help to control ICP and prevent secondary hypoxic brain damage. In the meantime, she should be given oxygen, her blood pressure should be supported, if necessary, to maintain cerebral perfusion pressure, and mannitol +/− frusemide should be given to decrease ICP after discussion with the neurosurgeons. Evidence of ongoing blood loss should be excluded and there may be time to exclude cervical spine injury clinically and radiologically. She should be cross-matched prior to theatre and craniotomy should be performed in less than 4 h from injury.

Further reading

Seelig JM et al 1981 Traumatic acute subdural haematoma: major mortality reduction in comatose patients treated within 4 hours. *New England Journal of Medicine* 304: 1511–1518.

3

A

Answer 3.3

a. The reconstructed three-dimensional bone views demonstrate an extensively fractured frontal complex with a fracture line extending into the right orbit. There is also fracture of the left orbital floor. The zygomatic arches appear intact, but little can be seen of the base of skull despite the rotation of the image. Disruption of the frontal sinuses make a compound fracture almost inevitable. Sinus content and air contamination of the brain and meninges are likely. The patient is at high risk of developing frontal contusions. The optic pathways, especially on the right, may have been compromised, as well as the olfactory nerve. These images are reconstructed from a volume of data which also provides thin axial sections and coronal reformations to further evaluate the extent of trauma.

b. The forced extension of her skull on her neck makes in-line stabilisation essential until her neck is cleared by an experienced neuro- or orthopaedic surgeon. No acute surgical intervention is warranted but this patient has a severe head injury with a poor prognosis and needs aggressive medical management. The severely disrupted frontal bones will almost act as a pressure-reducing valve for the rising intracranial pressure, and coning may not occur. The patient should be sedated, moderately hyperventilated ($P_aCO_2 = 4\text{--}4.5$), given mannitol +/– frusemide to decrease cerebral oedema, as well as antibiotics as she has a compound skull fracture. Cranial pressure monitoring should be instituted together with other measurements of cerebral perfusion such as jugular venous oxygen saturation. The first 24 h will prove critical from a cerebral perfusion point of view and with the likelihood of severe frontal lobe damage, craniotomy and frontal lobe excision may be life-saving. The status of her tetanus immunisation should be checked.

Early assessment of her eyes is important to determine if globe disruption has occurred with the added risk of sympathetic enophthalmitis. This information is provided from the same data as that used for the three-dimensional CT images.

Answer 3.4

a. His GCS is 7 (EI, M4, V2).

b. The CT scan shows a massive right-sided extradural haematoma with compression of both lateral ventricles and midline shift to the left.

c. Extradural haematomas arise from tears in dural arteries, usually the middle meningeal artery, and are often associated with linear skull fractures over the parietal or temporal areas. The incidence is about 1% of severe head injuries. The prognosis is generally good as the primary brain injury is not usually serious. However, secondary brain damage occurs rapidly due to raised ICP and may be rapidly fatal if the clot is not evacuated. This may require immediate measures to reduce ICP whilst a craniotomy is being prepared.

d. Extradural haematomata classically present as loss of conciousness immediately post-trauma, followed by a lucid interval and then a gradually decreasing conciousness level associated with the development of an ipsilateral fixed dilated pupil and contralateral hemiparesis. However, the presentation is often not classical and the patient may present in coma, as in this case. Less frequently, the hemiparesis may be ipsilateral to the clot.

e. Management in A&E is directed to excluding a more immediate threat to life, initiating measures to decrease ICP and transferring the patient safely to theatre. The only procedure to delay craniotomy would be to control life-threatening haemorrhage. It may be possible to perform a laparotomy and craniotomy simultaneously. If not already performed, blood should be taken for cross-matching, en route to theatre if necessary. If the patient has a GCS of 8 or less, immediate intubation is indicated to protect the airway and hyperventilation is initiated to a P_aCO_2 of 3.5–4 kPa to reduce ICP for a short period. If the patient is not hypovolaemic, mannitol +/– frusemide should be given to reduce ICP. If hypovolaemia is present and is causing hypotension, fluid resuscitation is imperative to restore circulating blood volume and thus maintain cerebral perfusion pressure.

Answer 3.5

a. There is marked superficial soft tissue swelling of the scalp. Multiple small petechial haemorrhages are seen in the brain with surrounding oedema. The diffuse pattern is illustrated by haemorrhages in the upper part of the brain stem and thalamus.
b. These appearances are consistent with severe shearing injury to the brain causing diffuse axonal injury and leading to shearing haematomas in the grey/white matter interface of the brain.
c. The right hemiparesis is due to the haematoma in the left thalamic area.
d. The prognosis is guarded. Severe diffuse axonal injury in adults, as in this case, usually has a poor neurological outcome. The damage caused by the initial injury is marked and even if secondary insult is avoided recovery will be limited. The prospect of full recovery of motor activity on the right is especially poor. The parents must be warned of this possibility as well as the likelihood of death.

Answer 3.6

a. In normal brain the blood flow is maintained at constant levels by the autoregulatory process. Following head injury this homeostatic mechanism is lost and blood flow becomes pressure-passive. Cerebral perfusion pressure (CPP) is a numerical indicator of this pressure-passive flow and reflects the effects of the competing forces in delivering blood to the brain, namely blood pressure and ICP. It is important to recognise that CPP is *not* an absolute measure of cerebral blood flow:

Cerebral perfusion pressure = mean arterial pressure − intracranial pressure

b. The cerebral perfusion pressure at 'a' is approximately 55 mmHg and that at 'b' is 5 mmHg.
c. Multiple options are available:

- mannitol
- hyperventilation
- frusemide
- cerebrospinal fluid (CSF) drainage via an external ventricular drain
- barbiturate coma
- decompressive craniectomy.

d. Intracranial pressure has equalled mean arterial pressure. CPP is zero. There is no blood flow to the brain.

Answer 3.7

a. Effacement of the basal cisterns, third ventricle and sylvian fissures indicate the presence of severe cerebral oedema. There is extensive loss of differentiation of grey/white matter in the cerebral cortex and poor visualisation of central grey matter (thalami, caudate nuclei). The midbrain is slightly flattened from side to side.
b. Such extensive loss of grey/white matter differentiation implicates global ischaemia or infarction. These changes are due to the severe hypoxic insult aggravated by subsequent cerebral oedema. The flattening of the midbrain is a reflection of the severity of cerebral oedema and may be a warning of the onset of tentorial herniation.
c. From this scan, tentorial herniation may be incipient. If complete, brain stem death is the inevitable consequence. If this does not happen, the global nature of the ischaemia on CT scan indicates the probability of profound and incapacitating brain damage. Recovery is unlikely and the patient may be

3

A

considered for organ donation, although the history of intravenous drug abuse may contraindicate this. A clear local policy for dealing with the sensitive issue of raising the possibility of donation and of gaining consent from relatives should be in place.

Answer 3.8

a. There is a large chronic subdural haematoma on the left with limited midline shift. There is no evidence of intracranial blood. Note the underlying atrophic change in the right hemisphere consistent with the patient's age.

b. This patient requires surgical drainage of the subdural haematoma. Whilst this is not immediately life-threatening, there is a degree of urgency because there are signs of neurological compromise at present. The prognosis following drainage is usually very good, and there are no major contraindications to this surgery, even in very unwell patients. Most commonly, these are drained by either single or multiple burr holes. The burr holes may be performed under local anaesthesia, but a general anaesthetic is usually more appropriate and allows a change of procedure if indicated in theatre.

c. The anaesthetic problems are related to her age, her level of confusion and the risk of a re-bleed following drainage. Some indication of her functional reserve can be gained from the history of her injury occurring whilst being engaged in a moderately strenuous activity – in this case, shopping. The routine monitoring for a craniotomy is necessary, especially for temperature changes. A technique that allows a rapid return to full consciousness is required and the recent volatile agents – sevoflurane or desflurane – and remifentanil have transformed our ability to achieve this.

Answer 3.9

a. Yes. The patient fulfils the two essential pre-conditions: he has irremediable structural brain damage; he is unresponsive and requires ventilatory support. It is essential to exclude other causes of coma. The patient must be normothermic. Drug intoxication must be excluded, as must endocrine/metabolic disturbances. The drug charts must be checked to ensure that an appropriate amount of time has elapsed for the excretion/degradation of sedating/neuromuscular blocking agents.

b. The essential feature of the apnoea test is to show that no respiratory movements occur after disconnection from the ventilator, whilst ensuring that the patient does not become hypoxic and that the P_aCO_2 rises to a level which will drive any respiratory centre neurones that may be alive. The patient requires pre-oxygenation with 100% oxygen for at least 10 min. The ventilation rate is reduced and arterial blood gases checked to ensure that P_aCO_2 is rising. The ventilator is disconnected and oxygenation maintained by direct insufflation of the lungs with 100% oxygen through a tracheal catheter placed at the carina of the trachea. The P_aCO_2 must rise above 6.7 kPa.

Further reading
Pallis C, Harley DH 1996 *ABC of Brain Stem Death*, 2nd edn. BMJ Publications, London.

Answer 3.10

a. This image is a three-dimensional reconstruction of a CT angiogram demonstrating the circle of Willis and the left and right middle cerebral arteries. There is a clearly visible aneurysm on the right middle cerebral artery. This would be compatible with a bleed in the territory of the right middle cerebral artery.

b. Immediate management involves sedation, intubation, moderate hyperventilation and supportive treatment on ITU. Intravenous nimodipine should be commenced. Consideration should be given to ICP monitoring or other form of intracranial perfusion monitoring. The CT scan should be repeated within 24 h, as she may require an external ventricular drain if hydrocephalus develops.

c. Treatment options are embolisation of this aneurysm under radiological control or clipping at craniotomy. Current opinion would suggest that neither option should be considered in a comatose patient until there is evidence of neurological recovery.

d. Surgical clipping of the aneurysm is the method chosen in this case. Aneurysm clipping at craniotomy may involve excessive blood loss, cerebrovascular system instability, air emboli and the effects of a prolonged procedure. These should be anticipated. Temperature, central venous pressure, intra-arterial and E_tCO_2 monitoring are mandatory. Monitors for auditory brain stem-evoked potentials may be required as well as EEG monitoring and occasionally a lumbar CSF drain. The ability to treat vasospasm with hypervolaemia, or a ruptured aneurysm with controlled hypotension, are common to both methods.

Answer 3.11

a. There is marked hyponatraemia. The haemoglobin is also low for a normal adult male, and in the absence of a cause for the bleeding suggests haemodilution. If the fall in sodium has been gradual over hours or days, there is unlikely to be any specific clinical features associated with the sodium level. Sudden changes may lead to coma and convulsions similar to that seen in the transurethral prostatectomy syndrome.

b. The urinary and plasma sodium concentrations and osmolarities are the essential investigations.

c. In the absence of mannitol or other osmotically active agents, the likeliest cause is an inappropriate secretion of antidiuretic hormone (ADH). A high urinary sodium and osmolarity would confirm the diagnosis. This is a recognised complication of head injury, subarachnoid haemorrhage or anterior fossa/pituitary surgery.

d. The treatment is water restriction to no more than 500 mL/day. Occasionally, hypertonic saline may be necessary but this should be given very slowly and the serum sodium checked hourly. This should not rise faster than 2 mmol/L per h to limit the risk of central pontine myelinolysis. Surgery should be delayed until the sodium has returned to a normal concentration.

Answer 3.12

a. Grading of the clinical status of patients with subarachnoid haemorrhage has been carried out according to a number of scales. Previously the Hunt & Hess grading was most widely used, but over recent years the World Federation of Neurological Surgeons Scale (WFNS) has become more commonplace as it is a clearly defined objective scale which utilises the Glasgow Coma Scale in association with neurological deficit (see table below).

b. Transcranial Doppler ultrasound is a non-invasive method of measuring blood flow velocity in cerebral vessels. Pulsed Doppler ultrasound at low frequency (2 MHz) is most commonly

WFNS grade	Glasgow Coma Score	Major focal deficit
1	15	Absent
2	13–14	Absent
3	13–14	Present
4	7–12	Present or absent
5	3–6	Present or absent

Major focal deficit = dysphasia/aphasia/hemiparesis/hemiplegia.

3

A

used and flow velocities are recorded through acoustic windows in the skull where the vault is thin. The anterior cerebral artery and middle cerebral artery are recorded through the squamous part of the temporal bone. The middle cerebral artery is usually located at a depth of about 55 mm from the surface of the scalp. Normal blood flow velocity in the middle cerebral artery is in the region of 55 cm/s. It is important to realise that flow velocity does not necessarily relate directly to volume blood flow.

c. (A) demonstrates a normal pattern with a mean velocity of approximately 50 cm/s. (B) demonstrates mean Doppler velocities in excess of 100 cm/s that are indicative of an increase in peripheral resistance and suggest vasospasm. In the absence of any symptoms to suggest further haemorrhage, it is likely that the development of the brachiofacial weakness is due to symptomatic arterial vasospasm, a recognised complication of subarachnoid haemorrhage.

Answer 3.13

a. The blush in the posterior occipital area is due to the highly vascular nature of this AVM. The limited numbers of feeding vessels, particularly when they are large, makes embolisation possible.

b. The second image – post-embolisation with glue – shows the marked reduction in vascular supply to the malformation. The result of this procedure is thrombosis of the AVM and the risk of adjacent ischaemic damage. There is a risk that the inevitable cerebral oedema will be of a magnitude to compromise cerebral function and close observation is essential for the first 48 h after embolisation.

c. Embolisation involves a different set of problems for the anaesthetist than, for example, routine craniotomy. Embolisation usually involves anaesthesia outside the operating suite, with limited patient access during the

procedure. The facilities, including the recovery area, should have been specially designed with these problems in mind. The patient should be ventilated during the procedure and monitoring should include end-tidal CO_2 and intra-arterial blood pressure. Cardiovascular stability is essential during the process of glueing to prevent a hyperdynamic cerebral circulation that may lead to the liquid glue passing through the malformation before setting. Hyperventilation and moderate hypotension may be necessary to reduce flow to a safe level. Once the embolisation has been performed, the patient should be restored to her pre-anaesthetic haemodynamic state and ideally woken up fully. This will allow the close observation of the patient that is necessary to identify the onset of a raised ICP or neurological deficit. Hypertension should be avoided because the hyperdynamic cerebral circulation may be enough to cause the glue emboli to move.

Further reading
Krivosic-Horber R, Leclerc X, Doumith S, Drizenko A, Frangie S, Pruvo JP 1996 Anesthesia and critical care for endovascular occlusion of ruptured intracranial aneurysms with electrically detachable coils. *Annales Françaises d'Anesthesie et de Reanimation* 15(3): 354–358.

Answer 3.14

a. The ultrasound scan shows ventricular dilatation. The CT confirms hydrocephalus with intraventricular blood lying in both posterior occipital horns. There is marked periventricular low density, indicating acutely raised ICP with transependymal passage of CSF.

b. Initiate regular head circumference measurements to document any rapid increases that may be due to excessive pressure from the hydrocephalus. Consult with the neurosurgical team. The hydrocephalus may require decompression with ventricular tapping through the enlarged anterior fontanelle.

In some cases this will control hydrocephalus and it may spontaneously arrest. Insertion of a ventriculoperitoneal shunt is not required at this early stage as the debris in the CSF from the intraventricular haemorrhage is likely to cause shunt valve malfunction.

c. Infection of the CSF is the most common and worrying complication of either ventricular tapping or shunting in this age group. Subdural haematoma or effusions can occur if the drainage is either too rapid or excessive. Overzealous drainage can lead to premature fusion of sutures in the infant.

On a longer term, the excessive drainage of CSF can lead to 'slit ventricles' where there has been almost complete drainage of the upper ventricles. This is not a benign state. The child is extremely vulnerable to changes in either intracranial blood or brain volume. Infusions of hypotonic fluids are particularly hazardous and can lead to cerebral herniation following even minor surgical procedures.

Further reading

Eldredge EA, Rockoff MA, Medlock MD et al 1997 Postoperative cerebral edema occurring in children with slit ventricles. *Pediatrics* 99: 620–630.

Answer 3.15

a. This is a three-dimensional reconstruction of a cranial CT scan of an infant. The abnormality is a prematurely fused left coronal suture. This contrasts with the clearly visible unfused right coronal suture. The incidence of craniosynostosis is approximately 1/1000 births. Surgical correction may be required to prevent raised ICP developing during infancy or for cosmetic reasons.

b. Apert's syndrome, after the Parisian paediatrician, Eugene Apert (1868–1940).

c. These cases present a considerable challenge to the anaesthetist. These children often have other problems such as congenital cardiac defects, especially VSD, raised ICP may be present, and intubation may be difficult due to the facial, especially maxillary, bone abnormalities. In addition, the usual timing of surgery is at about 6 months of age, with all other attendent problems at this age, such as size, hypothermia and vascular access. When the base of the skull or facial bones are involved, perioperative airway management may be difficult, and the use of a non-kinking endotracheal tube is mandatory. After complex procedures, the child will usually need to be admitted to a paediatric ITU. These children are at risk of direct cerebral trauma, venous air embolism and problems associated with intracranial hypertension. These operations are always prolonged, leading to problems of temperature control and hydration. Blood loss may be considerable, a mean of 91 ± 66% of the patient's red cell volume in one series. Ongoing blood loss estimation is essential, involving both weighing swabs but also frequent measurements of packed cell volume. Normovolaemic haemodilution and intraoperative red cell salvage have both been advocated. Clotting factors and even platelets are often required. Intra-arterial blood pressure monitoring is advisable, and urinary catheterisation and central vascular access are essential.

Further reading

Meyer P, Renier D, Arnaud E, et al 1993 Blood loss during repair of craniosynostosis. *British Journal of Anaesthesia* 71(6): 854–857.

Uppington JW, Goat VA 1987 Anaesthesia for major craniofacial surgery: a report of 23 cases in children under four years of age. *Annals of the Royal College of Surgeons of England* 69: 175–178.

Answer 3.16

a. The scan shows enlarged ventricles consistent with hydrocephalus. There is a left ventricular catheter and valve assembly in the left parietal region consistent with a ventricular shunt

3
A

device. The appearances suggest shunt malfunction/blockage.

b. The management of the respiratory arrest is straightforward. Support of the airway and oxygenation are immediately necessary because it has to be assumed that this a result of the very high intracranial pressure leading to herniation. As his history includes active vomiting he should have his trachea intubated to prevent any further aspiration. Hypoxic damage is highly likely unless oxygen delivery can be restored and ICP reduced using hyperventilation to reduce cerebral blood volume, and osmotically active agents such as mannitol 0.5 g/kg. Once stability has been achieved he must have an emergency shunt revision, even if this is simply to insert an external ventricular drain. Needle aspiration of the shunt system by an experienced neurosurgeon may be life-saving.

Answer 3.17

a. This scan shows cerebellar tonsillar descent. The tonsils appear impacted in the foramen magnum and there is a large syrinx present in the cervical spinal cord.

b. The Chiari malformation describes herniation into the spinal canal of the cerebellar tonsils (type 1) or the hind brain, vermis and IV ventricle (type 2). In adult life, the presentation is usually that of the associated syringomyelia or syringobulbia. If hydrocephalus occurs, presentation is often earlier.

c. Type 2 Chiari malformations may be associated with meningomyeloceles. Alternatively, they may present in infancy with hydrocephalus or brain stem dysfunction. In the absence of hydrocephalus, types 1 or 2 may present in later life with neck pain, occipital headaches and ataxia, together with symptoms and signs of syringomyelia, characteristically arm weakness with small muscle weakness, loss of tendon reflexes, dissociated sensory loss and a Horner's syndrome.

d. This patient requires cerebellar decompression which is accomplished by decompression of the foramen magnum. This is performed in the prone position. Adequate room should be ensured to allow diaphragmatic expansion with ventilation and to minimise hypotension due to decreased venous return from the legs. Positioning problems of the prone position include prolonged pressure on peripheral nerves, producing postoperative paresis, as well as pressure on the eyes which can cause blindness postoperatively. The eyes should be securely taped to avoid damaging the conjunctivae and not be in contact with any surface that may expose them to excess pressure. The cervical spine should be positioned carefully to avoid hyperextension, avoid carotid artery obstruction and allow free venous drainage via an unobstructed jugular venous system. Careful cardiovascular monitoring is essential in case brain stem cardiovascular reflexes are elicited and postoperative monitoring should be adequate to detect a developing haematoma in the brain stem.

Answer 3.18

a. This patient will need to be loaded with intravenous anticonvulsants. It is unlikely that he will have been taking regular medication and unless loading doses are prescribed a therapeutic concentration will take too long to be achieved.

b. The scan shows a brain abscess in the left frontal lobe. The post-contrast CT shows a well-circumscribed lesion in the frontal lobe with 'ring' enhancement and surrounding low density consistent with brain oedema. There is a gas bubble within the abscess cavity. The radiological appearances are suggestive of a sinugenic brain abscess caused by spread of infection from frontal sinusitis. Abscesses can present clinically in a variety of ways, ranging from headache due to raised ICP, focal neurological signs, systemic illness with meningism and, in about 25% of cases, generalised epilepsy.

c. Prompt surgical treatment by needle aspiration of the abscess through a burr hole will allow decompression of the abscess and provide microbiological diagnosis. Until the causative organisms are known, treatment with broad-spectrum antibiotic therapy should be instituted, including specific anti-anaerobic therapy. Steroids can be used to reduce brain oedema.

Answer 3.19

a. The patient is at risk of cerebral hypoxia with untreated status epilepticus. Immediate intubation/ventilation and administration of anticonvulsants is needed.

b. The scan shows the typical appearances of an interhemispheric parafalcine subdural empyema on the left side. There is an enhancing fluid collection, which is widening the interhemispheric fissure.

c. The recent history of upper respiratory tract infection may be relevant; the infection may be sinugenic in its origin. Treatment with broad-spectrum antibiotics should be initiated (including anti-anaerobes). Treatment with steroids can be initiated if there is suspicion of raised ICP. Immediate referral to a neurosurgeon is mandatory.

d. Subdural empyema is a life-threatening condition, with mortality approaching 30%. Surgical intervention (either craniotomy or burr holes) will be needed to decompress the empyema.

Answer 3.20

a. There is a large, dense, well demarcated mass to the left of the midline in the posterior parieto-occipital region. This is surrounded by an extensive hypodense region of cerebral oedema. There is midline shift to the right. This is a massive left parafalcine meningioma with surrounding cerebral oedema and pressure effects.

b. The contrast scan demonstrates marked enhancement of the tumour. This reflects its marked vascularity, as is typical of meningiomas. Large meningiomas may infiltrate the overlying vault and lead to catastrophic bleeding on raising the bone flap, or even on drilling the pilot burr holes.

c. This tumour is in the posterior occipital area of the brain and is classically slow-growing. Due to the gradual onset, many patients disregard early symptoms and signs, often attributing them to getting older.

d. Meningiomas arise from arachnoidal cells in the meninges, often indenting the underlying brain or spinal cord, and are classically benign, although some may erode into dura and bone. Excision is usually curative. Rarely, anaplastic or malignant meningiomas occur. Some meningiomas present problems with their position, as in this case, or due to their large size. In this example, treatment involves craniotomy and excision of tumour; however, this is a large tumour and may therefore involve extensive blood loss, which should be anticipated. This particular meningioma lies adjacent to the superior sagittal, straight and transverse sinuses, which may make surgery particularly hazardous. Preoperative angiography is important to demonstrate its vascular relationships and to assess whether preoperative embolisation to decrease its blood supply is possible. Extensive oedema of the brain is already evident. This may worsen intra- and postoperatively and consideration should be given to maintain adequate cerebral perfusion pressures and ICP monitoring and pressure-lowering manoeuvres. Sedation and ventilation in intensive care may be required postoperatively.

Answer 3.21

a. The scans show a scout image and an axial CT with a stereotactic biopsy frame in situ. They also show a deep-seated left parietal tumour consistent with metastasis or malignant glioma.

b. The delivery of a general anaesthetic to a distressed patient, especially one with a stereotactic frame in place, is no easy task. It should not be delegated to an inexperienced anaesthetist. Examination of the patient and obtaining an appropriate anaesthetic history are likely to be limited, and key investigations may be lacking. The decision to agree and proceed has to be balanced against the likely risks of a poorly prepared patient and also the need for a tissue diagnosis of a potentially highly malignant tumour. The positioning of the frame may interfere with pre-oxygenation and affect positioning of the head during intubation. Despite many frames having an indented lower front bar, direct visualisation of the vocal cords during laryngoscopy may prove impossible. The placement of the patient onto the supporting headrest for the stereotactic frame may involve marked neck flexion and this may be inadvisable if there is a history of cervical disease. Surgery is usually swift if the operating team are familiar with the coordinates and system, but there may be delays if a cytological smear result is awaited to confirm a successful biopsy.

Answer 3.22

a. These show a pituitary adenoma with chiasmal compression. The close relationship with the cavernous sinus and the optic chiasm are obvious.
b. The visual field loss is a bitemporal hemianopia due to chiasmal compression.
c. The biochemistry demonstrates mild hypopituitarism. The rise in the prolactin level is due to compression of the pituitary stalk. The markedly elevated random growth hormone is a worry and indicates a diagnosis of acromegaly.
d. Clinical examination is important in order to look for the somatic features of acromegaly. A detailed assessment of the airway, including the tongue and jaw, is essential. The airway may be

compromised by the excessive soft tissue and lead to severe obstructive sleep apnoea. Overnight oximetry will provide a rapid insight into the presence of sleep apnoea. Maintenance of the airway on induction of anaesthesia and tracheal intubation may be difficult, and skilled help and appropriate airway aids are essential. The postoperative recovery may prove challenging if nasal packs completely seal the nasal airway.

An ECG and CXR are indicated to assess for cardiomegaly and conduction defects. The associated risk of diabetes should be monitored by a random serum glucose and urinalysis.

Further reading
Seidman A, Kofke WA, Policare R, Young M 2000 Anaesthetic complications of acromegaly. *British Journal of Anaesthesia* 84(2): 179–182.

Answer 3.23

a. There is an enhancing mass in the left cerebellopontine angle associated with a cystic component consistent with an acoustic neuroma. Acoustic neuromas are readily demonstrated by MRI; invasive air meatography is no longer required.
b. This is commonly called an acoustic neuroma, but it is in fact a Schwannoma arising from the Schwann cells of the neural sheaths of the VIIIth cranial nerve and is properly called a neurilemmoma or neurinoma. Bilateral Schwannomas have been described in association with neurofibromatosis type II.
c. This is a benign tumour and is usually very slow-growing. Bilateral acoustic neuromas have been found in association with von Recklinghausen's neurofibromatosis. Treatment is by surgical excision and is usually curative.
d. The surgery is often prolonged and difficult and anaesthetic problems are those of infratentorial surgery. Infratentorial surgery may be performed in the prone, lateral (park bench) or, rarely, sitting position. The lateral 'park bench' position is particularly suitable for surgery around the cerebellopontine

angle. Using this position, one must be careful not to exert too much traction on the upper arm, which may cause injury to the brachial plexus, and avoid excessive rotation of the neck impairing venous drainage. The duration of surgery may be extremely prolonged with attendant problems of fluid balance, temperature control and the occasional need for postoperative ventilation due to slow recovery especially of airway reflexes. Blood loss may also be significant due to the vascular nature of the tumour and the difficult access to the tumour. This should be anticipated. As with all surgery involving the infratentorial region, autonomic instability and arryhthmias may occur due to surgical manipulation of the vagus nerve. Hypertension may result from stimulation of the trigeminal nerve. In addition to careful cardiovascular monitoring, pharmacological agents to counteract these changes should be to hand. EMG monitoring of facial nerve function or brain stem-evoked potentials may be used during infratentorial surgery to identify any perioperative loss of function.

Answer 3.24

a. The MRI scans show a cystic cerebellar tumour with an enhancing nodule in its wall. The features are characteristic of a cerebellar haemangioblastoma. The vascular nature is evident in the contrast-enhanced scan.
b. Yes. The patient has intermittent tachycardia, which indicates that the association of a haemangioblastoma with phaeochromocytoma may be present.
c. Haemangioblastomas can be inherited as part of the Von Hippel–Lindau syndrome. It is important to enquire about relevant family history. Questions regarding the tachycardia, such as the occurrence of palpitations or past history of hypertension, are needed. Family history of anaesthetic problems may also be helpful.

d. Having raised the possibility of underlying phaeochromocytoma, it is prudent to defer surgery until the diagnosis has been confirmed or refuted. Institute regular pulse/blood pressure assessments and request 24-h urinary vanillylmandelic acid (VMA)/catecholamine measurements.

Answer 3.25

a. The MRI shows a pineal region tumour with secondary obstructive hydrocephalus due to obstruction of the aqueduct. These are very deep-seated tumours and it can be very difficult to avoid damage to normal surrounding brain structures. The close relationship to the midbrain and the thalamic structures can be seen.
b. The supracerebellar approach can best be achieved by the use of the sitting position. This is still used in some centres despite the major anaesthetic risks. The extreme head-up position makes air emboli through open venous sinuses almost inevitable, and has led many centres to abandon it. The patient must be fully monitored as for craniotomy – invasive blood pressure, central venous pressure, temperature, urinary catheter, oxygen saturation, ECG – but should also have some means of detecting air emboli. The movement of the patient from the supine into the sitting position should be gradual because of the risk of extreme postural hypotension under anaesthesia. Lower body compression suits are useful both to prevent this and to raise venous return in the event of an air embolism. Doppler probes around the neck recording flow through the jugular venous system are useful to identify the air bubbles traversing the veins and allow the anaesthetist to increase thoracic venous pressure above atmospheric by PEEP and to increase venous return by pressurising the compression suit, and the surgeon to flood the wound with warmed saline. The Doppler is of limited utility in

3

A

differentiating between small, clinically insignificant, bubbles and a large catastrophic air embolus. The placement of the central venous catheter into the right atrium to allow aspiration of any air is only occasionally effective and cannot be relied on as a therapeutic manoeuvre in the face of a large embolus.

ORTHOPAEDICS AND TRAUMA

BASIC PRINCIPLES

A fracture may appear as a black (lucent) line in a plain radiograph when the bone fragments are separated or, less commonly, a white line when the fragments are impacted or overlapping. Some vascular markings, accessory ossicles, epiphyses and growth plates can cause confusion, so a good knowledge of anatomy and access to experienced help are vital.

Many fractures and some dislocations cannot be detected using a single view, so it is standard practice to request two views, usually taken at right angles to each other, e.g. standard cervical spine (c-spine) views include PA, lateral and open mouth. This chapter will concentrate on aspects of the management of multiple trauma of most relevance to anaesthetists and intensivists.

THE CERVICAL SPINE

Usually three basic views are obtained (Figs 4.1–4.3):

- AP (Fig. 4.1)
- lateral to include the top of T1 body (Fig. 4.2)
- open mouth 'peg view' to show the C1–C2 articulation (Fig. 4.3).

An additional swimmer's view may be required to delineate the upper thoracic and lower cervical vertebrae (Fig. 4.4).

Post-trauma, 70% of detectable abnormalities will be seen on an adequate lateral radiograph, whilst the three views together (Figs 4.1–4.3) have a quoted sensitivity for cervical spine fractures of 92%. Various other views such as 'trauma obliques' have also been described which may improve sensitivity to 95%. Remember

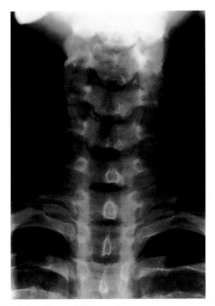

Fig. 4.1 Normal AP c-spine.

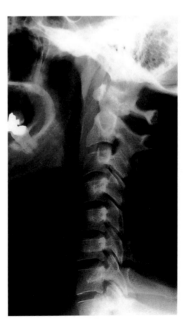

Fig. 4.2 Normal lateral c-spine.

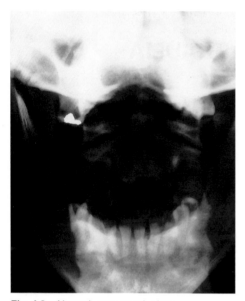

Fig. 4.3 Normal open mouth view.

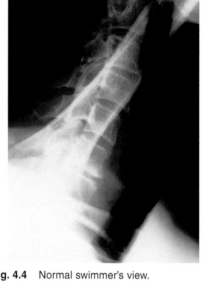

Fig. 4.4 Normal swimmer's view.

that 10% of patients with a cervical fracture will have another fracture somewhere in the vertebral column. In an unconscious patient, three normal and adequate plain radiographs together with CT scans of the craniocervical and thoracocervical junctions will exclude 99% of unstable injuries.

Possible spinal injuries include the following:

- *Atlanto-occipital dislocation.* Fortunately rare, this is invariably a fatal injury because of the resulting damage to the brain stem.
- *Atlas fracture (C1).* About 5% of all acute spinal fractures are at C1. 40% of C1 fractures are also associated with a fracture of C2. The Jefferson fracture is a burst fracture of the body of C1 where both the anterior and posterior rings are disrupted. The usual mechanism of injury is axial loading with the head in a relatively neutral position, e.g. a heavy weight falls on the head. It is not often associated with spinal cord injury but it is unstable.
- *C1 rotatory subluxation.* This is an uncommon injury most likely to be seen

in children or patients with rheumatoid arthritis, sometimes after only minor trauma. The presenting complaint is of persisting rotation of the head.
- *Axis fracture (C2).* This represents about 18% of all acute fractures; 60% of these involve the odontoid peg and 20% are 'hangman's' fractures. This is an unstable fracture of the posterior elements of the body of C2, i.e. the pars interarticularis, usually as a result of an extension injury.
- *C3–C7 fractures and dislocations.* Because of the vulnerability of the axis and more mobile lower cervical spine, C5 is the site of most cervical spine fractures, and subluxation of C5 on C6 is the most common level. The likelihood of spinal cord injury increases if facet dislocations occur, from 80% (30% complete) with a unilateral facet joint dislocation to 100% (84% complete) if bilateral.
- *T1–T10 fractures and dislocations.* Axial loading with flexion causes anterior wedge compression injuries, but the rigid rib cage makes most of these fractures stable. True vertical axial compression causes burst fractures, where fragments may encroach on the cord, particularly

since the thoracic canal is relatively narrow for the size of the spinal cord. Fracture dislocations are relatively uncommon from T1 to T10, but commonly result in complete spinal cord deficit. Chance fractures are vertebral fractures caused by acute flexion, e.g. caused by a lap belt in a back seat passenger. The fracture begins posteriorly and proceeds anteriorly through the vertebral body or intravertebral disc. This fracture is associated with retroperitoneal and abdominal visceral injuries and is named after CQ Chance, a radiologist.

- *T11–L1*. The thoracolumbar junction is particularly vulnerable because it forms a fulcrum between the mobile lumbar spine and the relatively immobile thoracic spine. Fractures most commonly occur as a result of hyperflexion and rotation and are commonly unstable. They are particularly vulnerable to rotational movement, so log-rolling should be performed with extreme care.
- *L1–S5*. Fractures in these areas generally only involve the cauda equina as the adult spinal cord usually terminates at around L1.

In assessing any patient with potential spinal injury, consider the mechanism of the injury, history and clinical findings before you allow yourself to be reassured by normal plain films and maintain a cautious approach to removing cervical spine restraints. Be particularly careful when treating patients with a lot of neck pain and muscle spasm, and children. These groups may have major ligamentous injury, instability and the potential for permanent cord damage despite normal plain films. Spinal cord injury without radiographic abnormality is often termed 'SCIWORA'.

Films should be examined in a systematic way. One method is alphabetical, and taught on the Advanced Trauma Life Support Program for Doctors of the American College of Surgeons and involves:

- adequacy and alignment
- bony abnormality and base of skull

- cartilage and contours
- disc space
- soft tissue.

The normal lateral c-spine

Adequacy
The base of the skull, all seven cervical vertebra and the top of the body of T1 must be clearly visible on a lateral cervical film. If all seven cervical vertebrae are not seen, the film may be repeated with one of the following:

- using a higher penetration technique
- while the patient's shoulders are pulled down
- using a swimmer's view
- using trauma oblique views.

If a satisfactory view still cannot be obtained, CT scanning may be required. MRI scanning gives important information regarding spinal cord injury but remains problematic in a patient with multiple injuries.

Alignment
Four lines have been described:

- anterior vertebral bodies
- anterior spinal canal
- posterior spinal canal
- spinous process tips.

The lines should be smooth unbroken curves. The only exception is the line along the posterior spinal canal where a small posterior step at C2 may occur normally, particularly in children. This step should be no more than a 2 mm gap between the C1–C3 line and the base of the C2 spinous process.

Loss of alignment of the posterior aspect of the vertebral bodies suggests dislocation, and narrowing of the vertebral canal suggests spinal cord compression. The spinous processes should be roughly equidistant, should converge to a point behind the patient's neck and should not fan outwards.

If you do find a step in the curves, look for overriding of the vertebral bodies. Note that:

- no vertebral fracture + 25% override suggests unifacetal dislocation – a stable injury
- no vertebral fracture + 50% override suggests bifacetal dislocation – an unstable injury
- a vertebral fracture + > 3.5 mm override indicates instability.

Bones

Trace the outlines of the vertebral bodies. Below C2 they should be the same size and shape. Look carefully at the pedicles, facets, laminae and transverse and spinous processes. Teardrop fractures may be caused by hyperflexion or hyperextension and are usually unstable injuries. A compression fracture of a cervical vertebral body of more than 25% is likely to be unstable.

The outline of the odontoid peg should be closely applied to the posterior aspect of the arch of C1. The normal distance between the bones at this point should be:

- 3 mm or less in adults
- 5 mm or less in children.

Cartilage, contours and disc space

The intervertebral disc spaces should be of uniform height. A widened disc space suggests a severe spinal injury. Angulation of > 10° between adjacent vertebral body end-plates is a sign of traumatic instability.

Soft tissue

Soft tissue at the front of the vertebral bodies has a characteristic shape and width at various levels. Note that:

- soft tissue opposite C1–4 should be less than 7 mm or approx. 30% of the width of the vertebral body
- soft tissue opposite C5–C7 should be less than 22 mm or approx. 100% of the width of the vertebral body.
- only 50% of patients with a bony or ligamentous injury show soft tissue swelling.

Soft tissue swelling may be particularly difficult to interpret in children who may have adenoidal enlargement, and may be crying or holding the neck flexed. An increased interspinous distance may indicate torn interspinous ligaments and a likely spinal canal fracture at that level.

The normal AP cervical view

The spinous processes should lie in a straight line and be equally spaced. A unilateral facet joint dislocation will cause one vertebra to rotate on another, altering the alignment. A space 50% wider than the one immediately above or below suggests an anterior cervical dislocation.

The normal open mouth or peg view

The odontoid peg should be clearly seen and not obscured by overlying teeth. A well-fitting semi-rigid cervical collar will restrict mouth opening and may need to be removed for adequate open mouth views (or for intubation). If so, manual in-line cervical stabilisation should be maintained.

Fractures of the odontoid peg may be mimicked by overlapping soft tissue shadowing, causing thin dark lines (Mach bands). If in doubt, ask for help! The space on either side of the peg should be equal and the lateral margins of C1 and C2 should be in alignment. If the spaces on either side of the peg are unequal, but the lateral margins of C1 and C2 remain in alignment, then the cause is most likely to be rotation of the neck. If the lateral masses of C1 overhang the lateral margins of C2, then suspect a burst (Jefferson) fracture.

THE CHEST X-RAY

The AP CXR is the single most important investigation in a patient with thoracic trauma and should be performed within 10 min of a patient's arrival at the resuscitation room. Interpretation of the CXR is discussed in detail in Chapter 1; however, a trauma-based system of interpretation may also be used.

Adequacy and alignment

If an adequate inspiration has been taken, five anterior ribs and 10 posterior ribs should be seen above the level of the hemidiaphragm. If the film is adequately centred, the medial ends of the clavicles should be equidistant from the vertebral spinous processes. Trace the natural curve of the ribs and thoracic cage looking for steps.

Bones
Look along the ribs for fracture lines and cortical discontinuity or disruption of the trabecular pattern. Check all the other bones visible, including thoracic spine, clavicles and humeri.

Cartilage and joints
Look at all joints visible on the radiograph, particularly the sternoclavicular joint (dislocation often being associated with injury to the brachiocephalic vein).

Soft tissue
The AP projection may make the vascular markings more prominent in the superior lung fields and make the mediastinum appear artificially wide. However, vascular markings and lung translucency should be equal on both sides. The mediastinum should remain central and not contain free air. The left hilum remains 1–2 cm above the right and the aortic knuckle should be well defined. Each hemidiaphragm should have a smooth contour. Look for abnormal lucency or opacity in the pleural, mediastinal, subcutaneous and subphrenic spaces and decide if this is due to air or fluid which is pulmonary, pleural, involving chest wall or due to artefact.

THE PELVIS

In 94% of cases, a correct diagnosis can be made from an anteroposterior (AP) radiograph of the pelvis. In the remainder, further plain views or CT scanning may be needed.

Adequacy and alignment
The whole pelvis should be visible. The symphysis pubis should line up with the midline of the sacrum. The pelvic brim and the two obturator foramina should be

smooth, uninterrupted circles. Shenton's line should be a smooth curve traced from the superior aspect of the obturator fossa along the inferior aspect of the femoral neck.

Bones
Look at the trabecular pattern of the pelvis and femurs and the outer edges of the bones to check for interruption. Check that the sacral foramina have smooth borders and are symmetrical. Make sure there are no bony fragments or overlapping bones.

Cartilage
The hips and sacroiliac joints should be symmetrical. All joints should be inspected for disruption of the articular surfaces, discongruity and widening of joint spaces.

Soft tissues
Look at the fat and soft tissue planes both inside and outside the pelvis. You may be able to detect large haematomas, which should alert you to the presence of fractures or major vascular damage. Abnormal gas shadows may indicate damage to the pelvic organs.

FACIAL VIEWS

Basic radiographs
- The occipitomental (OM) view is a tilted up frontal radiograph. Compare the two sides and look for soft tissue abnormalities and fluid levels. In addition, three lines may be traced to help diagnosis. Line 1 runs between the lateral margins of the orbits through the frontal sinuses; line 2 runs between the zygomatic arches along the inferior rim of the orbit; and line 3 runs along the inferior border of the zygomatic arch, crossing the floor of the maxillary antrum.
- Lateral radiograph.
- Orthopantomogram (OPG). This is a tomographic view taken with a moving beam to 'unwrap' the entire mandible. The mandible can be regarded (like the pelvis) as a rigid bony ring, meaning that it is likely to fracture in two places.

LeFort classification

Rene LeFort (1829–1893), a professor of surgery in Paris, dropped rocks onto the faces of cadavers and described a series of middle third of face fractures as a result of his experiments. CT scans give much better information on complex facial fractures than plain X-rays, but the true LeFort classification may not be obvious until surgery.

- *LeFort I.* This is a horizontal fracture of the maxilla, passing above the floor of the nose, involving the nasal septum and mobilising the palate. The fracture segment can rotate about a vertical axis and be displaced laterally or posteriorly.
- *LeFort II.* This is a pyramidal fracture. It begins at the upper part of the nasal bone, crosses the medial wall of the orbit, the lateral wall of the antrum and then posteriorly through the pterygoid plates. This creates a mobile segment which can rotate or be displaced posteriorly. The force necessary to create a LeFort II fracture can be sufficient to extend it into the base of the skull.
- *LeFort III.* The fracture line separates the midfacial skeleton from the base of the skull. The whole of the midface becomes mobile and is usually distracted posteriorly to form the 'dish-face' deformity. There is frequently an associated base of skull fracture.

FURTHER READING

American College of Surgeons Committee on Trauma 1997 *Advanced Trauma Life Support®* *Manual*, 6th edn. American College of Surgeons, Chicago.

Grande CM, Smith CE 1999 Trauma. In: *Anesthesiology Clinics of North America.* WB Saunders, Philadelphia.

Raby N, Berman L, de Lacey G 1995 *Accident and Emergency Radiology – a Survival Guide.* WB Saunders, London.

Skinner DB, Driscoll P, Earlam R 1996 *ABC of Trauma.* BMJ, London.

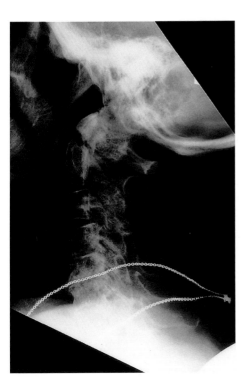

QUESTIONS

Question 4.1

A 70-year-old lady falls down a flight of stairs during a party. On admission she is complaining loudly of neck, chest and ankle pain and smells strongly of alcohol. She has pulled off the cervical collar that the paramedics applied because she felt it was choking her and making her arms hurt. Her c-spine X-ray was obtained with difficulty and is shown.

a. Describe the lateral c-spine radiograph.
b. Should the cervical collar be reapplied?
c. This lady also has a bimalleolar ankle fracture. Can she be taken to theatre for open reduction and internal fixation once she is sober?
d. List potentially unstable c-spine injuries.

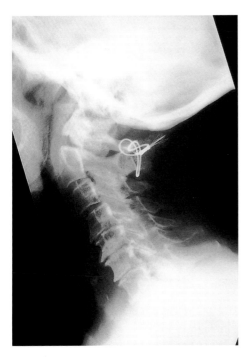

Question 4.2

The same lady who presented in Question 4.1 undergoes surgical stabilisation of this fracture, but presents 4 months later for elective repair of an umbilical hernia. She has no neck pain, but you request a c-spine X-ray.

a. Describe this c-spine X-ray.
b. What are the implications of this for the proposed surgery?
c. What plan of action do you recommend?

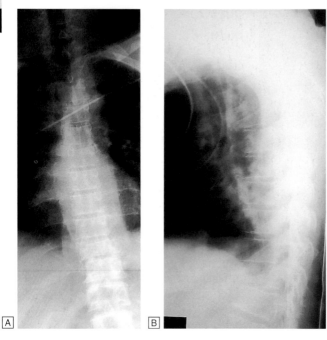

Question 4.3

A 42-year-old man was crossing the road when he was struck at high speed by a van. On admission he is unconscious with a GCS of 7/15. He is intubated, ventilated and a CT scan of his head shows a diffuse head injury. His thoracic spine X-rays are shown (A, B).

a. Describe the radiographs shown.
b. Is the main injury shown likely to be stable?
c. What precautions must be taken in the ITU?

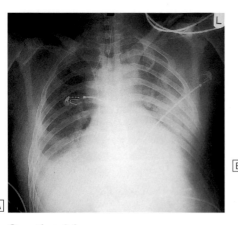

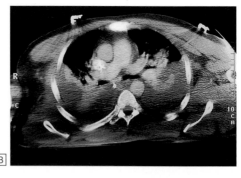

Question 4.4

The patient in Question 4.3 is ventilated in the ITU, but within 8 h of admission his oxygenation deteriorates. His CXR (A) and chest CT (B) are shown.

a. Describe the changes on this CXR.
b. Describe the changes on the CT scan of his chest.
c. What treatment do you recommended?

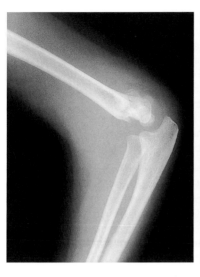 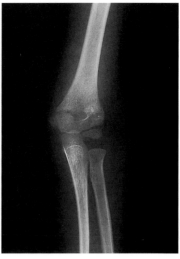

Question 4.5

A 6-year-old child falls off a bicycle and lands on her left arm. On examination her elbow is swollen and very tender. The orthopaedic registrar diagnoses a fracture and wants you to anaesthetise her first on the trauma list. She ate a hamburger and chips for lunch at 12.30 h, 30 min before the accident, and it is now only 14.00 h. Her X-rays are shown.

a. Describe these films.
b. Why have you been asked to put this girl first on your list?
c. Assuming cooperation, how should motor and sensory function be assessed?
d. How should you apply preoperative starvation guidelines for children in this case?

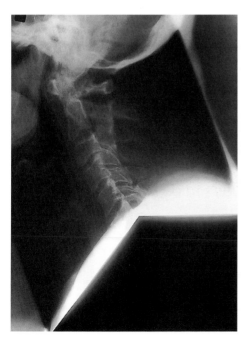

Question 4.6

A 38-year-old man drives a car into a wall at high speed and has a GCS of 10/15. His c-spine X-ray is shown.

a. Describe this c-spine X-ray.
b. What is the problem with this radiograph and what will you do next?
c. Describe the measures you should take when excluding a c-spine injury in an unconscious patient on ITU.

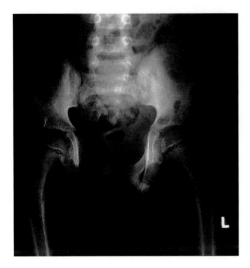

Question 4.7

An 8-year-old boy falls off his bicycle and under a truck. When admitted to hospital, he is drowsy and pale, with a respiratory rate of 40/min, a heart rate of 160 beats/min and a blood pressure of 40/20 mmHg. He feels icy cold and his capillary refill time is over 7 s. There are tyre marks across his abdomen, which is visibly becoming more distended. His pelvic radiograph is shown.

a. What would be the normal heart rate and blood pressure for this child?
b. Describe a classification of clinical signs and blood loss in children. What percentage of his blood volume do you estimate has been lost?
c. What fluids are you going to give this boy, and how will you decide what quantities to give?
d. What can you diagnose from the pelvic radiograph and what immediate treatment do you recommend?

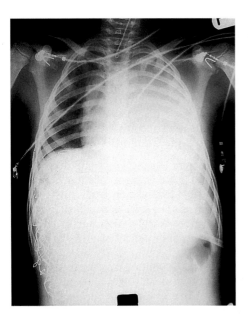

Question 4.8

The same child in Question 4.7 undergoes an emergency laparotomy, packing of liver laceration and application of a pelvic external fixator. Towards the end of the procedure, oxygenation deteriorates and examination of the chest reveals reduced movement on the left side. A CXR is taken.

a. Describe this CXR and your differential diagnosis.
b. Outline your plan of treatment.

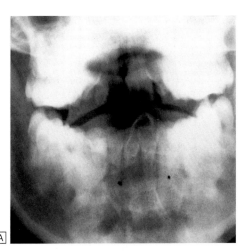

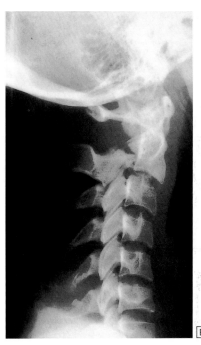

Question 4.17

An 18-year-old girl presents following a high-speed road traffic accident. She complains of severe neck pain and tingling in her legs. Her pulse rate is 80 beats/min, blood pressure 110/65 mmHg and she has a normal respiratory pattern. Her open mouth (A) and lateral c-spine radiographs (B) are shown.

a. Describe these films. Is this a stable injury?
b. Describe the immediate management of this patient.
c. How will you anaesthetise her for spinal stabilisation?

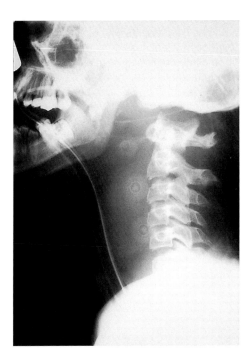

Question 4.18

A 17-year-old boy crashes a car into a wall at high speed. He is pulseless when found by the paramedics who bring him to A&E intubated and ventilated. After resuscitation, he has a pulse rate of 80 beats/min, blood pressure 96/45 mmHg, with no respiratory or limb movement. His pupils are reactive, size 3 mm. His c-spine film is shown.

a. What is the diagnosis on the c-spine film?
b. Describe your management plan.
c. His parents ask to speak to you. What can you tell them?

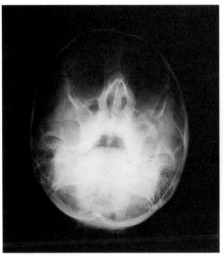
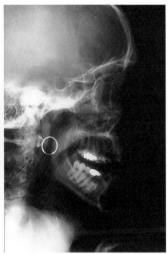

Question 4.19

A 21-year-old driver is involved in a head-on collision. His GCS is 14 and he insists on sitting up so that he can spit out blood from his mouth. His vital signs are stable and there are no other apparent injuries. Facial views are shown.

a. What injuries can be seen on the facial views?

b. In what ways may maxillofacial trauma affect the airway?

c. How would you anaesthetise him for surgery for these injuries?

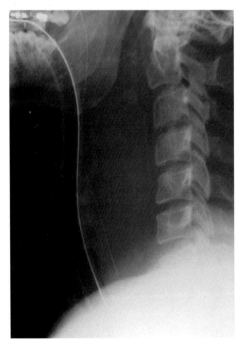

Question 4.20

An 18-year-old man is stabbed in the neck in a fight. He presents with airway obstruction, weakness of his left arm and leg, a dilated right pupil, but a GCS of 15. The anaesthetic SHO gives him a rapid-sequence induction but then finds he can neither intubate nor ventilate. You arrive and intubate him with a struggle, since the larynx appears deviated and oedematous. His lateral c-spine film is taken.

a. What is the problem demonstrated on this film?

b. What do you suspect as the underlying problem?

c. How would you have managed his airway?

d. What endotracheal tube would you have used?

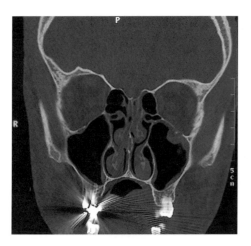

Question 4.21

A 17-year-old man is hit in the eye by a squash racquet. He has no other injuries. His CT image is shown.

a. What abnormality is visible on the CT image?
b. How should the eye be examined after trauma?
c. What surgery is proposed and what are the intraoperative anaesthetic considerations?

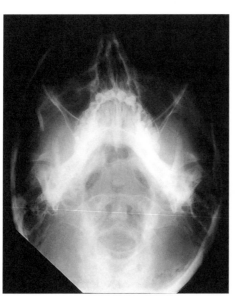

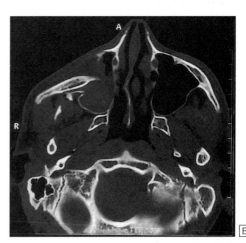

Question 4.22

A 32-year-old man is involved in a fight and presents the following morning with blurred vision in his right eye and a tender, swollen and painful face. His OM facial view is shown (A) with an axial CT scan (B). (Note: films are not from the same patient.)

a. Describe these radiographs.
b. What surgery will be proposed?
c. Why is this patient at risk of bradycardia during surgery?
d. Outline the anatomy of the trigeminal nerve.

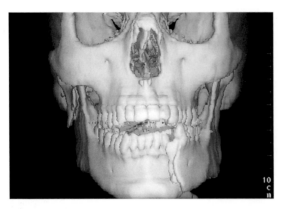

Question 4.23

A 23-year-old man is involved in a fight in a bar. He presents with mouth opening limited to 1 cm and a painful jaw. His radiograph is shown. He is scheduled for mandibular fixation.

a. What is this radiograph and what does it show?

b. How are you going to anaesthetise this man? Will he be a difficult intubation?

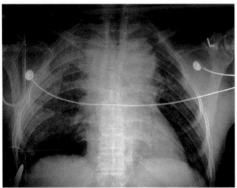

A

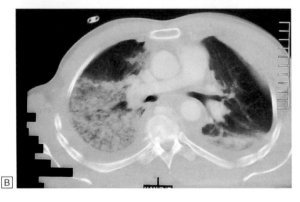

B

Question 4.24

A 50-year-old man was an unrestrained back seat passenger in a car which rolled over several times at speed when the driver tried to avoid a deer on the road. His CXR (A) and CT scan of chest (B) are shown.

a. Describe this chest film and CT scan. What is the diagnosis?

b. What clinical signs would make you suspect an aortic injury?

c. What signs on a chest film would make you suspect a traumatic aortic rupture?

d. How would you manage a patient with an aortic rupture and what is the prognosis?

e. What other injuries may be present?

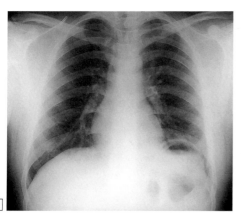
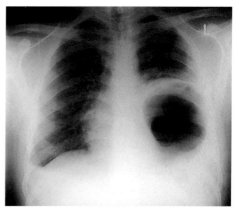

A

B

Question 4.25

A 25-year-old woman cyclist is hit by a car. She arrives in hospital complaining of mild chest pain. This settles over 72 h but then she re-presents 2 weeks later with mild chest pain and shortness of breath. Her initial chest film (A) and chest film 2 weeks later (B) are shown.

a. Describe these films.
b. What is the likely diagnosis and how would you confirm this?
c. What treatment does she need?

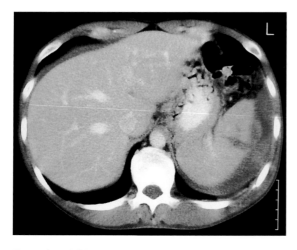

Question 4.26

A 16-year-old girl is hit by a bus. She complains of pain in her left femur, left-sided chest and abdominal pain. She has fractured the left 10th and 11th ribs on CXR. Her blood pressure is 90/45 mmHg and pulse rate 110. After intravenous fluid resuscitation, a CT scan of her abdomen is performed (as shown), following which she is transferred to orthopaedic theatre for femoral nailing. However, she becomes hypotensive, with blood pressure 50/30 mmHg, heart rate 145 beats/min and her CVP keeps falling.

a. Describe the CT appearances. What diagnosis has been missed?
b. What is the likely explanation for her blood pressure falling in theatre?
c. What does she need in the postoperative period?

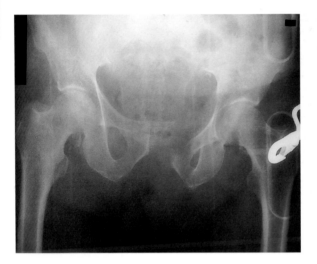

Question 4.27

A 42-year-old man is crushed by a fork lift truck. He presents fully conscious and in severe pain from his lower abdomen. He has a blood pressure of 90/45 mmHg and a heart rate of 128 beats/min. He has no neurological signs. His chest film is normal; his pelvic film is shown. An ultrasound of his abdomen does not show any bleeding.

a. Describe his pelvic film.
b. Why is major blood loss associated with pelvic fractures?
c. What needs to be done next?

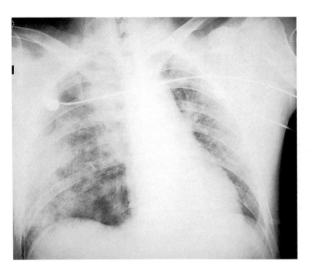

Question 4.28

A 58-year-old man is a pedestrian hit by a car. He presents with acute dyspnoea and central chest pain. His chest radiograph is shown.

a. Describe this chest film.
b. What should be done next?

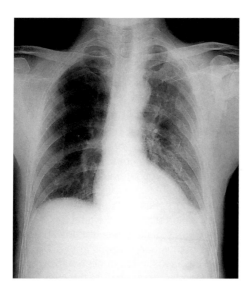

Question 4.29

A 48-year-old man falls off the roof of his house and presents with severe chest pain. His vital signs are stable and he has no other injuries. His arterial blood gases show a P_aO_2 of 26 kPa and a P_aCO_2 of 5.6 kPa on high-flow oxygen. You are asked to transfer him by ambulance to another hospital 10 miles way. His chest film is shown.

a. Describe this film.
b. What treatment would you initiate before transfer?
c. Discuss the pain management of rib fractures.

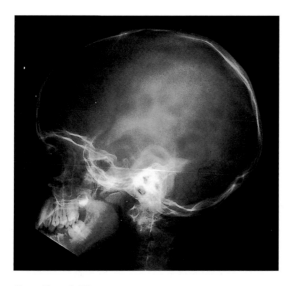

Question 4.30

A 9-year-old child presents having fallen out of her wheelchair and has facial lacerations, including full-thickness lip, requiring suturing under general anaesthesia. On examination she has a short neck with limitation of neck movement, but no pain. Her lateral skull X-ray is shown.

a. Describe two diagnoses identified from this film?
b. What specific problems may these diagnoses present for general anaesthesia?

ANSWERS

Answer 4.1

a. This is a lateral c-spine film. Views are inadequate as the vertebrae are only demonstrated to C6. There is artefact from a necklace. There is a transverse odontoid peg fracture with minimal displacement and surprisingly little prevertebral tissue swelling. Severe degenerative changes are present.

b. A properly fitting semi-rigid cervical collar should be reapplied because this lady has probably sustained an unstable cervical spine fracture.

c. The ankle fracture should be supported by a backslab plaster until the cervical fracture has been surgically treated, particularly since many ankle fractures need several days of elevation to allow soft tissue swelling to subside before surgical fixation.

d. Potentially unstable c-spine fractures include the following: basal peg fracture; Jefferson fracture of C1; C2 posterior arch fracture; hangman's fracture (traumatic spondylolisthesis of C2); hyperflexion 'teardrop' injury; hyperextension 'teardrop' injury; hyperextension fracture dislocation; bilateral facet dislocation.

Answer 4.2

a. This is a lateral cervical spine X-ray; the view is inadequate, only exposed to the body of C7. It shows surgical fixation of the posterior elements of C1 and C2. However, posterior displacement of the odontoid relative to C2 is slightly more marked than previously. Given that this film has been taken 4 months after the original injury, non-union should be considered, because the fracture is clearly visible and the edges are corticated.

b. The fracture may not be completely healed, even after this length of time. Although fibrous union may well have occurred, the neck should not be considered to be entirely stable, at least until further radiological investigations have been performed.

c. She requires a neurosurgical opinion regarding the stability of her neck and further radiology, CT or MRI, before consideration of her hernia surgery.

Answer 4.3

a. AP and lateral films have been taken of the thoracic spine. There is a crush fracture of T10.

b. Most of these injuries are stable, but there is a slight lateral shift of T10 relative to T11 and a right posterior 11th rib fracture, raising the possibility of associated posterior element injuries which may make the injury unstable.

c. This man is unconscious in the ITU and clinical assessment of his neurology is unlikely for many days. In the meantime, assume there is an unstable spinal fracture and ensure the patient is log-rolled when turned. Further assessment, which may include MRI, is unlikely to be possible until his condition is more stable.

Answer 4.4

a. This CXR is a supine AP film showing satisfactory positions of the endotracheal tube (ETT), nasogastric tube and right subclavian line. There is diffuse bilateral opacification of the lungs, with loss of both hemidiaphragms. He is likely to have severe pulmonary contusions, but the uniform opacification of the lung fields suggests pleural fluid collections.

b. The CT of the chest and thoracic spine is contrast-enhanced, shown by increased density of the superior vena cava. There are bilateral, very large pleural fluid collections of similar density to chest wall musculature. In the trauma setting, these are likely to represent haemothoraces.

c. The patient may benefit from chest drains. In fact, two chest drains were inserted in the fifth intercostal space in the midaxillary line and approximately 3 L of heavily bloodstained fluid were drained. His CXR post-chest drain insertion is shown (below) with marked

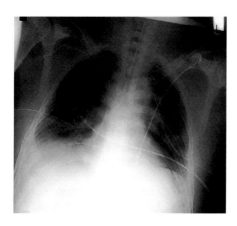

improvement in opacification of both lungs.

Answer 4.5

a. These are frontal and lateral elbow films taken of a skeletally immature child. There is a posteriorly displaced supracondylar fracture. There is also an elbow joint effusion, because the posterior and anterior fat pads are elevated (the anterior fat pad is difficult to see in this particular film). The effusion is likely to be a haemarthrosis.

b. This fracture can damage both nerves and arteries. The ulnar nerve runs behind the medial epicondyle. The posterior and anterior ulnar recurrent arteries run over the medial epicondyle, and the interosseous and radial recurrent arteries run around the lateral epicondyle and the neck of the radius. The brachial artery is a continuation of the axillary artery, and divides into the radial and ulnar arteries opposite the neck of the radius. Because of the risk of ischaemia and nerve damage, this fracture should be reduced as soon as is practical.

c. If the arterial supply has been compromised the hand may be pale, pulseless, painful, paraesthetic, paralysed and perishingly cold! Never wait for all of these symptoms to develop. Damage to the ulnar nerve at the elbow causes paralysis of flexor carpi ulnaris, the medial half of flexor

digitorum profundis, paralysis of the small muscles of the hand, except the muscles of the thenar eminence and the first two lumbricals (supplied by the median nerve), and adductor pollicis. The patient cannot make a fist, grip a sheet of paper placed between two fingers or grip a piece of paper between the thumb and index finger without flexing the terminal phalanx (Froment's sign). There will also be sensory loss over the anterior and posterior surfaces of the medial third of the hand, and the anterior and posterior surfaces of the little finger and half the ring finger.

d. Guidelines vary, but in general, for elective surgery expect children to be allowed solids and milky drinks until 4 h and clear fluids until 2 h before surgery. Since gastric emptying ceases after trauma, assume that the stomach is full, and will remain full, particularly if the child ate just before the accident. Transfer to theatre should not be delayed in the hope that gastric emptying may occur, and a rapid-sequence induction should be used.

Answer 4.6

a. This is a lateral c-spine X-ray. There is abnormal angulation at C3/4 and increased soft tissue swelling anterior to C5/6. The X-ray is inadequate as only the body of C6 is shown.

b. A further lateral c-spine X-ray should be performed with his arms pulled down by his sides to ensure penetration down to T1. This, in fact, shows an unstable C6/7 fracture dislocation (see figure below). If adequate plain views cannot be obtained then a CT scan may need to be performed down to the C7/T1 junction.

c. It may not be possible to exclude a c-spine injury completely in an unconscious ventilated patient on ITU. The gold standard of a clinical examination in a neurologically normal patient with no neck pain and no distracting injuries may never be achieved, particularly if there has been a severe head injury. This must be taken

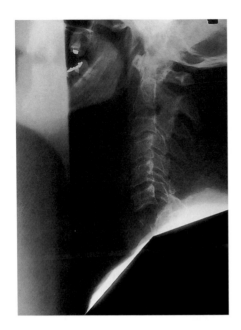

into account in the process of c-spine clearance in such patients.

If the three plain views are taken with CT scanning of the C1/2 junction, the C7/T1 junction (if it is unclear on plain films) and any suspicious areas, 99% of serious injuries will be excluded. Given the inherent risks of hard collars, with increases in ICP and pressure sores, many units will maintain a neutral neck position with sandbags and log-rolling.

Clearance is often then assumed once normal CT scans have been performed. Although this may miss 1% of injuries, it must be emphasised that complete clearance may never be accomplished in the unconscious ITU patient.

Answer 4.7

a. For an 8-year-old child who is not crying, normal heart rate would be 80–100 beats/min and systolic blood pressure 95–100 mmHg (estimate using the formula 80 mmHg + [2 × age]).

b. Children have an increased physiological reserve compared with adults, so vital signs may be only slightly abnormal despite considerable blood loss. Early diagnosis depends on feeling the temperature of the extremities, checking the capillary refill time (normally < 2 s) and looking for a depressed conscious level.

Classification of shock in children is detailed in the table below.

c. The child's weight may be estimated using the Oakley chart, or the following formula: weight (kg) = 2 (age + 4). In the UK, 4.5% albumin has been historically used during the initial resuscitation of children, rather than the exclusive use of crystalloids and blood. However, debate continues over the use of

	Class I < 15% blood volume	Class II 15–25% blood volume	Class III 25–40% blood volume	Class IV > 40% blood volume
Heart rate (beats/min)	↑10–20%	> 150	> 150	Tachycardia or bradycardia
Blood pressure	Normal	↓ Systolic pressure	↓↓ Systolic pressure	Severe hypotension
Pulse pressure	Normal	↓ Pulse pressure	↓↓ Pulse pressure	Absent peripheral pulses
Respiratory rate breaths/min	Normal	35–40/min	35–40/min	Starts to fall
Central nervous system	Normal	Irritable, confused	Lethargic	Comatose
Skin	Normal	Cool at edges, clammy	Cold, clammy, cyanotic	Pale, icy cold
Capillary refill time	Normal < 2 s	> 2 s	Very prolonged	Very prolonged

This child is likely to have lost nearly 40% of his circulating blood volume.

albumin and colloids. All fluids should be warmed to body temperature and given in 20 mL/kg aliquots in response to clinical signs initially and to central venous pressure once a line is inserted after initial resuscitation.

This child is in class III–IV shock and will require blood urgently. In a dire emergency O-negative blood can be given. If a wait of approximately 10 min is possible, then type-specific blood can be obtained, which should eliminate serious reactions due to ABO incompatibility. A formal cross-match will take a minimum of 45 min to provide blood, which is too long for the initial resuscitation of this child, but should be requested for later use in theatre. Seek advice from a haematologist about the use of coagulation products such as fresh frozen plasma, cryoprecipitate etc.

d. The pubic symphysis and left sacroiliac joints are both widened, in keeping with traumatic diastasis. Pelvic fractures can cause life-threatening haemorrhage, particularly in children. A senior orthopaedic surgeon should be asked to apply an external fixator in the resuscitation area if the child is not going to theatre immediately, although it is likely that this child will also require a laparotomy.

Further reading
Nadel S, De Munter C, Britto J, Levin M, Habib P 1998 Albumin: saint or sinner? *Archives of Disease in Childhood* 79: 384–385

Answer 4.8

a. This is a portable, supine film showing an endotracheal tube (ETT) and ECG electrodes. There are multiple radio-opaque filaments in the right upper quadrant in keeping with surgical packing of a ruptured liver. There is complete opacification of the left hemithorax, suggesting effusion, haemothorax or collapse. The possibility of a ruptured diaphragm must also be considered.

b. A ruptured diaphragm should have been noted at laparotomy. High intra-abdominal pressures created by the

packing of the liver laceration and closure of the abdominal wall may have forced fluid into the left chest with a contribution from left lung collapse. This could also be a massive haemothorax secondary to the initial trauma. In an emergency setting, it would be reasonable to insert a chest drain. Following this, 'bagging' the patient after the instillation of saline may shift mucus plugs and partly help to re-expand the lung. If this does not work, fibreoptic bronchoscopy should be performed, followed by a CT scan of the chest if the cause of opacification is still unclear. Rigid bronchoscopy may be required if a fibreoptic bronchoscope of sufficiently narrow diameter to fit down the ETT is not available.

Answer 4.9

a. This is a lateral c-spine film. It is an adequate view, with visualisation of the C7/T1 junction. Alignment is good, but there is prevertebral soft tissue swelling at the level of C7 with a fracture through the body of C7. This is a flexion teardrop fracture.

b. Flexion teardrop vertebral body fractures are often unstable.

c. He should be assumed to have a full stomach and a rapid-sequence intubation performed. A properly fitted hard collar will prevent adequate mouth opening, so it should be removed while a second assistant provides manual in-line stabilisation. Cricoid pressure is generally felt to be safe in unstable c-spine injuries to minimise the risk of pulmonary aspiration, but should be performed with the second hand supporting the back of the neck.

Further reading
McLeod ADM, Calder I 2000 Spinal cord injury and direct laryngoscopy – the legend lives on. *British Journal of Anaesthesia* 84: 705–709.

Answer 4.10

a. The chest film shows extensive bilateral pulmonary interstitial infiltrations, with an air bronchogram on the left side. An endotracheal tube and a right subclavian line are in satisfactory positions.

b. These radiographic findings are consistent with acute respiratory distress syndrome (ARDS). The principal pathology is of interstitial oedema and therefore the differential diagnosis includes fluid overload and left ventricular failure. Pulmonary fibrosis should also be excluded. Diagnosis is predominantly by the overall clinical picture, but clinical measurements (pulmonary artery occlusion pressure < 18 mmHg, cardiac echo demonstrating good left ventricular function) are useful.

c. The clinical picture in this case is of fat embolism syndrome (FES). This occurs in 3% of patients with a long bone injury and 10% of those with multiple trauma. Fat embolism characteristically presents as a triad of confusion, dyspnoea and petechial haemorrhages usually within the first 24 h following trauma. In addition, hypotension, right ventricular strain, thrombocytopenia, hypocalcaemia, pyrexia and hepatic and renal insufficiency are common. CXR findings are indistinguishable from those of ARDS, but the petechial rash occurs in 50% of cases and characteristically occurs over the anterior neck and the conjunctivae. Although the diagnosis is usually made on clinical grounds, this may be confirmed by identifying fat droplets in the urine or from bronchoalveolar lavage. Major and minor criteria have been established to support the diagnosis, with one major and four minor criteria needed to establish a diagnosis of FES.

Major criteria
- Axillary or subconjunctival petechiae
- Hypoxaemia (P_aO_2 < 8 kPa with F_iO_2 < 0.4)
- CNS depression disproportionate to degree of hypoxaemia
- Pulmonary oedema.

Minor criteria
- Tachycardia (HR > 110 beats/min)

- Pyrexia > 38.5°C
- Emboli observed in fundi
- Fat present in urine or sputum
- Sudden unexplained decrease in haematocrit or platelet count
- Increased ESR.

In addition to long bone fractures, FES may be caused by pancreatitis, burns, diabetes mellitus, liposuction, cardiopulmonary bypass and decompression sickness.

d. Mechanical and chemical theories have been used to explain FES:

- Torn marrow veins and disruption of marrow fat allow entry of fat droplets into the circulation, especially when the marrow cavity is exposed to increased pressure, e.g. time of trauma, femoral reaming. Droplets < 8 μm can pass through the pulmonary capillary bed and enter the systemic circulation – hence the fat deposits seen in eye, brain, kidney and liver. Pulmonary precapillary shunts and patent foramen ovale (probe patent in 20–35% of patients) allow systemic fat embolisation, especially if right heart pressures are high.
- Circulating free fatty acids (FFAs) deposited in the lung are directly toxic to pneumocytes, causing inflammation, increased capillary permeability and inactivation of surfactant, contributing to the development of ARDS.
- FFAs are thought to have a directly toxic effect on the brain, causing cerebral oedema.

e. Treatment is supportive. In particular, cardiorespiratory function, thrombocytopenia and hypocalcaemia should be monitored and treated appropriately. Depressed conscious level may require intubation, ventilation and occasionally intracerebral pressure monitoring to allow control of ICP. Nosocomial pneumonia is common. In the multitrauma patient, fractures should ideally be fixed within 24 h to minimise the risks of the syndrome. However, controversy exists about the timing of operative stabilisation of femoral fractures for patients with concurrent head and chest injuries.

Steroids, heparin, bicarbonate, dextran 40 and alcohol have all been advocated in the treatment of FES, but none has produced any convincing evidence of improved outcome.

Further reading

Bosse MJ et al 1997 ARDS, pneumonia and mortality following thoracic injury with a femoral fracture treated either with intramedullary nailing with reaming or with a plate. *Journal of Bone & Joint Surgery* 79: 799–809.

Hofmann S, Huemer G, Salzer M 1998 Pathophysiology and management of the fat embolism syndrome. *Anaesthesia* 53(suppl): 35–37.

Pape HC, Regel G, Tscherne H 1996 Controversies regarding fracture management in the patient with multiple trauma. *Current Opinion in Critical Care* 2: 295–303.

Answer 4.11

a. This is a supine AP CXR which shows a very wide mediastinum following trauma. There are no rib fractures.

b. The CT scan has been performed to investigate the wide mediastinum, particularly to diagnose a ruptured thoracic aorta. An arch aortogram has been described as the gold standard investigation to detect this condition, but the specialist personnel and facilities for this may not be rapidly available in many UK hospitals. The mediastinum is actually normal on CT scan, but a large left-sided occult pneumothorax is demonstrated on lung windows.

c. The treatment of occult pneumothoraces is controversial. Some authorities recommend observation using sequential CXRs, while others recommend chest drain insertion. If ventilation is required then a chest drain should be inserted.

Further reading

Brasel KJ, Stafford RE, Weigelt JA, Tenquist JE, Borgstrom DC 1999 Treatment of occult

pneumothoraces from blunt trauma. *Journal of Trauma* 46: 987–991.

Answer 4.12

a. This AP film demonstrates bilateral rib fractures, fifth to seventh (right) and fourth to eighth (left) and extensive subcutaneous emphysema. The other most obvious abnormality is that the armoured endotracheal tube (ETT) is lying in the right main bronchus. Bilateral chest drains, a right-sided subclavian line and a nasogastric tube are also in situ.

b. The ETT should be pulled back until breath sounds reappear on that side. The position may then be checked using bronchoscopy or a further radiograph. It would also be appropriate to change the ETT from the uncut armoured, low-volume, high-pressure cuffed tube to a conventional high-volume, low-pressure cuffed ETT to minimise tracheal damage.

Answer 4.13

a. This is an AP chest film; it is rotated and underpenetrated. The left lung field is opaque with a fluid level and the mediastinum is pushed across to the right. This implies the presence of a massive effusion, which in the context of trauma is likely to be a haemothorax.

b. The patient should sit up, and high-flow oxygen should be given and large-bore intravenous access secured. Analgesia

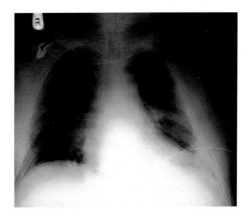

may be required. A chest drain, size 32 French or greater, should be inserted (his CXR post-chest drain is shown above). His tetanus status should be checked and intravenous antibiotics given. He should be referred to a cardiothoracic surgeon for possible thoracotomy if worsening surgical emphysema develops or blood loss from the chest drain is large (1500 mL immediately after insertion in an adult) or continues at more than 200 mL/h (or 3 mL/kg per h) for 2 h.

c. The chest drain directed towards the apex will drain air more effectively and the base fluid more effectively. The best sites are therefore in the midclavicular line in the second intercostal space anteriorly or the fifth space in the mid-axillary line, which is more commonly used. The drain acts on an underwater seal principle so that fluid or air can only escape under the fluid level and a separate vent in the top of the bottle permits this to take place. A purse string should be placed around the drain to permit easy control on removal. The drain should not be lifted unclamped above its insertion site, but should not be clamped during intra- or interhospital transfer. When the drain has stopped bubbling or draining more than 200 mL in 24 h, it can be removed. Sequential CXRs will confirm the recurrence of a pneumothorax or fluid.

Further reading

Clarke GM 1997 Chest injuries. In: Teik OH (ed) *Intensive Care Manual*, 4th edn. Butterworth Heinemann, Oxford.

Answer 4.14

a. The chest film is a well penetrated and centred AP view. There is a fractured left clavicle. An ETT is present, however the right subclavian line passes into the left subclavian vein. There is also a burst fracture of T6, which is visible on the chest film but is more clearly visible on the lateral thoracic spine film.

b. The spinal board is an extrication and immobilisation device, not a treatment

for a spinal injury. This is a very hard surface, putting the patient at risk of pressure sores. It should be removed as soon as the patient's condition permits, ideally within 30 min, but certainly by 2 h.

c. Although clues such as diaphragmatic breathing may be present, there are no pathognomonic features of spinal cord injury in unconscious patients. A high index of suspicion must be maintained in all patients whose mechanism of injury suggests a spinal injury. Examination of the entire length of the spine after the patient has been log-rolled (which must include removal of a cervical collar to examine the neck) may reveal bruising, swelling or a kyphosis, and palpation may detect malalignment of spinous processes or an increased interspinous gap. Hypotension with bradycardia may suggest a cervical or high thoracic cord injury.

A neurological examination may be performed as soon as the patient is sufficiently lightly sedated to respond to stimuli. This examination will naturally be limited, but may allow assessment of tone and reflexes (most important – abdominal, anal and bulbocavernosus), and response to painful stimuli. If a spinal cord injury is suspected, consult your local spinal injury centre for advice. The use of high-dose steroids continues to be controversial in acute spinal injury, but if they are given, this needs to be done within 8 h of the injury. The dose used is 30 mg/kg methyl prednisolone intravenously over 15 min, followed by 5.4 mg/kg per h for 23 h.

Further reading

Bracken MB, Shepard MJ, Collins WF et al 1990 A randomised, controlled trial of methylprednisolone or naloxone in the treatment of spinal cord injury. Results of the second National Spinal Cord Injury Study. *New England Journal of Medicine* 322: 1405–1411.

Answer 4.15

a. This is a barely adequate lateral c-spine film since the body of T1 is just visible.

There is a fracture dislocation of C5 on 6. This is easily seen once the lines of the anterior vertebral bodies are traced and an obvious step is demonstrated. This is likely to be unstable.

b. This man is in spinal shock. He has a slow pulse rate since he has impaired cardiac sympathetics (T2–4) and is unable to respond to a combination of blood loss from his compound fracture and profound vasodilatation due to his loss of sympathetic vasomotor tone.

c. Treatment should initially follow the ABC system as with any patient. Oxygen should be given and intubation may be required. Intravenous access should be secured, blood cross-matched, fluid given and primary and secondary surveys performed. Invasive arterial and central venous access is desirable and inotropes or vasocontrictors may be required. Steroids may be given depending on regional protocols.

Once stabilised, cervical traction should be applied and surgery for his compound femoral fracture addressed. Even with an apparent complete cord transection and total sensory loss, he still requires anaesthesia, since pain pathways often still persist from a partial transection or via autonomic pathways. Care should be taken with central nerve blockade in the acute spinal injury since changes in CSF pressure may potentially lead to worsening of spinal bleeding. In addition, his circulatory status is uncertain. General anaesthesia will necessitate either an awake fibreoptic intubation, with attendant problems of coughing with an unstable c-spine injury, or inhalation or intravenous induction maintaining in line stabilisation with the possibility of difficult intubation. Mean arterial pressure should be maintained to promote good spinal cord perfusion.

d. He should have reasonable respiratory function as the lesion is below the C5/6 level and diaphragmatic function should be preserved. Loss of intercostal and abdominal muscle function leads to a decline in functional respiratory capacity

and maximum inspiratory and expiratory pressures. Tidal volumes may be expected to fall by 60% and vital capacity to 1–1.5 L. With time these may increase to 50% of normal as intercostal tone recovers.

e. His breathing should be better lying down. When supine, the relaxed diaphragm is pushed into the chest by the abdominal contents. This gives it more room for excursion on inspiration, producing better respiratory function than in the sitting position.

Further reading

Baxendale BR, Yeoman PM 1997 Spinal injury. In: Goldhill DR, Withington PS, eds. *Textbook of Intensive Care*. Chapman & Hall Medical, London.

Answer 4.16

a. This film is inadequate as the body of C7 is only just visible. The spinous processes of C3 and 4 have been fractured and there is loss of the normal smooth lordosis of the c-spine. There is also a congenital abnormality of C1.

b. This injury may be stable, but will require a specialist opinion and CT or MRI. Surgery should be delayed until this has been obtained. It may be possible to perform suturing of the facial lacerations under local anaesthesia. If general anaesthesia is required, it would be prudent to take in-line c-spine stabilisation precautions throughout.

Answer 4.17

a. The film is inadequate as the C7–T1 is not visible. There is disruption of the spinolaminar line at C1–2. There are bilateral fractures of the pars interarticularis of C2. These features suggest a hangman's fracture, which is potentially unstable. In addition, the open mouth view shows a fracture through the odontoid peg.

b. She has a high spinal lesion. This is above cardiac (T2–4) and diaphragmatic (C3–5) innervation and she already has signs of incomplete cord injury. She is at high risk of spinal shock and respiratory compromise if the cord is further damaged by swelling or incorrect management of her cervical spine. She should be immobilised in a hard collar, sand bags and tape and log-rolled for procedures. Cervical spine traction should be performed as soon as practicable by an experienced spinal surgeon.

Subsequent management aims to prevent secondary cord damage. She should be managed in a critical care area to optimise oxygenation and perfusion of the cord and observed for signs of cardiorespiratory deterioration. Invasive monitoring is recommended. High-dose steroids may be considered.

c. Anaesthetic considerations include airway control, invasive monitoring, positioning and postoperative care and analgesia. Intubation may be awake or asleep, but traction and in-line stabilisation should be maintained throughout. Advantages of an awake intubation include cardiorespiratory stability, avoidance of a 'can't intubate, can't ventilate' scenario, reduced head and neck manipulation, ability to assess neurology post-intubation, and self-positioning (if required) of the patient on the operating table. However, intubation performed asleep is less distressing for the patient and avoids coughing or straining, which may lead to cord damage. The patient may present a difficult intubation given the need to maintain in-line traction and possible airway oedema.

All these patients are at risk of cardiovascular instability intraoperatively and invasive monitoring is required. Positioning must be taken with great care and with assistance from the spinal surgeon. Cord integrity may be assessed intraoperatively using evoked potentials. Postoperative care must be in a critical care area. Regional techniques beyond local infiltration are rarely appropriate for spinal surgery in high cord injured patients.

Answer 4.18

a. This shows a complete craniocervical dislocation. The cervical cord will be transected and the brain stem is likely to be irretrievably damaged. The film only extends to C6 and there is gross prevertebral soft tissue swelling.

b. This is invariably a fatal injury but there is a small possibility that this boy may still be conscious and paralysed, given his reactive pupils. Primary and secondary surveys should be performed and mechanical ventilation, fluid resuscitation and invasive monitoring established. Sedation should be instituted as soon as possible and he requires a CT scan of his brain.

c. Relatives must be told that this injury is almost universally fatal due to brain stem damage, and assured that he will be kept comfortable whilst treatment continues.

Answer 4.19

a. The facial views show fractures of the right zygomatic arch, right lateral orbital wall, bridge of nose, left lateral orbital wall and left body of maxilla. The lateral view shows the posterior extent of the bridge of nose fracture and posterior displacement of the midface. This pattern is suggestive of a LeFort II fracture.

b. Six specific airway problems may be associated with maxillofacial trauma:

- blockage of the nasopharynx by a fractured maxilla with posterior displacement
- blockage of the oropharynx if the tongue loses its anterior insertion after a bilateral anterior mandibular or symphyseal fracture, particularly if the patient is laid flat
- blockage of any part of the airway from the oral cavity to the bronchi by teeth, dentures, bone fragments, vomit, blood and other foreign bodies
- blockage of the airway by soft tissue swelling and oedema, which may lead to delayed airway problems

- bleeding from distinct vessels in open wounds or bleeding from injuries to the middle third of the face
- associated injury to the larynx or trachea is thankfully rare.

c. Most midfacial fractures do not present with obstruction or bleeding; indeed, surgery is usually delayed until the oedema has settled. In this elective context, intubation is rarely a problem, although with severe midface fractures, obtaining a seal for the facemask may be a challenge, and associated base of skull fractures may be present.

In the emergency situation, urgent airway control may be difficult if airway obstruction is present or bleeding is uncontrolled. If uncontrolled bleeding is the major problem, it may be necessary to perform a rapid-sequence induction for rapid airway control. If blood loss is less severe, or partial airway obstruction is present, an inhalational technique may be used. The left lateral or even prone position has also been recommended during induction to allow blood to drain away from the airway and allow the tongue to fall away from the larynx. Difficult intubation equipment, including facilities for needle cricothyroidotomy, should be on hand and a surgeon should be scrubbed and ready to create a surgical airway if required.

For elective fixation of severe midface fractures, a nasal tube is usually required to allow checking of occlusion. This should be placed under direct vision using a fibreoptic laryngoscope to avoid intracranial placement. The use of intermaxillary fixation (IMF) is fortunately declining, but if used the patient should be extubated awake and monitored postoperatively in a high-dependency area. Nasal airways may be of use post-extubation.

Further reading

Barham CJ 1987 Difficult intubation. *Baillière's Clinical Anaesthesiology* 1: 779–798.

Answer 4.20

a. There is massive prevertebral soft tissue swelling which in this case is likely to be blood. The film only penetrates to C7. There is an oral endotracheal tube in situ.

b. Massive bleeding in the neck has caused a deviated airway. He has a left hemiparesis which in the absence of other injury would imply a partially severed carotid artery.

c. This man had an obstructing airway with a probability of a 'can't intubate, can't ventilate' situation after intravenous induction. An inhalational technique would have allowed the possibility of wake-up in the event of an impossible intubation. An experienced surgeon should be scrubbed and standing by to perform a surgical airway. This may be performed asleep if an airway can be maintained spontaneously breathing or awake under local anaesthesia, although either option is hazardous. The patient may deteriorate too rapidly to permit either option. Urgent surgical exploration is required.

d. Due to the possibility of continued expansion of blood under pressure, an armoured ETT would have been preferable if time had permitted.

Answer 4.21

a. This is a coronal CT film which demonstrates a fracture of the orbital floor with protrusion of orbital fat and possibly inferior rectus muscle through the fracture into the maxillary antrum. This is known as a teardrop sign. This scan is usually performed with the patient prone and the neck hyperextended, so it cannot be done if there is suspicion of a spinal injury.

b. The eyes should be examined systematically. Visual acuity gives information on the overall integrity of cornea to cortex. Limitation of eye movements, diplopia or pupils at different levels imply trauma to the orbit with tissue entrapment. Abnormalities of direct, consensual or accommodation reflexes may indicate rising intracranial pressure; however, direct trauma to the globe or retrobulbar haemorrhage may also cause a fixed, dilated pupil. Proptosis (exophthalmos) suggests there is haemorrhage within the orbital walls, and enophthalmos suggests a fracture of the orbital wall. Periorbital swelling suggests a fracture of the zygoma or maxilla. Subconjunctival ecchymosis suggests direct trauma to the globe or a fractured zygoma. Trauma to the anterior chamber and fundus and the detection of papilloedema require the use of an ophthalmoscope. Advice should be sought from an experienced ophthalmologist.

c. Surgery for the correction of facial fractures may be prolonged and the airway should usually be secured. Repair of the orbit commonly provokes bradycardia due to manipulation of the globe, particularly whilst checking to ensure free movement of the recti muscles. This leads to stimulation of the oculocardiac reflex.

Further reading

Holmes SB, Carter JLB, Metefa A 2000 Lesson of the week: blunt orbital trauma. *British Medical Journal* 321: 750–751.

Answer 4.22

a. The OM view shows a depressed fractured right zygoma. The CT scan shows this more clearly, together with an opaque maxillary antrum, probably from bleeding. This is not visible on the plain film.

b. Proposed surgery will include elevation of the zygoma, which may also need fixation if not stable.

c. The patient is at risk of bradycardia from cranial nerve stimulation, in this case stimulation of the trigeminal nerve on lifting the zygoma. The trigeminocardiac reflex is well recognised and is similar to the oculocardiac reflex.

d. The trigeminal nerve is the largest cranial nerve. It supplies sensory fibres to:

- the skin of the scalp
- the skin of the face (except the angle of the mandible and the parotid gland)
- the mouth and teeth
- the nasal cavity
- the paranasal air sinuses
- proprioceptive fibres to the muscles of facial expression.

Motor fibres supply:

- the muscles of mastication
- tensor veli palatini – tightens soft palate
- tensor tympani – inserts on handle of malleolus.

There are three divisions of the trigeminal nerve:

- ophthalmic nerve – supplies the skin of the forehead, the upper eyelid, the conjunctiva and the side of the nose down to and including the tip
- maxillary nerve – supplies skin on the posterior part of the side of the nose, the lower eyelid, the cheek, the upper lip and the lateral side of the orbital opening
- mandibular nerve – supplies the skin of the lower lip, the lower part of the face, the temporal region, and part of the auricle.

Further reading

Lang S, Lanigan DT, van der Wal M 1991 Trigeminocardiac reflexes: maxillary variants of the oculocardiac reflex. *Canadian Journal of Anaesthesia* 38: 757–760.

Answer 4.23

a. This is a three-dimensional CT reconstruction of the mandible. It shows a fracture of the body of the left side of the mandible and a fracture of the right ramus.

b. Intubation is straightforward in most patients with fractured mandibles. Once asleep and relaxed, the mandible is often lifted out of the way on laryngoscopy since pain and muscle spasm contribute to limitation of mouth opening. Exceptions occur when swelling is marked and when the condyle or temporomandibular joint is involved in the fracture. In this case, the right-sided fracture impinges on the ramus, so you should prepare for a difficult intubation.

The choice is between an inhalational induction and intubation asleep or an awake fibreoptic intubation. A nasal ETT is required to allow surgical access and checking occlusion; a throat pack is recommended. Consider a nasogastric tube and prophylactic antiemetics. There is a small risk of airway obstruction in patients with fractured mandibles, particularly if severely swollen, bilateral or in intermaxillary fixation (IMF). Consider extubation awake, a nasopharyngeal airway in recovery, and oxygen for the first few postoperative nights. If placed in IMF, wire cutters should be freely available.

Further reading
Barham CJ 1993 Anaesthesia for maxillofacial surgery. In: Patel H (ed) *Anaesthesia for Burns, Maxillofacial and Plastic Surgery*. Edward Arnold, London.

Answer 4.24

a. The obvious abnormality on this AP chest film is a widened mediastinum. There is also a crush fracture of the seventh thoracic vertebrae and a fractured second rib on the right. The CT scan shows blood anterior to the thoracic spine with an obvious crush injury of the vertebra (seen as a white line anterior to the vertebra). This is the cause of the widened mediastinum. There is no evidence of aortic tear.

b. Diagnosis is difficult, 50% of patients will have no symptoms, 75% will have signs of external injury, 30% may have a paradoxical high blood pressure in the arms, 40% may have delayed peripheral pulses, 26% complain of chest pain, 30% have a systolic murmur and 10% complain of back pain.

c. In the context of a patient with a high-speed deceleration injury, aortic injury is suggested by:

- a widened mediastinum
- obliteration of the aortic knob
- deviation of the trachea to the right
- obliteration of the AP window (the space between the pulmonary artery and the aorta)
- depression of the left main stem bronchus
- deviation of a nasogastric tube (oesophagus) to the right
- pleural or apical cap
- small left haemothorax.

However, the chest film may be entirely normal in 7% of cases. A classical radiograph of aortic dissection is shown in Chapter 2.

d. About 85% are fatal at the scene. Of the 15% who survive to reach hospital, 40% do not survive the first 24 h. Patients who reach hospital tend to have an incomplete laceration near the ligamentum arteriosum, which tethers the aorta during deceleration; the adventitia is intact and contains the developing haematoma. Because this haematoma is contained, recurrent or persistent hypotension may be due to another site of bleeding. If the aorta ruptures into the left chest, this is a preterminal event unless the patient can be operated on within minutes.

The 'gold standard' for investigation of suspected aortic rupture is arch aortography, although valuable data may be rapidly obtained from spiral CT scanning or transoesophageal echocardiography. The patient will need treatment in a specialist centre.

Patients with a localised aortic haematoma with an intimal flap may be treated conservatively, often using β-blockers. These decrease the sheer stress on the wall of the aorta by reducing intraluminal pressures and rate of increase of the aortic pressure wave (dP/dt) after ventricular systole.

Surgical repair is through a left thoracotomy and will require bypass. Risk of paraplegia during clamping is 6–9%. The right radial artery should be used for intra-arterial monitoring since

4

A

the left subclavian artery may be involved or clamped. The left subclavian or internal jugular vein should be used for central venous access and a double lumen tube is required to provide one lung ventilation.

e. Approximately 8000 traumatic aortic injuries occur per year in the USA. They are often the result of high-speed deceleration and therefore other injuries are common, although most can wait until the aortic injury has been dealt with. Seventy-five per cent of patients have associated rib and sternal fractures, 66% have extremity or pelvic fractures, 50% have a head injury, 50% have significant pulmonary or cardiac contusions and 30% have abdominal injuries.

Further reading

Fabian TC, Richardson JD, Croce MA, et al 1997 Prospective study of blunt aortic injury: multicenter trial of the American Association for the Surgery of Trauma. *Journal of Trauma* 42: 374–380.

Answer 4.25

a. The first film (A) shows a gas bubble, apparently under the diaphragm. The second film (B) shows expansion of this to occupy half of the hemithorax.

b. This is likely to be a traumatic ruptured diaphragm with herniation of the stomach into the chest. A CT scan will help to differentiate between an intact but raised hemidiaphragm (e.g. from phrenic nerve paresis) and a ruptured diaphragm.

c. She needs urgent surgical repair of the diaphragmatic defect.

Answer 4.26

a. This CT scan shows free fluid in the abdomen together with a large laceration in the spleen. This represents a ruptured spleen.

b. She requires an immediate laparotomy and splenectomy. Follow a massive transfusion protocol. All fluids should be warmed using a high-pressure infusion

device and warming devices used in theatre. If hypotension persists, other diagnoses to consider include a tension pneumothorax (a chest drain must be inserted before artificial ventilation), intrathoracic bleeding or cardiac contusion.

c. She is at risk of pneumococcal infection post-splenectomy and should receive pneumococcal vaccine. This should be given at least 14 days after splenectomy, since before this a reduced antibody response is demonstrated. Prophylactic antibiotic therapy is required, usually phenoxymethylpenicillin (500 mg orally 12-hourly for adults), which should be continued after immunisation to cover serotypes not included in the vaccine. Revaccination is recommended every 6 or more years for adults (after 3–5 years in children under 10 years) after splenectomy. Her GP should be informed.

Further reading

BMA/RPSGB 2000 *British National Formulary*. British Medical Association and the Royal Pharmaceutical Society of Great Britain, London.
Consumer's Association 1998. Post splenectomy prophylaxis. *Drugs and Therapeutics Bulletin* 36(10).

Answer 4.27

a. There are displaced fractures of the pubic symphysis and left pubic ramus, associated with disruption of the left sacroiliac joint. This has created a large loose fragment (including the uninjured left hip) which is displaced inferiorly.

b. The bony pelvis is in close association with its blood supply. In addition to the potential for arterial bleeding after fracture, venous drainage from the pelvis is into the valveless portal system. Fortunately, bleeding from fractures to the pelvis may be contained within the retroperitoneal space and the development of tamponade from haematoma can at times prevent death.

The pelvis is a bony ring, so it usually breaks in two places. Lateral compression causes inward rotation of the hemipelvis with disruption of the sacroiliac joints, dislocation of the femur and acetabular fractures.

Anteroposterior compression drives the iliac wings and pubic symphysis apart, causing the 'open book' pelvic fracture which may double the volume of the pelvis in the adult. Posteriorly, damage occurs at the sacroiliac joints, placing the superior gluteal and lateral sacral arteries at risk. Vertical sheer injuries tend to displace the hemipelvis upwards in relation to the sacrum, which is likely to produce major vascular damage to the external iliac, superior gluteal and lateral sacral arteries.

It has been predicted that over 50% of patients with unstable pelvic fractures will need over 4 units of blood and over 30% may need over 10 units.

c. This patient needs urgent external fixation of the pelvis to control the haemorrhage. Fluid resuscitation should be performed at the same time. If there is ongoing evidence of blood loss, a laparotomy should be considered.

Further reading
Cryer HM, Miller FB, Evers BM et al 1988 Pelvic fracture classification: correlation with haemorrhage. *Journal of Trauma* 28: 973.

Answer 4.28

a. This is a poorly centred, underpenetrated AP film. There are multiple rib fractures on the right, with a large flail segment. There is also a large pneumothorax on the right. There is probably midline shift to the left, despite the poor rotation. Allowing for the obvious underpenetration of the film, there is obvious pulmonary contusion.

b. This patient needs a chest drain urgently. A large-bore i.v. cannula may be placed in the second intercostal space in the midclavicular line on the right whilst preparation is made for the formal chest drain placement. In the meantime, he should be sat upright and high-flow oxygen should be administered. He is likely to have suffered significant

pulmonary contusion and may also require artificial ventilation.

Answer 4.29

a. This chest film is well centred and penetrated. It shows multiple fractured ribs, scapula and clavicle on the left with surgical emphysema and pulmonary contusion.

b. The patient has multiple rib fractures and surgical emphysema and is at risk of developing a pneumothorax. He requires an intercostal underwater seal chest drain before interhospital transfer or artificial ventilation. A Heimlich valve system may be more convenient for transfer than an underwater seal drain. He should also receive adequate analgesia and subsequent observation prior to transfer. If he tires or arterial blood gases deteriorate, he may need artificial ventilation.

c. The principle behind the treatment of any pain should be to use an analgesic ladder starting with non-opioids, e.g. paracetamol, followed by weak opioid agonists, e.g. codeine, tramadol, then strong opioid agonists, e.g. morphine, often with the addition of other analgesics, e.g. NSAIDs.

Systemic analgesics all have side-effects, in particular opiates which may cause confusion, sedation, respiratory depression, nausea and constipation. Intravenous opiates should be titrated to effect initially and then preferably given by patient-controlled analgesia.

Fractured ribs may also be easily and effectively treated using nerve blocks, thus avoiding the side-effects of systemic analgesics altogether.

- *Intercostal nerve blocks* – safe and effective for two or three fractured ribs, but they need to be repeated.
- *Intrapleural anaesthesia* – introduces a catheter into the pleural space close to the plane of the intercostal nerves. This is a safe and effective block. The risk of pneumothorax is approximately 2%, but is particularly safe if a chest drain is in situ.

- *Thoracic paravertebral blocks –* involve injection of local anaesthetic ± catheter into the paravertebral space which then spreads to ipsilateral sympathetic and somatic nerves, epidural space and contralateral paravertebral space. This is an effective block with less risk of pneumothorax than intrapleural techniques and less risk of dural puncture than an epidural. However, there is a risk of misplacement, particularly into lung parenchyma and epidural, subarachnoid spaces.
- *Thoracic epidural –* this provides very effective analgesia using an infusion ± PCA technique. It may be technically challenging and there is a risk of dural puncture (contraindications include head injury, raised ICP and coagulopathy).

Further reading

Richardson J, Lonnqvist PA 1998 Thoracic paravertebral block. *British Journal of Anaesthesia* 81: 230–238.

Answer 4.30

a. This is a lateral skull X-ray of a 9-year-old child. There is a fluid level in the sphenoid sinus suggesting a base of skull fracture (hold the X-ray at 90° to see the horizontal fluid level more clearly). As an incidental finding, the posterior elements of the cervical spine are fused from C2 downwards, with preservation of the discs. This appearance is suggestive of Klippel–Feil syndrome, although juvenile chronic arthritis may produce similar fusion.

b. She has a base of skull fracture and therefore the potential for intracerebral bleeding. It would be prudent to observe her for 24 h before surgery and even consider a CT scan of brain, particularly if there is a history of loss of consciousness. Once it is thought safe to proceed with anaesthesia, she should be treated as if she has a head injury, intubated, ventilated to normocarbia, avoiding nitrous oxide, and observed closely postoperatively. A nasal ETT should not be used since she has a base of skull fracture.

The second problem of anaesthetic relevance is of Klippel–Feil syndrome. This is loosely applied to many forms of cervical fusion, although the original description by Klippel and Feil in 1912 consisted of a triad of short neck, low hairline and limited neck movement. This may be associated with neurological abnormalities as well as many associated malformations. Congenital fusion of the posterior elements of the cervical spine limits mobility to the C1/2 articulation. Although mostly affecting lateral movement, this may also severely limit both flexion and extension and a difficult intubation should be anticipated.

5

GENERAL ANAESTHESIA

INTRODUCTION

The data interpretation skills required for the daily practice of anaesthesia are those required of an acute perioperative physician. A broad knowledge of a wide variety of data is essential and this may also be presented in the FRCA exams. Much of this data is presented in other chapters. This chapter concentrates on airway assessment, biochemical and haematology abnormalities and sleep problems, subjects about which all anaesthetists should have a thorough knowledge. We will also present data on thromboelastography, an important subject which is rarely dealt with in standard texts. Questions are presented on a variety of other problems occasionally encountered in clinical practice and about which you may have to think on your feet, both in the examinations and in clinical situations.

AIRWAY PROBLEMS

Evaluation of the airway is largely a clinical problem and radiology only has a limited role. Causes of difficult intubation or ventilation of patients may be divided into:

- congenital causes, e.g. craniofacial dysostoses
- anatomical causes, e.g. receding jaw, prominent teeth, thick neck
- acquired causes, e.g. trismus, infection, tumour, arthritides etc.

Airway evaluation is performed daily by anaesthetists and a variety of clinical tests and rules of thumb exist in order to predict the difficult airway, such as the Mallampati and Patil tests and the Wilson five-point risk score (Wilson 1988). Unanticipated difficult intubation is usually due to temporomandibular joint (TMJ) dysfunction, airway distortion/narrowing and limitation of cervical spine mobility.

A variety of radiological rules of thumb exists to predict the difficult airway, such as mandibular length and a reduction in the atlanto-occipital gap; however, these are of limited use and obviously cannot be performed on all patients preoperatively. Appropriate radiology should be guided by clinical evaluation. Limited mouth opening necessitates an OPG with or without a CT to examine the TMJs. Limited cervical spine movement, severe rheumatoid arthritis, Down's syndrome or ankylosing spondylitis necessitate cervical spine X-rays and consideration of flexion/extension views if there is a risk of subluxation. Stridor, if time permits, necessitates a chest X-ray (CXR), thoracic inlet views, lateral cervical spine X-rays and often a thoracic CT scan depending on the site of the lesion. Spirometry and flow volume loops may also be performed to assess airway narrowing in these circumstances. Intrathoracic tracheal obstruction or deviation is a particularly difficult clinical situation and airway control may necessitate rigid bronchoscopy.

There is only a limited role for radiology in the emergency setting. Radiology should not be performed in the trauma setting until the airway is controlled. Epiglottitis is a clinical diagnosis and lateral cervical spine X-rays only serve to delay airway control. Radiology may be useful where the diagnosis is uncertain, e.g. a suspected retropharyngeal abscess. Each case of airway obstruction is different and clinical decisions need to be made in the light of the specific clinical circumstances.

POLYSOMNOGRAPHY

Polysomnographic data are commonly collected to investigate medical problems that occur during sleep. The number of physiological variables that are recorded depends on the medical condition. These recordings are usually monitored by technicians during the sleep period but can be remotely recorded. The variables may include EEG (electroencephalography), ECG, EMG (electromyography), EOG (electrooculography – eye movement), pulse oximetry, measures of breathing (e.g. respiratory plethysmography), position, digital video recording, sound and temperature. The errors from poor electrode placement, such as high impedance, will prevent accurate analysis of sleep stages, or they may simply fall off. Patient movement artefacts affect all non-invasive measurements of breathing and may result in changes in the amplitude of the signal. This can then be wrongly interpreted as real changes in tidal breathing, e.g. hypopnoea. The errors of pulse oximetry are well known. The size of the data set collected, especially if it includes high-resolution digital video, may exceed 20 gigabytes. Only samples of the study are placed in the clinical records, and the complete data set remains in the sleep unit.

There are three examples of simple polysomnographic data presented; each includes oximetry, heart rate and two channels of breathing – rib cage and abdominal signals. The timescales vary in each example.

THROMBOELASTOGRAPHY

Haemostasis is a complex dynamic process that incorporates interactions between platelets, pro- and anticoagulation factors. In the clinical situation, the distinct end-point of clot formation ultimately determines whether an individual has normal or abnormal haemostasis.

Common coagulation tests (PT, APTT, fibrinogen levels etc.) define specific deficiencies of the coagulation cascade and are often determined by the value at which the clotting process begins. These are extensively covered in other standard anaesthetic texts. In contrast, thromboelastography allows a quantitative measure of clot formation (from initial fibrin reaction through to clot retraction or lysis)

and provides information about several steps in the coagulation process. Furthermore, these measurements are made on whole blood rather than plasma, thereby monitoring the interaction between platelets, fibrinogen and the protein coagulation cascade.

Whole blood is placed in a cup that is being continually and slowly oscillated through an angle of 4°45'. A plastic pin attached to a torsion wire is immersed in the specimen and is closely opposed to the walls of the cup without direct contact. As clot formation occurs between the two surfaces, the pin becomes coupled to the motion of the cup and the two elements move in phase with each other. If a mechanical–electrical transducer monitors the movement of the torsion wire, the resulting signal can be converted into a graphical output (thromboelastogram, TEG) that may be recorded on heat-sensitive paper or computer readout. The TEG can then be analysed for quantitative measures that define clot formation.

The important values from the TEG are the R and K times, the alpha angle, maximum amplitude and LY30 rate (see Fig. 5.1). No value is a specific marker for a given coagulation disorder, but combinations of abnormal/normal values produce TEGs that are indicative of common coagulation abnormalities. In general, platelet dysfunction/depletion will decrease the rate of clot formation (K time) and ultimately lead to weaker clot strength (MA), whereas anticoagulants or clotting factor deficiencies have more widespread effects on clot formation and will affect all components of the TEG. Fibrinolysis is characterised by a continuous reduction in MA depicted in a LY30 time > 7.5%. Combinations of these abnormalities will lead to more complex TEG readings.

TEG analysis is relatively easy to perform and perioperative thromboelastography can guide 'point of care' haematological replacement therapy. It has been used effectively as part of algorithms to reduce unnecessary transfusion during cardiopulmonary bypass (CPB), liver transplantation and after trauma. It has

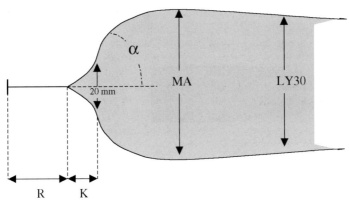

Fig. 5.1 Normal thromboelastogram.

also proved useful in general and paediatric surgery and may provide an indication of the safety of initiating epidural analgesia in those patients with abnormal platelet and coagulation tests.

Early difficulties of thromboelastography included control for intraoperative heparinisation, a lag period between taking the sample and obtaining TEG results and the need for temperature correction. However, many of these disadvantages have been addressed by addition of contact additives (e.g. Celite, tissue factor) and more advanced TEG technology and software. The addition of specific platelet antagonists may allow further delineation of the effects of platelets from the other factors important in clot formation. The TEGs presented in the questions are without the addition of Celite.

Normal TEG values are shown in the following table.

Value	Measurement	Normal values (Celite activated)	Normal values
R	Initiation of TEG to initial fibrin formation	10–14 mm	15–30 mm
K	Beginning of clot formation until amplitude = 20 mm	3–6 mm	6–12 mm
α angle	Acceleration of fibrin build-up and cross-linking	54–67°	40–50°
MA	Strength of formed clot	59–68 mm	50–60 mm
LY30	Rate of amplitude reduction 30 min after the MA	> 7.5%	MA – 5 mm

FURTHER READING

Mallett SV, Cox DJ 1992 Thromboelastography; A review article. *British Journal of Anaesthesia* 69: 307–313.

Ferk CM 1991 Predicting difficult intubation. *Anaesthesia* 46: 1005–8.

Rosenberg-Adamsen S, Kehlet H, Dodds C, Rosenberg J 1996 Postoperative sleep disturbances: mechanisms and clinical implications (review). *British Journal of Anaesthesia* 76(4): 552–559.

Whitten CW, Greilich PE 2000 Thromboplasty: past, present, and future. *Anesthesiology* 92(5): 1223–1225.

Wilson ME et al 1988 Predicting difficult intubation. *British Journal of Anaesthesia* 61: 211–216.

5
Q

QUESTIONS

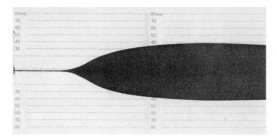

QUESTION 5.1

A 55-year-old man undergoes hepatic transplantion for alcoholic liver disease. Blood loss is estimated at 4500 mL and he is transfused 12 units of blood and 4 units of fresh frozen plasma (FFP). A TEG is performed one hour after graft reperfusion.

a. What does this TEG show?
b. How will you decide on the appropriate treatment?

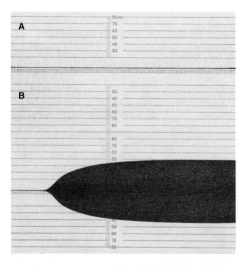

Question 5.2

A 62-year-old man undergoes a coronary artery bypass graft (CABG). He is given 40 000 units of heparin going onto bypass. He has a single internal mammary artery graft to the left anterior descending artery and comes off bypass easily. Protamine is administered. Two TEGs are performed, as shown in A&B: B has added heparinase.

a. Describe each TEG.
b. What treatment do you recommend?

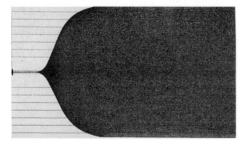

Question 5.3

A 72-year-old man is anticoagulated with heparin following the diagnosis of a pulmonary embolus following hip replacement. After 5 days of heparin treatment it is noted that his platelet count has fallen to 38×10^9/L. He has also had a cerebrovascular accident and developed a right hemiparesis. A TEG is performed, and is shown.

a. Describe this TEG. What does this imply?
b. What may be the underlying diagnosis?

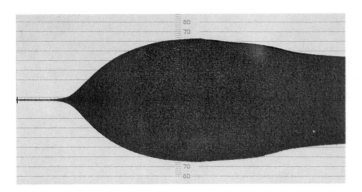

Question 5.4

A 62-year-old man undergoes repair of thoracic aortic aneurysm. He receives 30 000 units of heparin going onto bypass. Blood loss is estimated at 6000 mL and he is given 16 units of blood and 8 units of FFP. Protamine is administered coming off bypass and the TEG shown is performed.

a. What does this TEG show?

b. What does this imply and what treatment do you recommend?

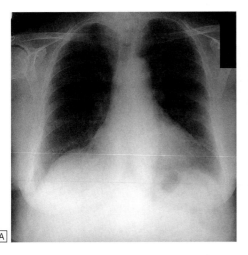

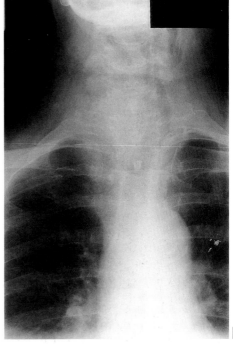

Question 5.5

A 42-year-old patient is scheduled for thyroidectomy. She has normal mouth opening and is Mallampati grade 1. Her CXR (A) and thoracic inlet (B) views are shown.

a. Describe these X-rays.

b. Are there any further investigations that you would consider?

c. Discuss the anaesthetic management of this patient.

d. Describe three causes of airway obstruction post-thyroidectomy in the immediate postoperative period?

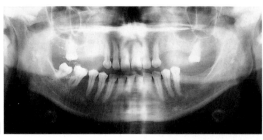

A

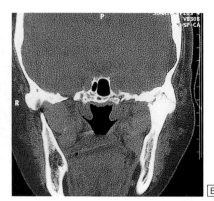

B

Question 5.6

A 48-year-old woman presents for mastectomy. She is generally fit and well, but her mouth opening is limited to about 3 mm. This has been getting worse for about 10 years but she has not sought medical advice and has lived on a liquid diet. An OPG (A) and CT scan (B) are performed.

a. Describe the changes seen on these X-rays.
b. What is the diagnosis?
c. What is this often associated with and can it be corrected?
d. Describe how you will anaesthetise this lady.
e. Describe how you would perform an awake fibreoptic intubation.

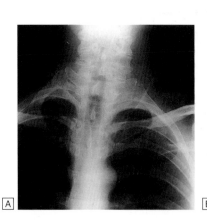

A

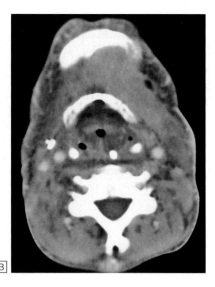

B

Question 5.7

A 62-year-old man presents with stridor 6 months following a radical neck dissection for carcinoma of the floor of the mouth and is scheduled for urgent palliative tracheostomy. His neck is fixed in flexion from previous radiotherapy and his trachea is palpable only with difficulty. His thoracic inlet X-ray (A) and CT scan (B) are shown.

a. Describe these X-rays. What is the diagnosis?
b. Outline how you propose to anaesthetise him for his tracheostomy.
c. What are the indications for an awake fibreoptic intubation?

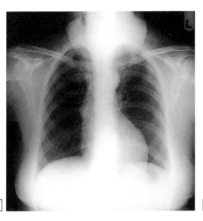 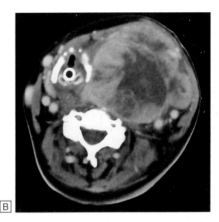

Question 5.8

A 68-year-old woman presents with acute stridor. She is tired, short of breath at rest, has audible stridor and cannot manage full sentences. Her CXR is shown (A), together with an axial CT slice, post-intubation, at the level of the larynx (B).

a. Describe the CXR and the CT scan.
b. What is the likely diagnosis?
c. Outline your immediate plan of management for this lady including how you would have secured the airway.

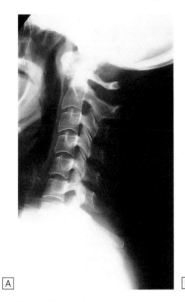 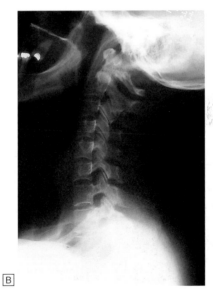

Question 5.9

A 58-year-old woman with rheumatoid arthritis is scheduled for laparotomy for large bowel obstruction. She has mouth opening limited to 2 cm and cervical spine movement limited by pain. Her c-spine X-rays are shown (A, flexion; B, extension).

a. Describe the changes on these X-rays.
b. Describe the anaesthetic options for this lady.
c. List five ways in which rheumatoid arthritis may affect the airway.
d. List other effects of rheumatoid arthritis which may have implications for anaesthesia.

5

Q

Question 5.10

A 28-year-old man presents for inguinal hernia repair. He has mild asthma, but is otherwise well. Routine blood results are performed and the house officer contacts you as he is concerned over his liver function tests (LFTs), which are as follows: alanine aminotransferase (ALT), 32 IU/l; alkaline phosphatase, 67 IU/l; aspartate aminotransferase (AST), 41 IU/l; bilirubin (total), 33 μmol/l; bilirubin (conjugated), 3 μmol/l; albumin, 49 g/l; prothrombin time, 14 s.

a. Describe the biochemical abnormality.
b. What do you think may be the underlying abnormality?
c. How will this affect your anaesthetic management?

Question 5.11

A 12-year-old adopted girl of African origin presents for cholecystectomy due to repeat episodes of gallstone colic. She appears well, but gives a history of repeated hospitalisation with abdominal pain and had her spleen removed 2 years previously, although her foster parents do not know why. Her full blood count and liver function tests are as follows:

FBC		LFTs
Hb	9.8 g/dl	ALT 32 IU/l
MCV	82 fl	Alk phos 67 IU/l
MCHC	27 g/dl	Albumin 49 g/l
WBC	11.6×10^9/l	AST 41 IU/l
Platelets	468×10^9/l	Bilirubin (total) 53 μmol/l
Reticulocytes	12%	

a. Describe the results shown.
b. What do you think is the underlying diagnosis and what might a blood film show on microscopy? How might the diagnosis be confirmed.
c. Describe your anaesthetic technique and how the cholecystectomy should be performed.

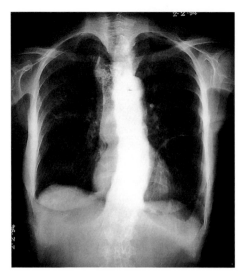

Question 5.12

A cachectic 76-year-old lady presents for total hip replacement. She has always been thin with a poor appetite and often finds it difficult to swallow food with severe heartburn for which she takes oral antacids. She has been a life-long heavy smoker and occasionally wheezes but adamantly refuses regional anaesthesia. Her CXR is shown.

a. Describe this CXR.
b. What do you think is the diagnosis?
c. Why is there no gas in the stomach?
d. How will this affect the conduct of your anaesthesia?

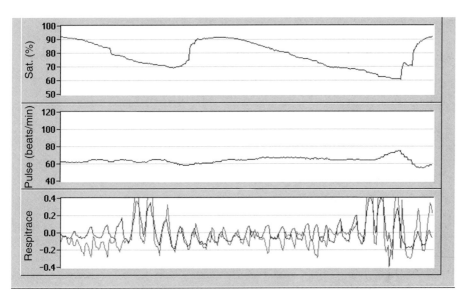

Question 5.21

A 50-year-old long distance lorry driver is involved in a single vehicle accident at 02.00 h (7 h ago). He is scheduled for fixation of bilateral femoral shaft fractures. On examination, he is grossly obese with a body mass index (BMI) of 44. He is drowsy but has no external sign of head injury with a normal head CT scan. He is cyanosed with a raised JVP and there is evidence of right ventricular enlargement on ECG and CXR. Pulse oximetry on air is 87%. Admission full blood count showed haemoglobin of 18 g/dL. His medical notes include this printout of 1 min of a polysomnographic recording.

a. What is the underlying diagnosis?
b. What is the 'ideal' BMI, and how is it calculated?
c. Describe the anaesthetic implications of this condition.
d. What is the normal treatment of this patient's medical condition?

5

Q

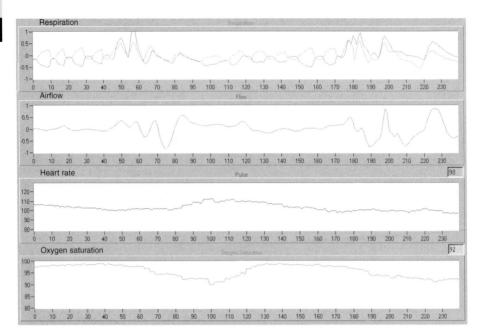

Question 5.22

This 2-year-old boy is admitted for routine tonsillectomy. Although he is small, he has become hyperactive through the day, but he no longer plays football with his friends. There is a note from the district nurse that he has occasional enuresis, which had not been present for some years. One of his brothers was a 'cot death' at about the same age, and the family are very anxious about any operations and the risks of another tragedy.

His mother gives you the history that he snores terribly loudly, but that he occasionally has sudden quiet periods. He sweats a lot at night, prefers to sleep on his side with his head back, and is very restless if he moves onto his back. His sleep studies are shown.

a. What initial steps would you take before proceeding to surgery?
b. What investigations do you think should be performed?
c. What are the risks to this child from anaesthesia?

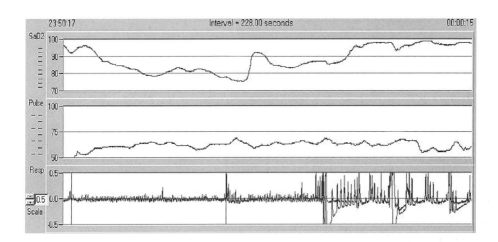

Question 5.23

A 31-year-old man has been admitted for surgery on a fractured humerus following a fall at home. He is currently being investigated for progressive weakness and has a brother with similar symptoms in another part of the country. He had cataract surgery almost 15 years ago under general anaesthesia with no identified problems. The chart shown is in his neurological notes, but there is no accompanying correspondence.

He appears sleepy with noticeable ptosis and balding. He can walk unaided for over 100 yards, but gets tired going up hills. He often wakes up throughout the night feeling breathless but has no chest pain or other symptoms of chest disease. He has poor muscle tone generally and cardiovascular examination is normal (10-min chart).

a. What is this investigation?
b. What is a likely diagnosis?
c. How will this affect your anaesthetic management?
d. How will you manage his postoperative pain?

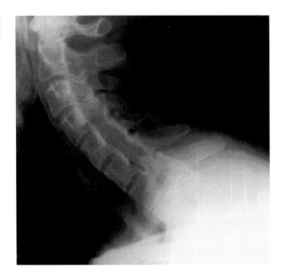

Question 5.24

A 30-year-old man is admitted to hospital for an elective open cholecystectomy. He describes severe early morning stiffness, since the age of 22, for which he has been undergoing physiotherapy. He is on diuretics for mild heart failure. He has limited neck movement and cannot look to the side. He has a lateral neck X-ray in the notes (shown here), and a review of his serum autoantibodies rules out rheumatoid arthritis.

a. What is the diagnosis?
b. What complications may occur with this condition?
c. Summarise your anaesthetic plan.
d. What are the postoperative risks?

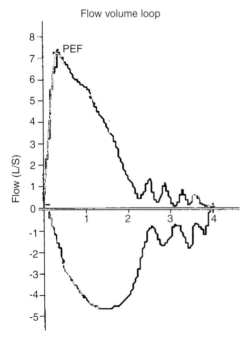

Flow volume loop

Flow (L/S)

PEF

Question 5.25

A 65-year-old man is admitted for TURP because of increasing prostatism. He is mildly demented and appears to be breathless at rest. Increasing respiratory effort causes him to develop mild stridor. He appears to be slow and to have limited involvement in the consultation you have with him.

He has been seen by the local neurologist and chest physician recently because of his breathlessness and progressing dementia. There is a pulmonary flow/volume loop record in his medical notes, which is shown here.

a. What is the likely diagnosis?
b. What are the implications of the flow/volume loop?
c. How can this condition affect your delivery of anaesthesia?
d. What is your priority in the postoperative period?

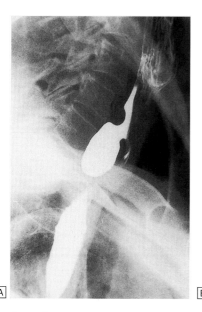
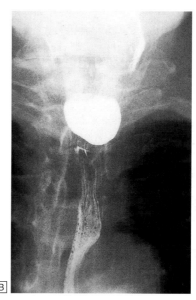

A   B

Question 5.26

A 68-year-old lady is scheduled for a panendoscopy on your ENT list. She has a history of increasing problems with swallowing and describes regurgitation following meals. There is a palpable mass in her neck. The two images (A, B) are from a gastrografin sequence you find in the notes.

a. What is the diagnosis?
b. What further questions would clear the diagnostic picture?
c. What precautions would you take during induction of anaesthesia?
d. What is the likely procedure that the surgeons are considering, and what are the postoperative anaesthetic implications?

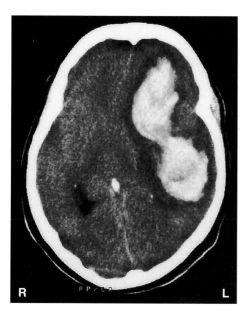

R   L

Question 5.27

A 67-year-old man is admitted to casualty with a sudden onset of loss of power on his right side and altered consciousness. He has been treated for many years for hypertension but has not seen his GP for over a year and has not collected his medication. He has had a CT scan, one image of which is shown. He is waiting to be admitted for a total hip replacement because of pain and limitation of movement on walking.

a. What does the image show?
b. Describe his initial management and any interventions that may be of benefit.
c. Once he has recovered from this event, how long should elective surgery be delayed for and why?

Question 5.28

A 77-year-old lady is scheduled for a total hip replacement (THR) on your elective orthopaedic list. She appears to be slightly confused and does not seem to remember what you have explained to her regarding the operation tomorrow. You plan to use a combined general/regional technique (your normal preference) and as part of departmental policy seek her consent to this. You note that she has seen the geriatricians last week and find the following scored record in her notes.

Score	Section	Task
	Orientation	
4		What is – the year, season, date, day, month?
2		Where are we? Country, county, town, hospital, floor
	Registration	
3		Name three objects – 1 s to say each, then ask to patient to recall all three. Repeat until the patient has learnt all three. Count and record trials
2		Serial 7 s – one point for each correct. Stop after five correct. Alternatively–spell 'world' backwards
3		Ask for the three objects repeated above – give an example of each
	Language	
3		Name a pencil and watch
2		Repeat the following 'no ifs, ands, or buts'
1		Follow a three-stage command: 'Take a paper in you right hand, fold it in half, and put it on the floor'
3		Read and obey the following: 'Close your eyes', 'Write a sentence', 'Copy a design'
23	Total score	

a. What is this test and what is the significance of this score?
b. How will this affect her signing your consent form?
c. What modifications would you make to your anaesthetic plan?
d. What drugs would you specifically avoid?

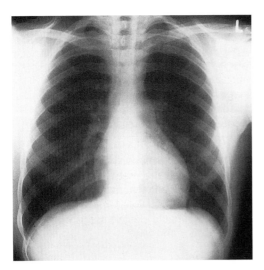

Question 5.29

A 28-year-old man is scheduled for inguinal hernia repair on your list. He has a blood pressure of 190/100 mmHg. His chest film is shown.

a. Describe this chest film.
b. What is the diagnosis?
c. What are the associations of this condition?
d. Can his blood pressure be corrected?

To be completed **Regularly,** at least 4 hourly, by nurse or patient

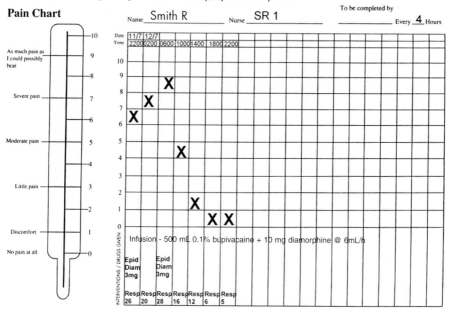

Pain Chart

Name __Smith R__   Nurse __SR 1__

To be completed by _____ Every __4__ Hours

Question 5.30

A 47-year-old man has been observed following his total cystectomy for a bladder tumour. He is 55 kg in weight and wasted due to his disease, and has been a heavy smoker for most of his life. He has an epidural in place and you are asked to review him urgently because his oxygen saturation is 87% and he is difficult to rouse. His pain chart is shown.

a. Comment on the medication used.

b. What is the likely problem and why has it happened?

c. What would be the effects of adding adrenaline to the bolus doses?

d. How will you manage this situation, and what changes would you institute in response to this?

ANSWERS

Answer 5.1

a. The TEG shows long R; long K time; reduced MA; reduced angle.

b. All TEG components are abnormal, suggesting deficient clot formation. The likely problem is major clotting factor deficiencies/dysfunction or the presence of an anticoagulant. A heparin-like compound is often present after reperfusion of the grafted liver which responds to protamine therapy. A confirmatory TEG repeated with and without commercially available heparinase pin/cup combinations would define the deficiency and suggest either protamine or clotting factor treatment.

Further reading

Bayly PJ, Thick M 1994 Reversal of post-reperfusion coagulopathy by protamine sulphate in orthotopic liver transplantation [see comments]. *British Journal of Anaesthesia* 73(6): 840–842.

Chapin JW, Peters KR, Winslow J, Becker GL, Skinner H 1993 Circulating heparin during liver transplantation. *Transplantation Proceedings* 25(2): 1803.

Answer 5.2

a. TEG A has no discernible clotting, suggesting severe coagulopathy or complete anticoagulation. TEG B with added heparinase is normal (MA borderline).

b. These are two TEGs run in parallel on the same patient. The first clearly demonstrates no clot formation. The second has been performed on the same blood sample with added heparinase and this shows almost complete reversal of the clotting defect. This demonstrates the presence of heparin. The treatment is therefore more protamine.

Answer 5.3

a. There is a short R and K time; large angle and MA; no fibrinolysis. This TEG demonstrates hypercoagulable blood.

b. Hypercoagulable states may occur in a variety of clinical conditions, both congenital and acquired. Inherited reasons include antithrombin III deficiency, protein C deficiency and protein S deficiency. Acquired reasons may range from malignancy, immobilisation, oral contraceptives, anticardiolipin syndrome, excess infusion of clotting factors and hyperviscosity states. He should be investigated for an underlying cause of a predisposition for thrombosis. In this case, the treatment with heparin, falling platelet count and evidence of thrombosis all point to heparin-induced thrombocytopenia and thrombosis syndrome (HITTS). Management involves stopping heparin therapy and considering treatment with aspirin and warfarin.

Further reading

Hunter JB, Lonsdale RJ, Wenham PW, Frostick SP 1993 Heparin induced thrombosis: an important complication of heparin prophylaxis for thromboembolic disease in surgery. *British Medical Journal* 307: 53–55.

Answer 5.4

a. This TEG shows R short; K borderline; MA normal; LY30 > 5 mm. It demonstrates normal clot formation followed by significant fibrinolysis.

b. This implies a lack of fibrinogen and the treatment is therefore with cryoprecipitate.

Answer 5.5

a. This is a PA CXR which is well centred and penetrated. The heart is enlarged. The trachea is seen to be tortuous. The thoracic inlet view shows significant deviation of the trachea in the neck, which is presumably pushed across by the goitre.

b. This lady should have already been investigated for thyroid function and may have already had an ultrasound with or without biopsy of the thyroid. From an anaesthetic point of view, you need to know the extent of airway obstruction, the degree of deviation of the trachea and any intrathoracic extension of the mass. The CT scan will help in this context. Simple tests of airway obstruction also include stridor on forced expiration, or expiration on exercise and flow volume loops.

c. Two problems are presented. She has a large heart on CXR which may suggest a cardiomyopathy. This will require cardiac assessment preoperatively, which should include echocardiography. Depending on this result, invasive monitoring or pulmonary artery catheterisation may be required intraoperatively.

  The most important consideration is the potential for difficult intubation and a difficult airway to maintain. Regional anaesthesia for thyroidectomy is possible (but difficult) and needs great cooperation on behalf of both patient and surgeon. Assuming that general anaesthesia is performed, the choice is between an inhalational induction and muscle relaxation only after controlled ventilation and an awake fibreoptic intubation. The larynx may be deviated and the subglottic trachea narrowed. Difficult intubation equipment should be at hand and an armoured endotracheal tube (ETT) used.

d. Although much discussed, airway obstruction is fortunately rare post-thyroidectomy but may occur from a variety of causes. Obstruction immediately post-extubation implies either bilateral vocal cord obstruction from bilateral recurrent laryngeal nerve injury or tracheal collapse due to tracheomalacia as a result of compression from a large, usually malignant, thyroid mass. Over the next few hours bleeding may also lead to obstruction and necessitate immediate removal of the clips. Laryngeal oedema may also occur in the subsequent 48 h, but usually settles with nebulised adrenaline.

Answer 5.6

a. The OPG shows severe bony ankylosis of the left TMJ. Compare this with the smooth outline of the right TMJ. This is highlighted on the CT scan where the bony fusion is well demonstrated.

b. The diagnosis is severe TMJ ankylosis.

c. This may be idiopathic, but is commonly associated with trauma to the mandible earlier in life. This may have been a fracture, or may have been minor trauma, long since forgotten. It can be surgically corrected by the use of a temporalis muscle flap used to line the glenoid and act as a meniscus. Prosthetic joint replacements have lost popularity after several expensive lawsuits in the USA.

d. This lady presents a considerable airway challenge for general anaesthesia. This is bony fusion of the joint and she will not gain any mouth opening from muscle relaxation on induction of general anaesthesia. Options are to consider performing the mastectomy awake under regional anaesthesia or to induce general anaesthesia, either by inhalational induction or after an awake fibreoptic intubation.

  The technique selected depends on the experience of the anaesthetist and the acceptability of awake techniques by the patient. Regional anaesthesia is best provided by a thoracic epidural. This is possible, but analgesia and muscle relaxation for axillary node sampling may be incomplete. Inhalational induction of anaesthesia and nasal intubation, either blind or using a fibreoptic bronchoscope, is possible, but if airway obstruction or nasal bleeding develops, this could be life-threatening. Awake fibreoptic intubation has the advantage of the patient maintaining her own airway at all times, bleeding in particular presenting less of a problem. Intravenous induction of anaesthesia may be quickly established once the trachea is intubated. The patient should subsequently be extubated awake at the end of the procedure; a nasopharyngeal airway may be useful in recovery and she should be initially cared for postoperatively in a high-dependency environment.

e. There are many techniques of anaesthetising the airway for an awake fibreoptic intubation, ranging from nebulised lignocaine to specific nerve blocks. The upper airway is easily anaesthetised using 2% lignocaine sprays to the nose, oropharynx and gargles, followed by packing the nose with ribbon gauze soaked in Moffat's solution (cocaine and adrenaline), which helps to vasoconstrict as well as anaesthetise the nasal mucosa. The rest of the airway can be anaesthetised using lignocaine 2% in a spray-as-you-go technique.

Additional helpful techniques include a transtracheal injection of 2% lignocaine to help anaesthetise the subglottic trachea and vocal cords, and blockade of the superior laryngeal nerve, either externally at the level of the hyoid cartilage or by using Krause's forceps soaked in lignocaine in the piriform fossae.

Further reading

Popat M 2000 Teaching and training fibreoptic intubation in Anaesthesia. *CPD Anaesthesia* 2: 66–71.

Answer 5.7

a. The first film is a thoracic inlet view on which the most obvious abnormality is a severe narrowing of the trachea to 2–3 mm. The CT scan confirms severe narrowing of the airway to 2–3 mm at the subglottic level. Given the clinical history, this is likely to be due to direct tracheal invasion from recurrence of his squamous cell floor of mouth carcinoma.

b. This man presents a considerable risk of total airway obstruction during general anaesthesia. The technique of choice is a tracheostomy under local anaesthesia as long as space exists on CT evaluation. A tracheostomy may be technically difficult if the neck is fixed in flexion from radiotherapy fibrosis and the trachea may even be impalpable from tumour recurrence. If general anaesthesia is considered, the patient should be anaesthetised in theatre, with an experienced surgeon scrubbed and ready to perform a tracheostomy if the airway is lost. An inhalational induction should be performed. A nasopharyngeal airway may be of help as obstruction develops; cocaine paste applied to the nasal cavity pre-induction may help to reduce bleeding. If intubation proves impossible, a tracheostomy may be performed whilst spontaneous breathing is maintained. Direct invasion of the airway and larynx from tumour, leading to severe airway obstruction, should generally be regarded as a contraindication to awake fibreoptic intubation due to the risk of total airway obstruction on manipulation of the larynx.

c. Indications for an awake fibreoptic intubation include an anticipated or proven difficult intubation from anatomical distortion or pathology, e.g. trismus from dental abscess, goitre or c-spine injury; also, patients in whom ventilation post-induction may be difficult (e.g. morbid obesity) and patients in whom it is difficult to apply a facemask or preoxygenate with external frames applied to the head and neck. It may also be useful for emergency surgery where there is an increased risk of inhalation of gastric contents during conventional induction, particularly in a difficult airway. However, acute airway obstruction from oedema or tumour should be regarded as a relative contraindication due to the potential for total airway obstruction in an awake patient.

Further reading

Mason RA, Fielder CP 1999 The obstructed airway in head and neck surgery. Editorial. *Anaesthesia* 54: 625–628.

Answer 5.8

a. The obvious abnormality on this CXR is a large mass arising in the neck but extending into the chest with severe deviation of the trachea to the right. The trachea also appears narrowed down to the level of the carina. The cardiac outline, lungs and bony outline appear normal. The CT scan shows a large cystic mass in the left side of the neck which is deviating the trachea across to the right.

b. A large cystic mass arising at this level in the neck and increasing in size over many months is likely to be a thyroid carcinoma.

c. Oxygen should be administered and the use of heliox may help to relieve the acute symptoms of breathlessness. The airway should be secured, but in order to do this the level of the obstruction should be identified by CT scanning if the patient is able to lie flat. Airway control will be hazardous in such cases and experienced ENT help should be sought at the outset.

In this case, the CXR suggests a narrowed and deviated trachea extending well below the sternal notch. CT scanning in such cases is helpful in gauging the tracheal diameter, level of stenoses and whether a tracheostomy can be placed below the lesion. The level of most significant obstruction in this patient was subglottic but did not extend into the chest. The first decision to make is whether intubation of the trachea is possible. If it is not, then the safest option is to perform a tracheostomy under local anaesthesia. In fact, a tracheostomy in this case may not be technically feasible, since the trachea is markedly deviated and may not even be palpable in the neck. Assuming general anaesthesia is attempted, what is the safest technique? The important distinction here is between a tumour producing stridor involving the larynx and obstruction lower down in the trachea.

If tumour mass involves the larynx, then awake fibreoptic intubation is contraindicated due to the possibility of producing total airway obstruction on manipulation of the vocal cords. In this case, inhalational induction of anaesthesia should be performed in the operating theatre with the surgeon scrubbed and prepared to perform an emergency tracheostomy if the trachea

cannot be intubated or if the patient develops airway obstruction. Equipment for difficult intubation should be available and the use of nasopharyngeal airways may overcome upper airway obstruction as anaesthesia deepens.

In contrast, if the obstruction is lower in the trachea, the fibreoptic bronchoscope may be extremely useful. In practice, with obstruction of the mid-trachea, intubation of the trachea itself is rarely a problem, and although manipulation of the tube beyond the obstruction may be difficult, it is rare in practice not to have space to pass a 7 mm ETT. In most cases, therefore, inhalational induction of anaesthesia is the technique of choice, although if there is concern over malignant tracheal invasion, then awake fibreoptic intubation may be useful.

An additional piece of equipment that may be useful in both scenarios is the rigid ventilating bronchoscope that might be able to ventilate past the obstruction. Visualisation of the larynx whilst awake with either the fibreoptic bronchoscope or fibreoptic nasendoscopy by the ENT surgeon may be useful in helping to determine feasibility of intubation and involvement of the larynx in the disease process.

Further reading

Gray AJG, Hoile RW, Ingram GS, et al 1998 The Report of the National Confidential Enquiry into Perioperative Deaths 1996/1997. NCEPOD, London

Mason RA, Fielder CP 1999 The obstructed airway in head and neck surgery. Editorial. *Anaesthesia* 54: 625–628.

Answer 5.9

a. These are lateral c-spine X-rays, one taken in flexion and one in extension. The obvious abnormality is marked atlantoaxial subluxation. The gap anterior to the peg is about 8 mm on flexion. This should be less than 3 mm in an adult and 5 mm in children. There are remarkably few other changes of rheumatoid arthritis.

b. She has an unstable c-spine and is not only at risk of cervical cord compression on c-spine manipulation but also airway obstruction on induction of general anaesthesia and regurgitation of gastric contents on induction. It may be possible to avoid these complications altogether by performing the laparotomy under regional anaesthesia, either combined spinal epidural (CSE) or continuous spinal or epidural anaesthesia. However, this is sometimes also difficult in rheumatoid arthritis due to distorted anatomy, calcification of ligaments and narrow interspaces.

  If general anaesthesia is necessary, the stomach should be emptied using a nasogastric tube and suction. Intravenous induction of anaesthesia is relatively contraindicated, due not only to the potential for difficult intubation but also to the difficulty in maintaining the airway. The choice of anaesthetic techniques is between an inhalational induction whilst the neck is stabilised in traction and two-handed cricoid pressure performed or an awake fibreoptic technique. An awake fibreoptic technique should be regarded as the technique of choice as it will not run the risk of airway obstruction or excessive c-spine manipulation and runs a low risk of pulmonary aspiration in the emergency setting.

c. Rheumatoid arthritis may affect the airway by limitation of mouth opening from TMJ involvement, limitation of cervical spine movement, potential for atlantoaxial subluxation, mandibular hypoplasia and airway obstruction from calcification of laryngeal synovial joints.

d. Rheumatoid arthritis is a multisystem disorder and it is important to be aware of the potential complications that may present to the anaesthetist. Pulmonary effects include diffuse fibrosis, pleural effusions, fibrotic nodules, and restrictive ventilatory defects from costochondral involvement. Renal failure may develop because of amyloidosis or vasculitis; congestive cardiac and angina may develop; and a normochromic,

normocytic anaemia is usual. Distorted anatomy has implications for both the performance of regional and peripheral nerve blocks as well as pressure points and patient positioning on the operating table. In addition, the effects of drug treatment, e.g. steroids and NSAIDs, should be considered. Gold may produce renal damage and bone marrow suppression, and in addition penicillamine may produce a myasthenic state.

Answer 5.10

a. The liver function tests show a mild unconjugated hyperbilirubinaemia. They are otherwise normal.

b. The presence of a mild unconjugated hyperbilirubinaemia in an otherwise fit patient with normal liver function suggests a diagnosis of Gilbert's syndrome. This is a familial condition with an incidence of around 1% of the population. The exact method of inheritance is unclear. The syndrome embraces a heterogeneity of biochemical defects, but the result is reduced hepatic uptake, intracellular binding and conjugation of bilirubin. Bilirubin levels often rise when the patient has a reduced calorie intake, frequently precipitated by acute illness. Haemolysis and splenomegaly may also be present in some patients, but the syndrome is essentially benign and the patients have otherwise normal liver function.

c. Hepatic function is essentially normal in these patients and they should be treated normally during anaesthesia.

Answer 5.11

a. This full blood count (FBC) shows a mild hypochromic normocytic anaemia with a borderline raised platelet count and white cell count. The raised reticulocyte count and raised bilirubin in the face of normal LFTs implies increased red cell turnover and a chronic haemolytic anaemia.

b. This is a typical picture of sickle cell

anaemia with a chronic haemolytic state. She is likely to have had her spleen removed from splenic infarction during a previous sickle cell crisis and she now has gallstones from increased red cell turnover. A blood film might show sickled erythrocytes and the diagnosis may be confirmed by a sickling test, and a haemoglobin electrophoretic pattern will show an absence of HbA with a preponderance of HbS and variable HbF.

c. Anaesthesia should be conducted to minimise the risk of precipitating a sickling crisis. This most commonly takes the form of vaso-occlusion which may be precipitated by infection, dehydration, hypoxia and cold. Hypoxia is the commonest problem postoperatively and some authors recommend supplemental oxygen for as long as 48 h. Shivering postoperatively serves to increase oxygen requirements and should be avoided. The patient must be well hydrated intraoperatively and actively warmed to normothermia. Pain will lead to increased oxygen consumption and should be treated aggressively. At the same time, care must be taken not to oversedate, which may also lead to hypoxia. Regional techniques would therefore appear ideal, but there has been some suggestion that their use may lead to more postoperative complications in sickle cell disease.

Sickle cell patients are prone to infection, partly because of functional hyposplenism, and these should be treated aggressively. A laparoscopic technique of cholecystectomy may reduce postoperative respiratory complications in these patients. Patients with sickle cell trait rarely present clinical problems postoperatively, since sickling only occurs under extreme physiological stress.

Further reading

Esseltine DW, Baxter MR, Bevan JC 1988 Sickle cell states and the anaesthetist. *Canadian Journal of Anaesthesia* 35(4): 385–403.

Koshy M et al. 1995 Surgery and anesthesia in sickle cell disease. *Blood* 86(10): 3676–84.

Answer 5.12

a. This is a PA CXR. The patient is very thin and the lung fields are overinflated with horizontal ribs and flat diaphragms consistent with chronic obstructive pulmonary disease (COPD). The other abnormality is a speckled soft tissue widening of the upper mediastinum with a fluid level, which is obvious if you look between the clavicular heads. There is no air in the stomach.

b. This lady has background changes of COPD. The main abnormality is the abnormal appearance of the upper mediastinum. This is widened with the appearance of speckled matter. This looks similar to faeces because like faeces this is a mixture of solid, liquid and gas and has a fluid level. These appearances are typical of achalasia. This is a chronic and progressive obstruction to the lower oesophageal sphincter resulting from the degeneration of the ganglion cells of the myenteric plexus or vagal nuclei resulting in failure of relaxation of the sphincter. The oesophagus becomes dilated and acts as a reservoir for food. Repeat pulmonary aspiration may be common.

c. Since gas rises above fluid, it does not pass into the stomach. As the fluid level is too high, only liquid seeps past the oesophageal sphincter.

d. If this lady insists on a general anaesthetic for her hip replacement, she should be treated as if she had a full stomach and is at high risk of pulmonary aspiration on induction. The oesophagus may be partly emptied by the gentle passage of a nasogastric tube and the contents aspirated. Antacid premedication may be given, although the contents do not usually have gastric secretions. The effects of prokinetics are variable and may only serve to increase the tone of the lower oesophageal sphincter. A rapid-sequence induction should be performed and a cuffed ETT used. The patient should be extubated awake in the left lateral position. Regional blockade may be considered for postoperative analgesia, since opiate-induced drowsiness may worsen the risk of pulmonary aspiration.

Further reading

Creagh-Barry P, Parsons J, Pattison CW 1988 Achalasia and anaesthesia. *Anaesthesia and Intensive Care* 16(3): 371–373.

Answer 5.13

a. The rhythm strip shows a sinus baseline tachycardia of 120 beats/min. There is no normal sinus arrhythmia and there is no change in heart rate during a Valsalva manoeuvre. This implies a severe autonomic neuropathy.

b. She is dizzy on standing due to postural hypotension. Patients with autonomic neuropathies are unable to maintain their blood pressure on standing, since the ability to respond with a tachycardia, increased stroke volume or vasoconstriction is impaired. There is often a baseline tachycardia due to loss of vagal tone.

c. As many as 60% of all diabetics have evidence of an autonomic neuropathy. It is often unrecognised but may be associated with increased perioperative mortality and morbidity. If severe, this has been associated with profound hypotension in response to drugs used during induction of anaesthesia and cardiorespiratory arrest during or shortly after anaesthesia. Cardiovascular response to surgical haemorrhage will be impaired and there is also an increased risk of sleep apnoea and gastric stasis. In addition, many of these patients will have undiagnosed cardiac ischaemia since anginal pain is not transmitted. Although in theory regional anaesthesia must be used with caution in these patients, since cardiovascular responses are impaired, in practice they are commonly used and have specific advantages. Awareness is maintained, hypoglycaemia may be noted earlier,

the stress response may be reduced and the patients may be able to reinstitute their usual diabetic regimen earlier in the postoperative period.

d. Diabetes affects every organ system. Some chronic effects include myocardial and peripheral ischaemia from macroangiopathy, retinopathy, nephropathy, hypertension, neuropathy, cataracts and impaired immune response and poor tissue healing. Impaired metabolic response to trauma or surgery is common and leads to decreased response to insulin. Therefore diabetics often require more insulin in the perioperative period than usual.

Other specific problems in association with anaesthesia include impaired response to hypoxaemia, aggravation of hyperglycaemia by hypoxaemia and hypercapnia via catecholamine release, precipitation of vitreous haemorrhage from hypertensive swings, postoperative renal failure and intraoperative cardiovascular instability. Hartmann's solution (compound lactate solution) should not be used as infused lactate is rapidly converted to glucose.

Further reading

Horton JN 1994 Anaesthesia and diabetes. In: Nimmo WS, Rowbotham DJ, Smith G, eds. *Anaesthesia*, 2nd edn. Blackwell Scientific Publications, Oxford.

Answer 5.14

a. The classical triad of confusion, bradycardia and hypotension post-TURP is known as the TUR syndrome.

b. This occurs in approximately 7% of all TURPs and is due to absorption of prostatic resections fluid, usually glycine, under pressure via the open venous sinuses of the prostate during resection. As much as 20 ml of fluid may be absorbed per min of transection. Fortunately, the incidence appears to be decreasing due to improved surgical techniques. Clinical effects are secondary to fluid overload and hyponatraemia. Patients may develop transient hypertension due to rapid fluid absorption, followed by pulmonary and cerebral oedema. Bradycardia and cardiovascular collapse then intervene due to the cardiac effects of a rapidly developing hyponatraemia.

Treatment consists of obtaining haemostasis and terminating surgery if still in progress, fluid restriction, forced diuresis with a loop diuretic such as frusemide, and inotropes or vasoconstrictors to maintain perfusion pressure. The mortality associated with rapid falls in sodium to less than 120 mmol/L is around 50%. Under such circumstances, the use of hypertonic saline may be considered. However, its use is controversial and the rate of rise of serum sodium should not exceed 2 mmol/h.

c. This is often regarded as 130 mmol/L by many authors since this is the level below which cerebral oedema may develop. However, the evidence for this level is largely theoretical and it is much more important to consider the patient's clinical situation and to avoid sudden changes in serum sodium levels.

d. The risk of TUR syndrome may be reduced in several ways. Many patients who present for surgery may be hyponatraemic from diuretic treatment and this may be amenable to treatment preoperatively. Duration of surgery should be kept to a minimum, usually below 1 h, and the lowest hydrostatic pressure used. Resection may be superficial, avoiding deep veins, and the use of lasers may reduce the presence of open sinuses. Regional anaesthesia is often recommended as the technique of choice for TURP. This allows communication with the patient and thereby gives early warning of the development of hyponatraemia by the development of confusion. At this point, surgery may be terminated and the patient treated with diuretics before the serum sodium drops further.

Further reading
Reed PR, Kaplan JA 1989 Transurethral resection of the prostate. In: Reed PR, Kaplan JA, eds. *Clinical Cases in Anesthesia*. Churchill Livingstone, New York.

Answer 5.15

a. This is a lateral cephalograph, which is an orthodontic film and is reproduced to scale. The marker at the nose is 1 cm wide, and the two markers at the ears are there to confirm that this is a true lateral. They should appear as concentric circles as seen in this image.

b. The lower airway boundaries can clearly be seen, with the tongue anteriorly, the posterior pharyngeal wall and the uvula shadow above. The hyoid bone is also visible. The lower airway at this point should be in excess of 7 mm, and it is less than 2 mm in this film. She has marked retrognathia – compare the anterior border of the maxilla with that of the mandible – and this is contributing to her narrow airway. She is likely to be very difficult to intubate (especially with cricoid pressure in place). She may well have sleep apnoea from the referral pattern in her case notes.

c. The urgency of her surgery makes prolonged preparations unacceptable and the most likely technique to safely secure her airway would be an awake fibreoptic intubation. This should be performed by an anaesthetist experienced in the technique and sedation should be minimised in light of a full stomach.

Alternative methods of induction require cricoid pressure and preparation for a difficult intubation. Providing ventilation can be maintained with cricoid in place, there will be time to use other adjuncts to intubation such as bougies or an intubating laryngeal mask.

The risks to her airway will remain in the immediate and delayed recovery phases of her management. The use of regional blockade, i.e. epidural (if possible in light of probable sepsis), for postoperative pain control would be helpful, but she needs to be monitored for both oxygenation and respiratory obstruction for the first three nights following surgery. This would usually best be achieved in an HDU or critical care setting.

Further reading

Riley R, Guilleminault C, Herran J, Powell N 1983 Cephalometric analyses and flow-volume loops in obstructive sleep apnoea patients. *Sleep* 6(4): 303–311.

Answer 5.16

a. He is positive for MH sensitivity to halothane, but not caffeine. This is described as $MHE_{(h)}$ (equivocal). Such patients should be treated as MH-susceptible. The caffeine test may be negative in 14% of patients who test positive to halothane; this may be refined further in the future by the use of ryanodine testing. The false-positive rate has been estimated at 6% using normal volunteers. The false-negative rate is effectively nil.

b. With the rapid advancement of molecular genetics from polymerase chain reaction techniques, the genetics of MH have proven to be extremely complex. Early studies found linkage to the ryanodine receptor on chromosome 19, but now marked genetic heterogeneity has been noted. In practical terms, inheritance should still be thought of as autosomal dominant inheritance with variable penetration.

c. This is autosomal dominant and therefore his immediate first-degree relatives, Wednesday, Pugsley, Letitia, Gomez and Morticia, all stand a 50% risk of MH susceptibility. His uncle Fester has a 25% risk at the moment since we do not know if it is Gomez or Morticia who is positive. If it proves to be Morticia, then there is a 50% chance that Fester will be positive, since he is her brother.

Further reading

Hopkins PM 2000 Malignant hyperthermia: advances in clinical management and diagnosis. *British Journal of Anaesthesia* 85: 118–128.

Answer 5.17

a. This is a PA CXR. The most obvious abnormality is bilateral pulmonary plethora. Hilar vascular markings are prominent, but these decrease toward the periphery until there is little evidence of lung markings around the periphery of the lung. This is described as peripheral pruning. Additionally, the cardiac outline is enlarged and the pulmonary knuckle is prominent. This CXR is compatible with pulmonary hypertension.

b. The physical findings are those of pulmonary hypertension. The parasternal heave reflects right ventricular hypertrophy. The pulsatile JVP may reflect forceful atrial contraction or a regurgitant tricuspid valve in the face of high right-sided pressures. The systolic murmur may reflect increased pulmonary flow or the presence of an underlying shunt, such as a ventriculoseptal or atrial-septal defect. The loud second heart sound reflects pulmonary valve closure in the presence of pulmonary hypertension.

c. She has evidence of pulmonary hypertension on her CXR and clinical findings agree. This may be primary pulmonary hypertension, which is idiopathic, or secondary to an underlying intracardiac shunt. She needs a cardiology assessment, specifically including echocardiography.

d. If this lady has a significant underlying intracardiac shunt, she may be considered for corrective surgery for this and will require cardiac catheterisation for assessment. If the diagnosis is a small shunt or primary pulmonary hypertension, then the main principle of anaesthesia is aimed at decreasing pulmonary vascular resistance whilst maintaining a normal peripheral vascular resistance. The patient should be kept warm, intravascularly well filled (requiring central venous monitoring) and well oxygenated perioperatively. Unfortunately most drugs that dilate the pulmonary circulation also cause peripheral vasodilatation which may catastrophically increase the shunt fraction. Selective pulmonary dilatation is therefore usually achieved by local delivery of drugs and may be combined with an infusion of vasoconstrictors to maintain peripheral vascular tone. The administration of high concentrations of oxygen may reduce pulmonary vascular resistance by up to 50%. Inhaled nitric oxide (NO) may also be useful to decrease pulmonary vascular resistance in this situation.

Answer 5.18

a. The ABGs show a combined respiratory and metabolic acidosis.
b. The ECG shows sinus rhythm at 90 beats/min, prominent P wave in lead II, right axis deviation (+120°), prominent R waves V1–3 with ST-segment depression and T wave inversion. These are consistent with right ventricular hypertrophy and strain.
c. This is an AP film which is underpenetrated and poorly centred. There is marked cardiomegaly and pulmonary plethora. An ETT is present, as is a Swan–Ganz catheter, which is not in a correct position and appears kinked.
d. This patient has pulmonary hypertension with right ventricular hypertrophy and strain. She was hypoxic preoperatively, probably from an intracardiac shunt, and her CXR shows marked cardiomegaly. She has worsened with positive pressure ventilation. This all implies a right-to-left shunt (Eisenmenger's syndrome, ES). The underlying problem is likely to be a ventricular septal defect (VSD) but could also be an atrial septal defect (ASD) or patent ductus arteriosus.

Patients with ES run a high perioperative risk. She required a cardiology assessment, including echocardiography and cardiac catheterisation, before surgery was contemplated.

Current treatment should now be directed at lowering pulmonary artery pressures and restoring systemic perfusion, i.e. decreasing pulmonary vascular resistance and maintaining a normal peripheral vascular resistance. Inhaled nitric oxide has been used successfully during anaesthesia for ES patients and inhaled prostacyclin has also been advocated. Fortunately, peripheral vascular resistance is usually maintained during laparoscopic procedures; however, a strategy such as using dobutamine as an inotrope and pulmonary vasodilator together with noradrenaline (norepinephrine) to peripherally vasoconstrict may theoretically be of benefit. Maintenance of low airway and intra-abdominal pressures will help to minimise increases in pulmonary vascular resistance. Most importantly she should be kept warm, well oxygenated and intravascularly optimised throughout the perioperative period.

Further reading

Sammut MS, Paes ML 1997 Anaesthesia for laparoscopic cholecystectomy in a patient with Eisenmenger's syndrome. *British Journal of Anaesthesia* 79: 810–812. (Correspondence *British Journal of Anaesthesia* 1998, 81(2): 296–298.)

Answer 5.19

a. This man is severely hypokalaemic and also has a mildly elevated sodium, chloride and bicarbonate. The high bicarbonate suggests a mild metabolic alkalosis. Although hypokalaemia is common in hypertensive patients, with the severity of this hypokalaemia and the metabolic alkalosis in such a young man on no routine medication, the diagnosis is likely to be primary hyperaldosteronism (Conn's syndrome).
b. This endocrine disorder stems from the hypersecretion of aldosterone, from adrenal hyperplasia (40%), adrenal adenomas (60%) or rarely carcinomas, and represents 1% of all hypertensive patients. The effects are those of chronic mineralocorticoid excess. The

5

A

primary effect is to increase sodium reabsorption from the kidneys, in exchange for an increased potassium, magnesium and hydrogen ion loss. This leads to a high total body sodium with an expansion in the extracellular fluid volume (ECF), severe, occasionally debilitating hypokalaemia and a metabolic alkalosis. The increase in ECF manifests itself clinically as hypertension. The rise in plasma sodium is only slight and ECF volume rarely rises sufficiently to cause oedema. This may be because atrial natriuretic peptide excretion increases, which serves to increase sodium excretion.

c. No, elective surgery should be delayed. The risks of anaesthesia are related to the hypertension and the biochemical abnormalities. The hypertension may be malignant. In addition to sodium and water retention, aldosterone acts as a vasoconstrictor, sensitises the myocardium to catecholamines and may produce fibrosis. The profound hypokalaemia reflects a massive total body potassium depletion and may lead to muscle weakness, interaction with muscle relaxants, tetany from alkalosis and associated hypocalcaemia and cardiac arrhythmias in association with the hypomagnesaemia.

d. Diagnosis rests on demonstrating elevated plasma aldosterone, by renal vein sampling if necessary, and CT or MRI to look for tumours of the adrenal glands. A rare form, genetically inherited, may be dexamethasone-responsive. Medical treatment centres on the use of antihypertensives, particularly spironolactone. Unilateral or bilateral adrenalectomy may be required and may be performed laparoscopically. Efforts should be made to restore serum potassium preoperatively. Invasive monitoring is required intra-operatively since the patient may be on many antihypertensive drugs and bradycardias and hypotension is to be expected. Replacement mineralocorticoid therapy may be required postoperatively.

Further reading

Winship SM, Winstanley JHR, Hunter JM 1999 Anaesthesia for Conn's syndrome. *Anaesthesia* 54: 564–574.

Answer 5.20

a. Techniques include hypotensive anaesthesia, avoiding venous congestion and the use of vasoconstrictors. These are not very practical in the emergency situation. A 'cell saver' may be acceptable and certainly should be discussed with the patient prior to surgery. The use of aprotinin and tranexamic acid can reduce fibrinolysis and should be employed routinely.

b. This man is severely anaemic with an iron-deficient picture. He has low platelets and prolonged clotting with a low fibrinogen indicating a disseminated intravascular coagulation (DIC) picture.

c. Under normal circumstances you would transfuse with red cells, fresh frozen plasma, cryoprecipitate and consider a platelet transfusion.

d. You must not administer blood or blood products to competent patients against their will. The prohibition of blood is a deeply held belief. If wishes are documented in advance in front of witnesses, this constitutes an advance directive and must be taken into account. In the elective case, the anaesthetist may refuse the case but should try to find a colleague to undertake it. In an emergency, the anaesthetist is obliged to provide care and respect the patient's wishes.

e. Elective mechanical ventilation ensures optimum oxygen delivery until a safe haemoglobin is reached. The use of intravenous iron, folinic acid and erythropoietin are indicated to try to restore the haemoglobin. One patient has survived a leaking aneurysm with a haemoglobin of 2.8 g/dL. Early nutrition is advisable. Ongoing use of aprotinin or tranexamic acid may be considered.

Further reading

Association of Anaesthetists 1999 *Management*

of Anaesthesia for Jehovah's Witnesses. Alresford Press, Hampshire.

Baker CE, Kelly GD, Perkins GD 1998 Perioperative care of a Jehovah's witness with a leaking aortic aneurysm. *British Journal of Anaesthesia* 81: 256–259.

Answer 5.21

a. The printout confirms the diagnosis of severe obstructive sleep apnoea (OSA), with falls in saturation to nearly 60%. The bottom traces are recordings of rib cage and abdominal movement. Normal breathing would overlay the traces, and increasing paradox from the obstruction can clearly be seen. The arousal and recovery of the airway can be seen by the increased, in-phase, tidal volumes taken after the periods of desaturation. These obstructions can occur 600–800 times every night, and have both clinical and behavioural effects. The desaturations cause pulmonary hypertension and lead to right heart failure. The repetitive arousal leads to sleep deprivation and severe daytime hypersomnolence. The very sleepy lorry driver is 20 times more likely to be involved in a serious single driver accident.

b. BMI is the weight (kg) divided by height (m) squared. The normal range is 22–25 (44 is morbidly obese).

c. These patients have profoundly depressed hypoxic and hypercarbic drives, even when awake, and are extremely sensitive to opiate or benzodiazepine medication. Respiratory arrest has been caused by such drug therapy. They are also prone to severe pulmonary vasoconstriction if they become hypoxic. This may cause right heart failure on induction. They may prove very difficult to intubate, but because of the poor autonomic control, they must be ventilated perioperatively. Combined regional and general anaesthetic techniques are the most suitable in this case, and the continuation of a regional form of postoperative analgesia is very desirable.

Extubation should only occur when that patient is fully awake and orientated, because fatal airway obstruction can occur if there is any residual muscle weakness or limitation in upper airway tone.

d. Treatment of adult patients with severe OSA is by nasal CPAP (continuous positive airways pressure). The machines are compact and pre-set by the sleep investigation unit to that patient (this means they are rarely transferable between patients). The nasal masks are not disposable but are for single patient use. Elective patients will bring their CPAP machines with them, and they should use it immediately once in the recovery room. Treatment with CPAP improves the autonomic dysfunction after about a fortnight of use. This is the minimum time to delay elective surgery if you make the diagnosis.

Answer 5.22

a. This is a child with a history very suggestive of severe OSA. He should not proceed to surgery until he has been fully investigated as a matter of urgency. Transfer to the nearest paediatric sleep unit is important to reach a diagnosis and gauge its severity. It is rare for children to desaturate as profoundly as adults on oximetry, but they develop pulmonary hypertension and right heart failure much more rapidly.

b. Investigations should include an overnight sleep study, including oximetry, airflow, measures of breathing and either direct observation or video recording of positioning. Transcutaneous and end-tidal capnography also have their advocates. This sleep study confirms obstructive sleep apnoea, with periods of increased respiratory effort associated with decreased airflow and followed by desaturation. Movement arousal is a characteristic of paediatric obstruction, and this can be difficult to separate from artefact if there is no observation of the child available. Sleep position also provides valuable information because such children will either lie on their sides with full extension of the head on the neck, or adopt a kneeling posture (Salaam position) to protect their airway from obstruction. Any movement from these positions results in marked obstruction and arousal.

Echocardiography is very helpful in identifying the status of the right ventricle (over 25% of young children with severe OSA have right ventricular wall movement disorders, and up to 5% have right heart failure).

c. The risks to these children include loss of airway on induction and rapid oxygen desaturation and heart failure. Removing the tonsils and adenoids is often curative, but because there is no gain in airway dimension until the oedema resolves, they remain at high risk in the immediate recovery phase. They should be monitored in a paediatric critical care area overnight. Opiates have been used but NSAIDs are probably the safest form of analgesia.

The smaller the child on presentation for adenotonsillectomy, the more likely he or she is to have severe OSA, and the more vigilant the anaesthetist needs to be. A history of loud snoring and periods of silence is pathognomonic of sleep apnoea in children and must be actively investigated prior to surgery.

Answer 5.23

a. The graph is a 10-min sample from a sleep respiratory data set.
b. The fall in oxygen saturation over several minutes (the bars identify the apnoea to last 228 s) and the lack of respiratory effort confirm a diagnosis of prolonged central apnoea. (The small oscillations on the respiratory trace reflect stroke volume measurements by the plethysmography.) There is a short period of breathing before another respiratory pause, but no evidence of the post-apnoea hyperventilation usually seen after obstructive events. This leads to a diagnosis of a severe impairment of the normal autonomic control of

breathing, and that the normal daytime breathing is dependent on a higher 'behavioural' drive.

c. The diagnosis is most likely to be either a myotonia or a muscular dystrophy, and muscle biopsy and genetic screening may be needed to reach a firm diagnosis. Mental retardation is present in up to 25% of patients with myotonia, with implications for obtaining consent.

There is a high risk of cardiac involvement, with conduction problems in about 50% of patients. Cardiac ejection fraction may fall below 40% because of a direct reduction in myocardial contractility. Profound hypotension on induction may occur.

Respiratory muscle weakness predisposes towards sputum retention. They also have a greater risk of regurgitation and aspiration because of poor tone in the pharyngeal muscles. Endocrine function is affected and there is an increased risk of diabetes.

The site of the injury makes it difficult to provide regional analgesia alone, and a combined regional and general anaesthetic technique is indicated. Suxamethonium is most likely to result in contractures that are not responsive to neural or neuromuscular blockade. Equally they have an increased sensitivity to the non-depolarising relaxants. There are also risks related to the very poor control of breathing identified in the sleep chart. Controlled ventilation is imperative during any sedative or general anaesthetic. Hypothermia and the shivering response must be avoided.

d. Analgesia with NSAIDs and an indwelling central nerve catheter to administer local anaesthetic drugs are probably the safest measures. Certainly, the prolonged central apnoea cautions against potent opiates.

Answer 5.24

a. The likeliest diagnosis is severe ankylosing spondylosis. It occurs mostly in males with an incidence between

1:2000 and 1:1000. It usually presents with low back pain after sitting for a while. Immobility progresses with an adoption of a flexed posture that becomes fixed over time. There is rigidity of the vertebral column but it is also very brittle and easily fractured.

b. The complications that can occur with ankylosing spondylosis most commonly include iritis. An anterior uveitis occurs in almost a third of patients, usually unilateral. Rarely it may be severe, leading to glaucoma and blindness. Atlantoaxial subluxation also frequently occurs and may lead to cord damage during intubation.

There is damage to the aortic valve leading to incompetence and regurgitation. This may lead to left ventricular hypertrophy, angina and conduction defects. This affects about 5% of patients and should be suspected in this patient. Respiratory function is usually well preserved despite the great reduction in chest wall movement. Compensation by the diaphragm maintains vital capacity in most patients.

Rarer complications include ulcerative colitis and amyloid.

c. The areas of concern include a potential difficult intubation in a patient with a rigid neck, but who may have atlantoaxial subluxation. Flexion/extension films may be necessary to explore this possibility. Luckily he does not need a rapid-sequence induction, because cricoid pressure may fracture his brittle cervical spine. He needs a cardiological opinion, and probably an echocardiograph, to define his cardiovascular compromise and may even require valve replacement prior to elective abdominal surgery.

d. Postoperatively he must resume his mobility exercises as rapidly as possible, and discussion with the surgeon about the possibility of a laparoscopic cholecystectomy should be raised.

Further reading

Popitz MD 1997 Anesthetic implications of chronic disease of the cervical spine (review). *Anesthesia & Analgesia* 84: 672–683.

Answer 5.25

a. The presentation is very suggestive of Parkinson's disease. This condition is not common, occurring in about 1:300–2000 patients, is a disorder of the basal ganglia, and has a triad of symptoms. They have a resting tremor of about 4 Hz, limited voluntary movement (including facial and skeletal muscles), and cogwheel rigidity seen in the increased resting muscle tone.

b. The flow/volume loop shows a 'sawtooth' pattern, indicating episodic collapse of the upper airway. This is likely to be due to poor bulbar muscle function and explains the stridor that occurs with increased inspiratory effort. This is a relatively common problem in patients with Parkinson's disease and should be sought in the history and examination. They are also prone to aspiration because of the poor tone, and because they also have poor chest wall power they are less able to cough effectively and clear secretions.

c. Preoperative care is largely related to identifying the pattern and timing of medication to prevent rigidity in the patient. This is often very individual and has been learnt by trial and error. It should be maintained until the very last moment before surgery. Management of the anaesthetic will focus on the avoidance of antidopamine effects that could precipitate an acute crisis. Specifically, antiemetic drugs are particularly prone to exacerbate Parkinsonism. Where the surgical procedure allows a purely regional anaesthetic technique, this is to be preferred, but sedation is hazardous with this pattern of upper airway instability and should be avoided. Aspiration remains a risk even whilst awake.

d. The most important element of postoperative care is to restart his oral medication as soon as possible. If this cannot be achieved, then parenteral apomorphine should be considered. The emetic effects are less than expected and respond to domperidone.

Further reading

Severn AM 1988 Parkinsonism and the anaesthetist (review). *British Journal of Anaesthesia* 61(6): 761–770.

Vincken WG, Darawy CM, Cosio MG 1989 Reversibility of upper airway obstruction after levodopa therapy in Parkinson's disease. *Chest* 96: 210–212.

Answer 5.26

a. This is a lady with a large pharyngeal pouch. The gastrografin can be seen to lie above the epiglottis, and the pouch remains filled after the residual gastrografin has been swallowed.

b. Closer questioning identifies that she regurgitates *undigested* food, and that if she massages her neck the lump disappears. This is pathognomonic of pharyngeal pouches. They are relatively uncommon but have important anaesthetic aspects.

c. The risk of regurgitation is extremely high, and cricoid pressure is specifically contraindicated because it empties the pouch into the airway. The opening of the pouch is always above the glottis, and aspiration is inevitable. Options to protect the airway include an awake intubation technique or induction in the sitting position. Emptying the pouch using soft catheters does not work. The major risk is of particulate contamination because the contents are not acidic. Recovery from anaesthesia for endoscopy is also hazardous because it may not be possible for the ENT surgeon to enter the pouch if its neck is narrow. Air may be trapped in the pouch even if the surgeon has aspirated most of the material, and there will still be some particulate food debris present. Bacterial contamination of the debris is common and this will exacerbate problems if aspiration does occur.

d. The definitive surgical treatment is to identify the neck of the pouch and close this, with removal of the diverticulum or pouch. If the pouch has been present for many years, it may be large enough to extend into the mediastinum.

Dissection of the pouch may be difficult from adhesions and there may be marked blood loss. The pharyngeal constrictors are involved in the repair and swallowing may be impaired in the immediate postoperative period.

Answer 5.27

a. The scan shows blood extending throughout the left hemisphere with an area of lucidity around it. There is some brain compression and midline shift. This is a typical picture of a cerebrovascular accident (CVA) secondary to a bleed. His uncontrolled hypertension is the most likely cause. The embolic form of CVA is less common and produces discrete areas of infarction but with no blood visible. The embolic form is also more often associated with transient ischaemic attacks.

b. He is at risk from increased intracranial pressure and from further, often transient, motor problems. Bulbar weakness and airway maintenance are the two most threatening complications. There is an indication to remove the blood clot to reduce pressure and the vasospasm caused by the bleed. Careful observation of his neurological status is essential, and if there is a deterioration, intubation and ventilation may be required. However, the hypertensive response to intubation should be fully obtunded to prevent extension of the bleed. The cerebral perfusion pressure should be monitored and intervention with mannitol, diuretics or hyperventilation may be necessary.

c. Early rehabilitation is essential if recovery following the stroke is to be possible. Even so, he may be unable to become fully independent and the need for his hip replacement would have to be reviewed once his clinical progress had stabilised. The risk of a second CVA falls over the first month following the bleed and becomes clinically acceptable after 6 weeks. The risk of a second stroke is always higher than if there had been none, but providing rapid rises in blood pressure can be avoided, the risks are acceptable. He is unlikely to progress to surgery before 6–8 weeks have elapsed and would fall into a low-risk group.

Answer 5.28

a. This is a mini-mental state examination (the MMSE). It is a commonly used screening test for dementia in the elderly and is both reliable and repeatable. It takes about 10 min to use and scores a maximum of 30 points. A score of over 28 is probably normal, although lower scores are certainly related to poor mental function. Mild dementia is about 26–27, while moderate to severe dementia is 23–25. Scores below 22 are diagnostic of severe disease and these patients have almost no short-term memory processing.

b. A score of 23 indicates that she is unlikely to have the competence to understand your explanations about her anaesthetic management or pain control postoperatively. She is incapable, on this score, legally to sign her consent; equally no one else can sign for her. If the team believe that the operation is in her best interests, they may proceed and should keep her family informed of the decisions being made and the reasons behind them.

c. The evidence to support a change in anaesthetic technique is scanty, but patients who have a general anaesthetic for abdominal surgery do have a 25% incidence of postoperative cognitive dysfunction. There is some improvement over time but 10% are still affected after 3 years. Regional anaesthesia has a better record and may be the choice in this lady who appears still to be cooperative. A history of previous delirium or confusion after previous operations should be sought, because this indicates a high likelihood of a recurrence after her THR.

d. Prolonged use of pethidine should be avoided because the metabolite norpethidine is a CNS stimulant and proconvulsant. Atropine should be avoided because it crosses the blood–brain barrier and may cause a central cholinergic state.

Further reading

Folstein MF, Folstein SE, McHugh PR 1975 A practical method for grading the cognitive state of patients for the clinician. *Journal of Psychiatry Research* 12: 189–198.

Moller JT, Cluitmans P, Rasussen LS et al 1998 Prolonged post-operative cognitive dysfunction in the elderly. *Lancet* 351: 857–861.

Answer 5.29

a. This is a PA CXR which is well centred and overpenetrated. The aortic knuckle is prominent and there is obvious rib notching in the upper ribs bilaterally.

b. The diagnosis is coarctation of the aorta. Rib notching is secondary to dilated intercostal arteries acting as a collateral circulation to the lower aorta. The coarctation is well demonstrated in the MRI image shown below, where it may be seen as a narrowing of the arch with post-stenotic dilatation.

Coarctation

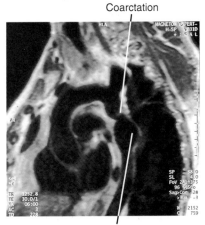

Post-stenotic dilatation

c. Associated features include a bicuspid aortic valve in 50% of cases, cerebral artery aneurysms and an increased incidence in males and certain syndromes, such as Turner's and

5
A

Noonan's syndromes. Presentation late in adolescence is usually from hypertension or diagnosed on CXR. Presentation may be rarely due to associated aortic valve disease or subacute bacterial endocarditis.

d. Coarctation of the aorta is a well recognised reversible cause of hypertension, particularly in young adults. Correction is via a thoracotomy involving aortic cross-clamping. This corrects the hypertension and improves life expectancy. Balloon angioplasty has been used as a less invasive treatment. Severe hypertension in the immediate postoperative period may be problematic.

Further reading

Boon NA 1996 Coarctation of the aorta as a cause of secondary hypertension in the adult. In: Weatherall DJ, Ledingham JGG, Warrell DA, eds. *Oxford Textbook of Medicine*, 3rd edn. Oxford University Press, Oxford, pp 2557–2559.

Answer 5.30

a. Diamorphine has been used in this case both as an infusion and as a bolus injection. Both speed of onset and offset of spinally acting opioids are related to lipid solubility. The more lipophilic opioids lead to rapid onset by diffusion and more rapid offset by vascular uptake. Diamorphine therefore has slow onset and slow offset and is unsuitable for repeat bolus injection which leads to accumulation and delayed respiratory depression, as in this case.

b. The problem is likely to be delayed respiratory depression following epidural administration of diamorphine, thought to occur as a direct result of opiates reaching the brain. This may occur 3–12 h after administration of diamorphine, in contrast to the earlier respiratory depressant effects associated with the more lipophilic opioids such as pethidine, which usually occurs within an hour of administration. In this case, repeated doses have been administered on a background of local anaesthetic and opiate infusion, leading to a delayed and cumulative respiratory depression. Since cephalad transport of opiates is thought to be responsible for respiratory depression, the more lipophilic agents should be safer. However, it has been shown that only 4% of epidurally administered opiate reaches the CSF, and the CSF concentration of lipohilic agents, such as pethidine, rapidly declines. It may therefore be a combination of spinal and systemic effects that is important.

c. The addition of adrenaline would only serve to prolong the effects of the opioids further, leading to worsened respiratory depression. In addition, adrenaline has a direct analgesic action of its own on the spinal cord.

d. This man requires urgent airway support. Oxygen should be given and naloxone given slowly intravenously. If he wakes then a naloxone infusion and management in a critical care area would be appropriate. If he does not wake up despite i.v. naloxone, then his airway should be secured with an ETT and he should be transferred to an ICU for respiratory support. Protocols should be in place, with opiate-based epidurals, that bolus doses of opiates are not given whilst on an epidural infusion other than standard patient-controlled doses administered through the PCA. These patients should all be monitored hourly, including conscious level and respiratory rate, and medical staff should be called at an early stage.

6

INTENSIVE CARE MEDICINE

INTRODUCTION

A wide-ranging knowledge of data interpretation is vital to the practice of intensive care medicine. This knowledge should cover all aspects of general medicine, general surgery, neurotrauma and paediatrics. Many of these aspects, in particular chest X-ray (CXR) interpretation, will be covered in other chapters in this book. This chapter will concentrate on specific data that underpin management of intensive care, namely the interpretation of arterial blood gases and cardiac output assessment.

THE INTERPRETATION OF ARTERIAL BLOOD GASES

Arterial blood gas analysis gives rapid and crucial information on disturbances in P_{O_2}, P_{CO_2} and acid–base disturbance. However, in order to interpret such data correctly, it is important to understand how these measurements are derived.

The blood gas machine

Measured variables

In the blood gas machine, pH (or [H$^+$] in nmol/L) is measured by the generation of a potential across a pH-sensitive glass membrane. Common causes of error include too much heparin in the sample syringe (the correct dose is 0.1 mL of 1 in 1000, e.g. the dead space of a syringe) and coating of the pH electrode with blood proteins. P_{O_2} (partial pressure of oxygen) is measured directly using the reduction of oxygen between a platinum cathode and a silver anode which generates a small current. Oxygen electrodes often underread slightly since oxygen is consumed around the cathode tip; this inaccuracy increases with increasing oxygen tensions. P_{CO_2} measurements are

achieved by allowing CO_2 to diffuse through a Teflon membrane, altering the pH of a test solution. These measurements are usually accurate, although the CO_2 electrode needs frequent changes due to holes appearing in the Teflon membrane or loss of silver coating on the reference electrode. Such frequent changes prevent blood protein coating of the electrode becoming a problem.

Haemoglobin (Hb) estimation is usually performed photometrically, but may be more accurately measured using a co-oximeter. In a co-oximeter, blood is haemolysed, which allows absorption spectroscopy at six to eight wavelengths to give an accurate measurement of total Hb, fetal Hb, oxyhaemoglobin, carboxyhaemoglobin, methaemoglobin and sulphaemoglobin.

These values are the only directly measured values from the blood gas machine. All other variables are derived, and therefore more open to error, and require careful interpretation.

Derived variables

Total or actual bicarbonate concentration is calculated by the blood gas machine using the Henderson–Hasselbach equation:

$$pH = 6.1 + \log_{10}\left(\frac{\text{arterial [HCO}_3^-]}{P_a\text{CO}_2 \times 0.03}\right)$$

This includes bicarbonate, carbonate and carbamate concentrations. Standard bicarbonate can be derived to assess the contribution of metabolic factors and ignore the contribution of CO_2. It does this by estimating the bicarbonate concentration that would be present if the P_{CO_2} was 5.3 kPa (40 mmHg), P_{O_2} 13.3 kPa (100 mmHg) and temperature 37°C. The base deficit is a way of quantifying the metabolic component of an acidosis as the amount of base that would have to be added to or subtracted from a litre of extracellular fluid to return the pH to a value 7.4 at a $P\text{CO}_2$ of 5.3 kPa at 37°C. Standard base excess is calculated to an in vivo state. Most blood gas machines also give the oxygen saturation. This is also a derived variable calculated on the assumption that the oxygen haemoglobin dissociation curve is normal. Some machines also calculate oxygen content, arguably of greater clinical relevance than the $P\text{O}_2$. However, such calculations usually assume that the Hb is normal and do not take into account the presence of abnormal haemoglobins such as carboxyhaemoglobin.

Analysis of acid–base disturbance

All enzyme systems have an optimal working pH. Disturbances in pH therefore lead to disruption of metabolism, which may be life-threatening. Other affected systems include molecular ionization (e.g. hypocalcaemia in alkalosis), distribution of ions across cell membranes (notably potassium) and the oxygen haemoglobin dissociation curve. Changes in pH are therefore resisted by the body with a sophisticated system of buffers. Other regulatory systems include the lungs altering $P_a\text{CO}_2$ by adjusting alveolar ventilation and, in the longer term, the excretion of acids or bases by the kidneys.

The main buffers in the body are carbonic acid/bicarbonate system, phosphates and proteins. Of these, the carbonic acid/bicarbonate system is the most clinically useful, mainly because it is easy to measure and is involved in renal and respiratory compensation:

$$H^+ + HCO_3^- \underset{\substack{\text{Ionic}\\\text{dissociation}}}{\Longleftrightarrow} H_2CO_3 \underset{\substack{\text{Carbonic}\\\text{anhydrase}}}{\Longleftrightarrow} CO_2 + H_2O$$

It may be seen that disturbances in acid–base balance may be modified by respiratory control over CO_2 and renal regulation via control over HCO_3^- excretion/re-absorption, excretion of ammonia and titratable acid.

The Henderson–Hasselbach equation may be rewritten as follows:

$$[H^+] \propto \frac{P\text{CO}_2}{[HCO_3^-]}$$

$P\text{CO}_2$ may therefore be plotted against $[H^+]$ and abnormalities of acid–base disturbance described in relation to this. This may be conveniently described in one graph (Fig 6.1).

Respiratory acidosis

Hypoventilation leads to a rise in $P\text{CO}_2$, which is followed by a rise in $[H^+]$. In the acute phase there may be a small rise in bicarbonate levels due to the dissociation curve (see above). In chronic states, renal retention of bicarbonate brings pH and $[H^+]$ to normal over 2–5 days. In this circumstance, the primary abnormality is a respiratory acidosis with a compensatory metabolic alkalosis. The most common cause for this is chronic obstructive pulmonary disease (COPD).

Respiratory alkalosis

Hyperventilation leads to a fall in $P\text{CO}_2$ and $[H^+]$. In the acute phase the bicarbonate concentration may fall slightly. However, if the hyperventilation becomes chronic (an uncommon clinical problem), renal compensation occurs which may produce a mild metabolic acidosis. Complete correction of acidosis is unusual in this situation. Acute hyperventilation is common due to anxiety, but chronic hyperventilation is more unusual and may be due to chronic hypoxaemia from altitude, type 1 respiratory failure, or is occasionally produced during artificial ventilation on ITU.

Metabolic acidosis

Metabolic acidosis results from excessive production of endogenous acids (e.g. lactic acid, ketoacids), loss of alkali (e.g. renal tubular acidosis) or from exogenous acid (e.g. methanol, salicylates). Compensatory respiratory alkalosis develops once the brain has sensed the rise in $[H^+]$ and hyperventilation is stimulated. Lactic acidosis may be divided into type A, resulting from tissue hypoxia, and type B, in which tissue perfusion and utilisation are normal. Causes of type B lactic acidosis

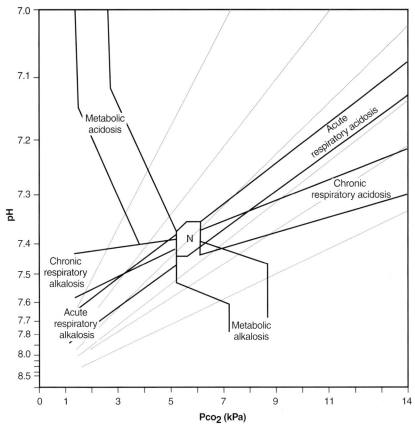

Fig. 6.1 The acid–base map in diagnosis and identification of acid–base disturbances. (Adapted with permission from Goldberg M et al, *Journal of the American Medical Association* 1973, 223: 269–275.)

include diabetic ketoacidosis, severe liver disease and methanol poisoning.

Anion gap
The anion gap is the difference between the sum of sodium and potassium minus the sum of bicarbonate and chloride and may be useful in the determination of the cause of a metabolic acidosis. This represents the unmeasured anions (sulphates, phosphates etc.) and is usually 6–12 mmol/L. If the acidosis is due to loss of base, then the anion gap will be normal, but a raised anion gap implies the presence of acid. This may be due to ketoacids, renal failure, lactic acidosis or the presence of exogenous (ingested) acids.

Metabolic alkalosis
This may be caused by the loss of acid

(commonly from the gut) or exogenous administration of alkali (e.g. milk–alkali syndrome). If the cause is unclear, a high urinary chloride may suggest hyperaldosteronism, Cushing's syndrome or severe potassium deficiency. A decrease in the extracellular fluid compartment results in the loss of hydrogen ions in preference to sodium reabsorption, and total body potassium deficiency results in loss of hydrogen ions in exchange for potassium. Respiratory compensation is severely limited and a P_{CO_2} over 6.5 kPa is rare, even in profound metabolic alkalosis. Once underlying factors are treated, acetazolamide may be considered.

How to interpret arterial blood gases
Initially, decide if an acidosis or alkalosis exists based upon pH, then look at the

CO_2 to decide if the respiratory component is the primary abnormality or a compensatory mechanism. If a metabolic acidosis exists and no cause is obvious, calculate the anion gap in order to look for unmeasured acid. However, any interpretation of arterial blood gases must be performed in clinical context in order to ascertain the primary abnormality. In addition, severely ill patients who are dehydrated, acidotic, severely hypokalaemic and in respiratory failure may have many processes occurring simultaneously. Most patients will also have been treated medically before referral to ITU. Consider how this may have affected the underlying abnormality. However, it is almost impossible to mask the underlying disturbance completely.

ASSESSMENT OF CARDIAC OUTPUT AND ORGAN PERFUSION

The assessment of cardiac output involves both clinical examination and monitoring techniques. These techniques are becoming increasingly complex and may be either invasive or non-invasive. They are not a substitute for clinical examination, which should focus upon the evaluation of vital organ perfusion.

The skin can be assessed rapidly for warmth and capillary refill. The central nervous system is particularly sensitive to a low cardiac output, resulting in an altered level of consciousness progressing to coma. Examination of the respiratory system may reveal alterations in respiratory rate or signs of pulmonary oedema, whilst urine output reflects renal perfusion (which is itself dependent upon cardiac output). Unfortunately, many other factors influence these clinical indicators and, hence, in critically ill patients additional information is frequently necessary. The measurement of heart rate and blood pressure is essential. Blood pressure is dependent upon both cardiac output and systemic vascular resistance (SVR). In its simplified form:

$$BP = CO \times SVR$$

where BP is blood pressure, CO is cardiac output, and SVR is systemic vascular resistance, thus making it impossible to assess cardiac output from blood pressure alone. This equation is of great significance as measurement of cardiac output with a known blood pressure allows us to derive vascular resistance (see below) and hence titrate therapy appropriately.

Non-invasive methods of assessing cardiac output have benefited from advances in technology. They are becoming increasingly reliable and frequently are used to follow trends rather than absolute values. They include echocardiography, Doppler and thoracic electrical bioimpedance.

Echocardiography uses ultrasound to examine the heart and great vessels. This has recently been extended by Doppler (to measure blood flow velocity) and transoesophageal techniques. They are gaining increasing popularity, and correlation with thermodilution-derived values is improving. Thoracic electrical bioimpedance lacks this accuracy in the majority of ventilated patients.

Invasive techniques usually involve thermodilution cardiac output measurements. Application of the Fick principle may be problematic in intensive care patients; however, modified techniques including a non-invasive carbon dioxide method have been reported. Pulse contour analysis examines the aortic pulse wave and requires calibration to estimate cardiac output. Transpulmonary indicator dilution is an additional technique of note, especially in paediatric intensive care practice. Lithium dilution appears to correlate well with thermodilution techniques and is gaining popularity.

At present, thermodilution cardiac output is considered to be the gold standard in clinical practice. A multi-lumen pulmonary artery flotation catheter (PAFC) is introduced into a central vein and advanced through the right atrium, right ventricle and then into the pulmonary artery. The balloon tip assists with catheter placement and causes it to wedge in the pulmonary artery. The pulmonary artery occlusion pressure (PAOP) is measured and can be used as a guide to left ventricular filling pressure. A fluid bolus of known volume and temperature is injected into the right atrium via the proximal lumen of the PAFC. This bolus mixes with blood returning from the periphery in the right ventricle and then enters the pulmonary artery. Any change in temperature, measured by a thermistor (4 cm from the tip of the PAFC), is dependent upon the cardiac output. This can be calculated using the Stewart–Hamilton formula (essentially using a plot of the temperature change with time and appropriate constants). The average figure obtained from multiple injection attempts throughout the respiratory cycle is then taken to be the cardiac output.

We can measure heart rate, right atrial, systemic and pulmonary arterial pressures directly. Now we are also able to estimate left atrial pressure and cardiac output. Hence, it is possible to derive pulmonary and systemic vascular resistances.

Normal values

CO (L/min)
$= HR \times SV$ 4–7
PAOP (mmHg)   6–12
SVR (dyn s/cm^5)
$= [(MAP - CVP) \times 80]/CO$ 900–1400
PVR (dyn s/cm^5) =
$[(MPAP - PAOP) \times 80]/CO$ 150–250

Measurement of height and weight allows for the calculation of body surface area and so we are able to index our measurements accordingly.

CI (L/min per m^2)
$= CO/BSA$ 2.8–4.2
SVR index (dyn s/cm^5 per m^2)
$= SVR/BSA$ 700–2600

Measuring haemoglobin concentration, arterial oxygen saturation and partial pressure enables calculation of the arterial oxygen content, and combined with cardiac output we can calculate oxygen transport variables:

C_aO_2 (mL/100 mL)
$= ([Hb] \times S_aO_2 \times 1.34) +$
$\quad (P_aO_2 \times 0.003)$ 18–20
$\dot{D}O_2$ (mL/min)
$= 10 \times C_aO_2 \times CO$ 640–1200

Furthermore, measurement of the mixed venous oxygen saturation using a fibreoptic oximeter at the end of the PAFC allows us also to calculate mixed venous oxygen content, oxygen extraction ratio and oxygen consumption:

C_vO_2 (mL/100 mL)
$= ([Hb] \times S_vO_2 \times 1.34) +$
$\quad (P_aO_2 \times 0.003)$ 13–15
Oxygen extraction
$= $ oxygen uptake/delivery   0.22–0.30
$\dot{V}O_2$ (mL/min)
$= 10 \times (C_aO_2 - C_vO_2) \times CO$ 100–180

Abbreviations
HR, heart rate; SV, stroke volume; PAOP, pulmonary artery occlusion pressure; SVR, systemic vascular resistance; PVR, pulmonary vascular resistance; MAP, mean arterial pressure; CVP, central venous pressure; BSA, body surface area; CI, cardiac index; C_aO_2, arterial oxygen content; C_vO_2, venous oxygen content; DO_2, oxygen dispatch; VO_2, oxygen uptake; S_aO_2, arterial oxygen saturation; P_aO_2, arterial oxygen tension; [Hb], haemoglobin concentration. P_vO_2, venous oxygen tension.

FURTHER READING

Goldberg M et al 1973 Computer based instruction and diagnosis of acid-base disorders. *Journal of the American Medical Association* 223: 269–275.
Webb AR, Shapiro MJ, Singer M, Suter PM (eds) 1999 *The Oxford Textbook of Critical Care.* Oxford University Press, Oxford.

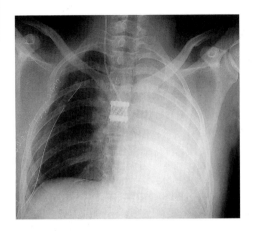

QUESTIONS

Question 6.1

A 19-year-old boy falls 3 m and suffers a T5 compression fracture. There is no neurological deficit. He undergoes a T5 vertebrectomy and Moss cage repair via a combined posterior approach and anterior thoracotomy. He is sent back to a surgical ward using patient-controlled analgesia for pain relief. Two days later you are asked for your opinion regarding ITU admission as he is hypoxic and breathless. On examination he has significant pain on coughing. There is decreased air entry on the left side of his chest. His CXR is shown. His ABGs breathing air are: pH, 7.49; base excess (BE), −3.1 mmol/l; P_aO_2, 7.2 kPa; P_aCO_2, 3.9 kPa; serum bicarbonate (Sbic), 28 mmol/L.

a. How do you interpret the ABGs?
b. Describe the CXR findings.
c. What is the differential diagnosis of opacification of the hemithorax? Why could this not be a large pleural effusion? What do you think is the diagnosis?
d. Why has this happened?
e. Outline a plan of treatment.

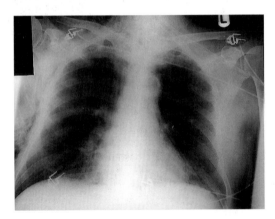

Question 6.2

A 73-year-old man presents with type 2 respiratory failure, secondary to long-standing COPD. He is ventilated and a tracheostomy performed as part of the weaning process. Unfortunately he pulls his tracheostomy out on day 3 and it is reinserted with difficulty. He immediately complains of severe dyspnoea and the tracheostomy is removed and reinserted using a bougie. His breathing improves but he now complains of central chest pain. His CXR is shown.

a. Describe the CXR.
b. What is the diagnosis? Is it life-threatening?
c. What clinical signs may be associated with this diagnosis?
d. Why has this occurred and what other pathologies may give rise to this condition?
e. Outline a plan of treatment.

Question 6.3

A 19-year-old student presents in casualty with a history of headaches, irritability and shortness of breath. His pulse is 90 beats/min, BP 135/86 mmHg and oxygen saturation 97% on room air. His chest is clear to auscultation. The casualty SHO brings his arterial blood gases to you for advice: pH, 7.48; P_{O_2}, 11.2 kPa; P_{CO_2}, 4.1 kPa; Sbic, 23 mmol/L; BE, −2.4; oxygen saturation (OxSat, measured by co-oximeter), 82%.

a. Describe the arterial blood gases.
b. What is the diagnosis? Explain why, and discuss the pathophysiology, clinical presentation and potential causes.
c. What treatment do you recommend?

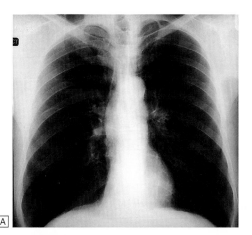

A

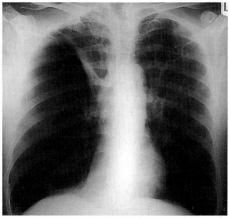

B

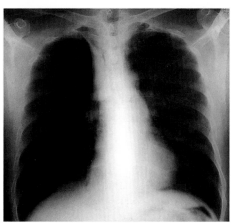

C

Question 6.4

A 45-year-old man presents with increasing shortness of breath. He has a long history of emphysema with marked exercise restriction. Clinical examination reveals a barrel-chested man, short of breath at rest, with scattered bronchi on auscultation, but decreased breath sounds on the left side. (A) is his CXR taken the previous year in the chest clinic, (B) is his CXR on presentation to ITU, and (C) is his CXR 24 h later and is associated with a rapid worsening in his clinical condition.

a. Describe the CXR in (A).
b. Describe the CXR in (B).
c. Describe the CXR in (C).
d. Describe the pathophysiology of this condition. What may be the underlying diagnosis?
e. He deteriorates and needs intubation and ventilation. Outline how this may be safely performed and what further therapeutic strategies are possible.

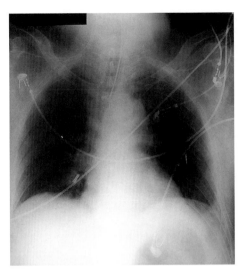

Question 6.5

A 55-year-old man is admitted to ITU following craniotomy for a massive meningioma. He was a grade 3 intubation at induction of anaesthesia. Surgery is prolonged and he is brought to ITU for overnight ventilation. This is his CXR on admission.

a. Describe this CXR. What is the abnormality?

b. How was this missed?

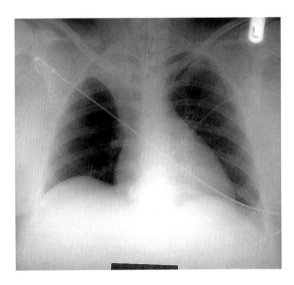

Question 6.6

A 32-year-old woman is brought to A&E unconscious with a GCS of 6/15. She is intubated and ventilated and a CT scan reveals a subarachnoid haemorrhage. She is brought to ITU for further treatment. A right internal jugular line is inserted and a CXR taken to ensure correct placement.

a. Describe the CXR. What is the diagnosis?

b. Why has this happened and what is the treatment?

c. In what age group does this often happen in ITU? Why?

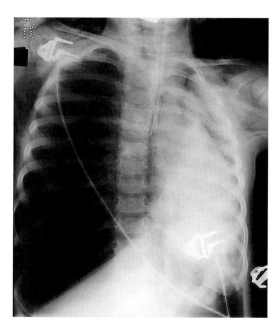

Question 6.7

An asthmatic 3-year-old girl is admitted to A&E with dyspnoea, tachypnoea, high pyrexia and bilateral expiratory wheeze. She is exhausted, cyanotic and requires intubation and ventilation. Initially the airway pressure is very high and she has to be hand-ventilated, but responds to nebulised salbutamol, steroids and aminophylline. However, after 10 min, her chest again becomes tight, wheezy and her oxygen saturation drops to 80% on 100% oxygen. A CXR is taken, as shown.

a. Describe the CXR. What is the diagnosis and why has this happened?
b. Outline a plan of treatment.
c. What clinical signs might you have expected on examination?

Question 6.8

An 18-year-old girl is admitted to A&E with increasing lethargy, somnolence and disorientation. She had complained of abdominal pain and tinnitus prior to admission. On examination she is pale, but not icteric, has a temperature of 38.2°C, pulse rate of 138 and BP of 96/49 mmHg. She eye opens to voice, localises to painful stimuli and talks incoherently. There are no localising neurological signs or evidence of trauma. Her pupils are 6 mm and reactive. A CT scan is reported as normal. Her blood results are as follows:

U & Es
Na, 143 mmol/l
K, 2.8 mmol/l
Cl, 101 mmol/l
Glucose, 7.8 mmol/l
Urea, 9.2 mmol/l
Creatinine, 128 µmol/l

ABGs
pH, 7.28
Po_2, 9.8 kPas
Pco_2, 3.9 kPas
Sbic, 19 mmol/l
BE, −10.9 mmol/l

a. What is her GCS?
b. Describe the arterial blood gases.
c. What is the anion gap and what do think is the diagnosis?
d. Describe the pathophysiology and outline a plan of treatment.

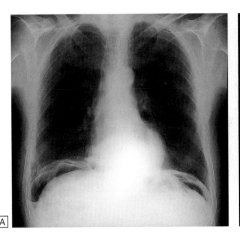
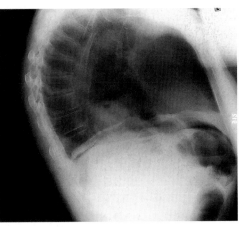

A B

Question 6.9

A 76-year-old man presented in a debilitated and confused state. He had had abdominal symptoms for 5 days prior to admission. He was acidotic and the other finding was blood glucose noted to be 2.9 mmol/l, which persisted after a glucose infusion. He was not on any medication and his CXRs are shown (A, B).

a. What two abnormalities do the CXRs show?
b. What explanation can you give for the low serum glucose?
c. What treatment of the low glucose would you recommend?

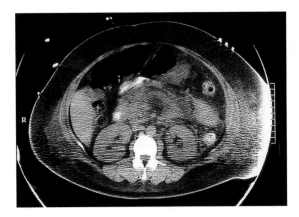

Question 6.10

A 42-year-old woman presents with a 7-day history of epigastric pain radiating to her back associated with vomiting. On admission she has a temperature of 38.5°C. A contrast-enhanced CT scan of abdomen is shown, and her blood indices are as follows: Hb, 10.9 g/dL; WCC, 26.1 × 10^9/L; platelets, 186 × 10^9/L; urea, 14.4 mmol/L; creatinine, 126 μmol/L; albumin, 24 g/L; calcium, 1.6 mmol/L; phosphate, 0.32 mmol/L; amylase, 1013 IU/L.

a. What two abnormalities do the contrast CT of the abdomen show?
b. What is the further plan of management?
c. Why does this patient have a low serum phosphate, and what difficulties are associated with it?

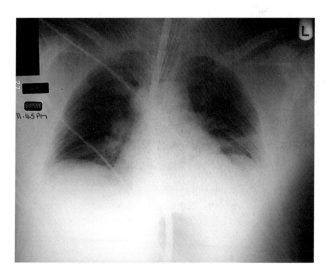

Question 6.11

A 50-year-old publican presents with a haematemesis. His blood pressure is 85/38 mmHg and he is confused. His conscious level drops and you are asked to see him for potential ITU admission. His CXR is shown. His full blood count is as follows: Hb, 7 g/dl; MCV, 108 fl; MCH, 28 pg; WBC, 16.9×10^9/l; platelets, $73\,000 \times 10^9$/l; prothrombin time, 26 s. His liver function tests are: bilirubin, 32 µmol/l; alanine aminotransferase, 272 IU/l; aspartate aminotransferase, 186 IU/l; alkaline phosphatase, 35 IU/l; albumin, 29 g/l; globulin, 48 g/l.

a. Interpret these blood results. What is the underlying diagnosis and what other blood results would you want to see?
b. Describe the CXR. Describe how the device shown should be used.
c. Outline your plan of management for this patient.
d. What is the prognosis?

Question 6.12

A 79-year-old man presents with a leaking aortic aneurysm. This is repaired in theatre and he receives 20 units of blood and clotting factors. Postoperatively he remains hypotensive. A pulmonary artery catheter is inserted and the following readings are made: pulmonary capillary wedge pressure (PCWP), 18 mmHg; pulmonary artery pressure (PAP), 50/35 mmHg; cardiac index, 1.7 L/min.

a. What are the functions of a pulmonary artery flotation catheter?
b. What is your interpretation of these findings? What are the sequelae?
c. What would you do next? What blood test may be relevant?

Question 6.13

An ill-looking middle-aged patient presents with a temperature of 39.5°C and a white cell count of 17×10^9/L. His pulse rate is 143 beats/min, blood pressure 90/60 mmHg and respiratory rate 43/min.

a. What are your working diagnosis, prognosis and initial steps in treatment?
b. What investigations would you perform initially?
c. The patient deteriorates – what is indicated next?

Question 6.14

A teenage girl presents with thirst, hyperventilation and polyuria. Her blood results are as follows: sodium, 125 mmol/l; potassium, 6.6 mmol/l; chloride, 100 mmol/l; urea, 9.8 mmol/l; creatinine, 126 µmol/l; random blood glucose, 40 mmol/l. *ABGs* – pH, 7.01; P_aCO_2, 2.6 kPa; P_aO_2, 15 kPa (air); bicarbonate, 8 mmol/l; BE, –18.9 mmol/l.

a. What is your immediate diagnosis?
b. Calculate the anion gap. What is the patient's prognosis?
c. What are the criteria you look for and what is your immediate treatment in the first hour?

Question 6.15

A patient weighing 35 kg with Crohn's disease is admitted to hospital for preoperative optimisation. Her blood results are as follows: sodium, 128 mmol/l; potassium, 3 mmol/l; urea, 15 mmol/l; creatinine, 50 µmol/l; magnesium, 0.48 mmol/l; albumin, 15 g/l; random blood glucose, 4 mmol/l.

a. How do you assess this patient's nutritional state?
b. What other aspects of general care need to be addressed?
c. What evidence exists for the benefits of nutritional support in critically ill patients?

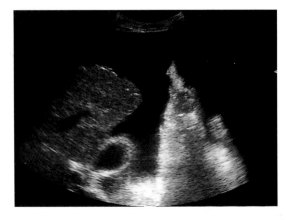

Question 6.16

A patient presents with a grossly distended abdomen and abdominal pain. An ultrasound scan of his abdomen is shown (above).

a. What abnormality does the ultrasound show?
b. What would you do next?
c. What problems do you anticipate?
d. What are the causes of this problem?

Question 6.17

A 66-year-old man presents with laboured breathing, blood pressure 90/40 mmHg and a pulse rate of 138 beats/min. His serum lactate is 12 mmol/l. His blood gases are as follows: *ABGs* – pH, 7.21; P_aCO_2, 2.3 kPa; P_aO_2, 7.1 kPa; Sbic, 14 mmol/l; BE, –12.2 mmol/l.

a. What acid–base disturbance is this? What diagnostic approach would you adopt?
b. What is the anion gap and its classification? Will it be raised or normal in this case?
c. What are possible common causes?

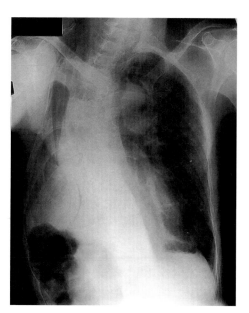

Question 6.18

A 78-year-old man presents in A&E with severe dyspnoea. He gives a history of TB when 26 years old. He has reduced air entry over the right side of his chest with an old thoracotomy scar. There are no added sounds on auscultation. His CXR is shown and his blood gases are as follows: pH, 7.14; P_aCO_2, 11.9 kPa; P_aO_2, 18.9 kPa; Sbic, 34 mmol/l; BE, −1.9 mmol/l.

a. Describe these blood gases.
b. Describe the CXR and interpret your findings.
c. Outline a plan of treatment.

Question 6.19

A 41-year-old man admits to taking an overdose of 40 paracetamol tablets 24 h ago. He now presents with vomiting and diarrhoea. His blood results are as follows: prothrombin time (PT), 110 s; activated partial thromboplastin time (APTT), 77 s; fibrinogen, 1.3 g/l; bilirubin, 138 µmol/l; alkaline phosphate, 77 IU/l; alanine aminotransferase (ALT), 6340 IU/l; creatinine, 285 µmol/l; urea, 15 mmol/l.

a. What do you do next?
b. He becomes agitated and acidotic with a pH of 7.1. What do you recommend?
c. What treatment do you propose and what is the prognosis?

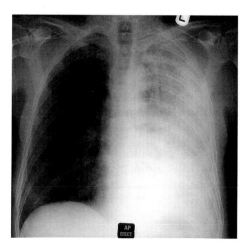

Question 6.20

A 74-year-old man with mild COPD presents with increasing confusion and immobility. On examination he is drowsy, flushed and pyrexial, with a temperature of 39.5°C. He is dyspnoeic at rest and auscultation of his chest reveals decreased air entry with bronchial breath sounds on the left side. His CXR is shown.

a. Describe the CXR.
b. What is the diagnosis?
c. List the likely causative organisms and their respective treatments.

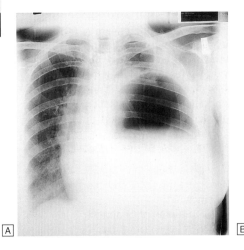

A

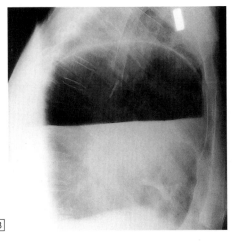

B

Question 6.21

A 69-year-old lady presented with intermittent epigastric pain for 3 months and severe dyspnoea for 24 h. AP (A) and lateral (B) CXRs are taken, but immediately following this she suffers an electromechanical cardiac arrest and is intubated.

a. Describe the AP and lateral CXRs.
b. What is the differential diagnosis and how might you confirm your probable diagnosis?
c. What immediate treatment do you recommend which may improve cardiac output?

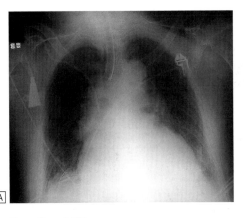

A

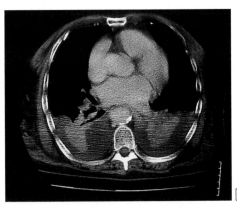

B

Question 6.22

A 57-year-old man with a history of dilated ischaemic cardiomyopathy is admitted with increasing dyspnoea. A CXR shows signs of pulmonary oedema and he is treated with oxygen and diuretics. Unfortunately within 24 h, he has a cardiac arrest, necessitating intubation and ventilation on ITU. Despite treatment for poor left ventricular function, his oxygen requirement remains between 60 and 80% after 5 days. At this stage, a CXR (A) and thoracic CT scan (B) are performed.

a. Describe the CXR.
b. Describe the CT scan.
c. What immediate treatment do you recommend?

Question 6.23

A 36-year-old man presents with abdominal pain and vomiting. Acute pancreatitis is diagnosed and treatment includes analgesia, nasogastric drainage and intravenous fluids. However, after 10 days he continues to vomit with large nasogastric aspirates. During this time, intravenous fluid intake is maintained with a fixed regime consisting of 2 litres of 4% dextrose saline and 1 litre of 0.9% normal saline per 24 h. By day 11 he has a depressed level of consciousness, is intermittently obstructing his airway and has no gag reflex. His pulse is thready, rate 126 beats/min and blood pressure 90/45 mmHg. His biochemical profile is as follows: *ABGs*: pH, 7.55; P_aO_2, 7.7 kPa; P_aCO_2, 6.2 kPa; bicarbonate, 38 mmol/l; BE, +12.8 mmol/l. *Electrolytes*: Na^+, 136 mmol/l; K^+, 2.7 mmol/l; Cl^-, 84 mmol/l; urea, 9.8 mmol/l; creatinine, 144 µmol/l; glucose, 8.4 mmol/l; urinary $[Cl^-]$, 8 mmol/l.

a. Describe this metabolic abnormality.
b. What is the cause of this abnormal biochemical state?
c. How should this patient be managed?

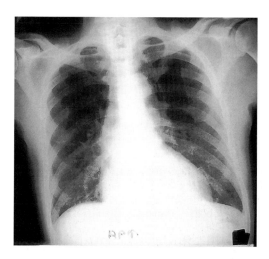

Question 6.24

A cachectic 73-year-old man with end-stage renal failure and type 2 (non-insulin-dependent) diabetes mellitus presents to the A&E department with confusion and a reduced level of consciousness. He is normally dialysed three times a week but is known to be poorly compliant with his restricted fluid regime. He has underlying chronic obstructive pulmonary disease, and is a life-long smoker.

On arrival at A&E he is comatose (GCS 7). His airway is clear, he is warm and well perfused, heart rate 130 beats/min, blood pressure 190/90 mmHg and respiratory rate 8 breaths/min. Oxygen saturation is 84% but rises to 99% with high-flow oxygen. Auscultation of his chest reveals bilateral inspiratory crepitations and a prominent third heart sound. He has no focal neurological signs and no signs of meningism. His CXR is shown (above). His biochemistry results are as follows: *ABGs* – pH, 6.9; P_aO_2, 22.4 kPa ($F_iO_2 = 0.6$); P_aCO_2, 13.1 kPa; Sbic, 16 mmol/l; BE, –9.6 mmol/l. *Electrolytes* – Na, 126 mmol/l; K, 5.2 mmol/l; Cl, 104 mmol/l; urea, 21.4 mmol/l; creatinine, 822 µmol/l; blood glucose, 9.6 mmol/l.

a. Describe his biochemical abnormality.
b. Describe the CXR.
c. What is the likely cause of his deterioration?
d. How would you manage this patient?

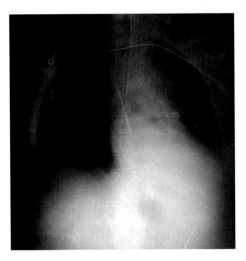

Question 6.25

A 58-year-old male patient undergoes an orthotopic liver transplant. A PAFC was inserted. This is technically difficult, and the pulmonary artery balloon bursts on inflation. A second catheter is inserted uneventfully and his pulmonary artery pressures are normal. The patient is transferred to the intensive care unit postoperatively. His immediate postoperative chest X-ray is shown. He is extubated and discharged to the HDU. However, 3 days later he develops acute hypoxic respiratory failure with bright red haemoptysis. His PT is 22 s and platelet count is noted to be $30 \times 10^9/l$.

a. Describe the CXR.
b. What is the cause of his deterioration?
c. How would you manage this patient?

Question 6.26

A 36-year-old male patient is admitted to the A&E department confused and agitated. He has a blood pressure of 58 mmHg systolic and a pulse rate of 138 beats/min. His family describe a 3-month history of malaise, mental confusion, anorexia and weight loss. He had recently complained of abdominal pain and had been vomiting. Over the preceding 3 days he had developed a fever. He has no previous medical history of note, takes no regular medications and no illicit substances. His electrolyte estimations are as follows: Na, 122 mmol/l; K, 5.8 mmol/l; Cl, 104 mmol/l; bicarbonate, 16 mmol/l; urea, 6.2 mmol/l; creatinine, 128 μmol/l; glucose, 3.1 mmol/l.

a. What clinical condition is likely?
b. What abnormal clinical findings may be present?
c. What further investigations are necessary?
d. What treatment should be instituted?

Question 6.27

A 21-year-old patient is admitted to a liver ICU 72 h post-paracetamol overdose. She had presented to hospital 36 h after her overdose. She is acidaemic and her PT is 108 s. Her level of consciousness rapidly deteriorates and she is listed for an urgent liver transplant. She is intubated and mechanically ventilated, yet her blood pressure progressively falls and she becomes anuric. A PAFC is inserted. The following haemodynamic measurements and derived figures are obtained: MAP, 52 mmHg; CVP, 12 mmHg; PCWP, 6 mmHg; cardiac index (CI), 6.1 l/min per m²; systemic vascular resistance (SVR), 340 dyn s/cm⁵.

a. What haemodynamic abnormality is demonstrated?
b. How should the patient be managed?

Question 6.28

A 74-year-old patient is admitted to hospital from her residential nursing home. She had become increasingly drowsy and confused over the previous 2 weeks, and now only responds to painful stimuli. Her previous medical history includes osteoarthritis of both hips and ischaemic heart disease. She takes regular paracetamol and isosorbide mononitrate. Her biochemical results are as follows: Na, 149 mmol/l; K, 3.9 mmol/l; urea, 8.3 mmol/l; creatinine, 154 µmol/l; glucose, 52 mmol/l; bicarbonate, 19 mmol/l; ketones, negative.

a. What is the diagnosis?
b. Estimate the osmolarity. What is the normal serum osmolarity?
c. Outline the pathogenesis of this condition.
d. How would you manage this patient?

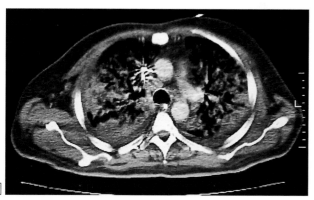

A

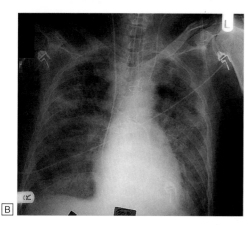

B

Question 6.29

A 46-year-old male patient undergoes triple-vessel coronary artery bypass grafting. On return to cardiac ITU he is hypotensive and returns to theatre where the internal mammary artery is found to be bleeding. This is sutured and he returns to ITU. During the perioperative period he receives 18 units of blood, 8 units of FFP, cryoprecipitate, 3000 ml of crystalloid and 2500 mL of colloid. The following day, his F_iO_2 rises to 0.8, with airway pressures of 46/10 mmHg. His CT scan of chest (A) and CXR (B) are shown. His clinical results are as follows: HR, 88 beats/min; MAP, 76 mmHg; PCWP, 10 mmHg; CVP, 12 mmHg; pH, 7.30; P_aO_2, 7.6 kPa; P_aCO_2, 7.8 kPa; BE, −5.8 mmol/l.

a. Describe the CXR and CT scan of chest.
b. What is the diagnosis?
c. What are the causes of this syndrome?
d. How should the patient be managed?

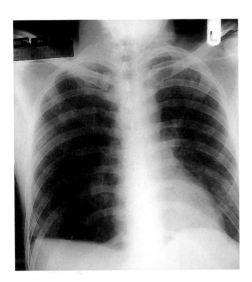

Question 6.30

A 19-year-old injecting drug user presents with a pyrexia of 40°C, rigors, BP of 60/30 mmHg and heart rate of 148 beats/min. He has a loud systolic murmur. His CXR is shown.

a. Describe the CXR.
b. What is the diagnosis and what do you think is the causative organism?
c. What other diagnosis do you suspect and what investigations will you perform?

ANSWERS

Answer 6.1

a. The ABGs reveal a respiratory alkalosis secondary to hypoxia. Hypoxic-induced hyperventilation (such as occurs at altitude) decreases the P_aCO_2 and may serve to increase the P_aO_2 (alveolar blood gas) equation, $P_AO_2 = P_iO_2 - P_ACO_2 \times (F_iO_2 + 1 - F_iO_2/R)$.

b. The most obvious abnormality on the CXR is complete opacification of the left lung field; no lung markings are visible. In addition, the mediastinum is pulled significantly to the left (look at the carina, right heart border and central line all pulled to the left). There is also a Moss cage at the T5 level, right thoracotomy with resection of the third rib, right-sided chest drain and right internal jugular central line.

c. Total opacification of the hemithorax is usually due to either pulmonary collapse secondary to bronchial obstruction (malignancy, mucus plugging or inhalation of foreign body, particularly in children) or pleural effusion (malignancy, TB, pneumonic empyema, haemothorax following trauma and, more rarely, cardiac failure, pneumonia, pulmonary infarction or hypoproteinaemia).

   In this case, the diagnosis is sputum plugging. This is because the mediastinum is pulled over to the side of the opacification due to underlying lung collapse. If this was a large effusion, the mediastinum would be pushed towards the normal lung, or at least remain midline if there was associated lung collapse together with an effusion (as may occur with a Ca bronchus). If this was a pneumonic process, one would expect to see an air bronchogram.

d. This may occur postoperatively secondary to a combination of restricted coughing because of pain, prolonged surgery allowing sputum to accumulate, and dry inspired gases (oxygen).

e. Treatment consists initially of humidification of inspired gases and improved pain control to assist with physiotherapy. The target for analgesia should be the ability to cough effectively without pain. In this case, this may mean more opiates or regional blockade, such as paravertebral blockade. If clinical signs and hypoxia persist, fibreoptic bronchoscopy is indicated, and if the patient tires despite this, ventilation may need to be considered. Sputum should be sent for culture. The CXR shown below was performed immediately after paravertebral blocks were performed and after a coughing fit which produced a large quantity of thick clear sputum. The left heart border is now a straight line. This is called a sail sign (as it resembles the sail of a ship) and indicates collapse/consolidation of the left lower lobe. The mediastinum is still pulled over to the left. After further physiotherapy, the left lower lobe also cleared.

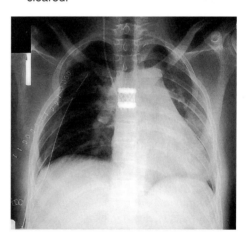

Answer 6.2

a. The most obvious abnormality demonstrated on this CXR is a ring outlining the aortic knuckle and a double shadow on the left heart border. There is also subcutaneous air demonstrated, particularly in the neck and the right side of the chest. Incidentally there is a tracheostomy in situ, which is difficult to see on this film, and opacification at the right base suggesting infection or aspiration.

b. The diagnosis is pneumomediastinum. This may present as chest pain. The ring around the aortic knuckle and along the left heart border is air within the mediastinum. This is also tracking subcutaneously. This is not immediately life-threatening in this case, as the cause of the air entering the mediastinum has resolved. If the tracheostomy had not been changed and more air was forced into the mediastinum, this may have led to a tension pneumomediastinum, which may drastically impair cardiac performance and lead to an electromechanical dissociation cardiac arrest.

c. Crepitus synchronous with the cardiac cycle may occur on auscultation (Hamman's sign).

d. This has occurred because the tracheostomy was changed too early before a reasonable track was established and a false passage was created where air was forced into the mediastinum. Little firm evidence exists to time the first change, but it is the author's practice to change at 7–10 days. A pneumomediastinum is usually caused by rupture of the oesophagus from any cause (neoplasm, trauma, spontaneous rupture during vomiting), although it may also occasionally occur in emphysema, amongst asthmatics and, rarely, in pregnancy during labour. It may also be associated with a pneumothorax or pneumoperitoneum.

e. Treatment is directed initially at stopping the cause of the pneumomediastinum, done in this case by replacing the tracheostomy. Mild cases usually resolve spontaneously. If associated with severe subcutaneous emphysema, subcutaneous incisions over the chest wall may allow air to escape. If severe, tension or associated with cardiac compromise, chest drains and rarely thoracotomy may be required.

Answer 6.3

a. The arterial blood gases show a mild respiratory alkalosis.

b. The diagnosis is carbon monoxide (CO) poisoning. There is mild hyperventilation and a marked discrepancy between the oxygen saturation on pulse oximetry, measured P_aO_2 with a blood gas machine and oxygen saturation measured by a co-oximeter which is markedly reduced, implying low oxygen carriage.

Carbon monoxide has a 240× greater affinity for haemoglobin than oxygen and forms carboxyhaemoglobin (CoHb), which does not release oxygen in the tissues. The absorption spectrum for CoHb is similar to oxyhaemoglobin, so that currently available pulse oximeters that use two wavelengths of light for analysis, cannot distinguish between them. Conventional arterial blood gas machines calculate S_pO_2 from the P_AO_2 and therefore will also be inaccurate in the presence of significant CoHb. The co-oximeter measures the oxygen saturation using four or more wavelengths of light, minimising inaccuracies due to CoHb, and therefore more accurately reflects oxygen carriage.

Significant levels of CoHb occur in smokers (up to 10%), fires in confined spaces, inhalational injuries and from poorly maintained vehicles or domestic gas appliances. This 19-year-old student may live in a house with a poorly maintained gas fire, well known to produce CO poisoning. Both pulse oximetry and arterial blood gas analysis will overestimate circulating blood oxygen content in such patients and a blood gas machine using a co-oximeter should always be used.

c. Symptoms usually arise from tissue hypoxia. They include headache, dizziness, confusion, abdominal and chest pain, nausea and vomiting, and in severe poisoning, coma, convulsions and cardiac arrest. Levels of CoHb may reach 10% in smokers and symptoms generally start at greater than 15%. Severe poisoning occurs with levels greater than 40%, and with levels greater than 50% mortality may be as high as 50%. Treatment is based on the administration of 100% oxygen and supportive measures. The half-life of CoHb at room air (F_iO_2, 0.21) is 240 min and this decreases to 90 min on 100% oxygen. The use of hyperbaric oxygen is controversial. Although the half-life of CoHb falls to only 20 min at 2 atm, there are logistical problems as well as potential problems with oxygen toxicity. Hyperbaric chambers are rarely close to A&E departments and by the time patients are transferred, CoHb levels will often be within safe limits.

Further reading

Moyle J 2000 Advances in pulse oximetry. *CPD Anaesthesia* 2000 2: 9–12.

Answer 6.4

a. The lung fields are overinflated and there is evidence of widespread severe emphysematous disease with giant bullae at both bases, particularly large on the right.
b. The CXR shows that the giant bulla at the right base is increasing in size.
c. The bulla has increased dramatically in size and is now pushing the mediastinum over to the left. This is a tension bulla. It is not a tension pneumothorax as lung markings may still be seen all the way to the periphery of the right lung field and no lung border is visible.
d. This man has giant bullous emphysematous disease. He is young and almost certainly will have α_1-antitrypsin deficiency. Alpha-1-antitrypsin is a serum protein that inhibits proteolytic enzymes that contribute to lung breakdown. Its deficiency leads to severe emphysema at a young age and often affects the lower zones. This man has presented with a tension bulla. Bullae form due to loss of elastin. This decreases elastic recoil and leads to a wide variety of time constants to expiration. A giant bulla such as this one expands rapidly as there is no time for complete emptying on expiration.
e. When establishing IPPV in patients with severe emphysema, adequate time

must be allowed in expiration to ensure emptying of alveoli with long time constants and airway pressures must be minimised to decrease risk of barotrauma. Non-invasive ventilation may be of benefit in lowering peak airway pressures, but in the situation of a rapidly expanding bulla this may only create a tension. If a tension bulla develops, it may be reduced by the insertion of a small chest drain. If this fails, intubation and ventilation usually involve a slow respiratory rate, low tidal volume and pressure-controlled ventilation. Oxygenation is rarely a problem and the use of permissive hypercapnia may allow these parameters. In this case, with a large unilateral tension bulla, it may be possible, although technically challenging, to ventilate the lungs independently using selective endobronchial intubation. The right lung may then be independently ventilated with a very slow respiratory rate, high-frequency ventilation or oxygen insufflation.

Once stabilised, lung volume reduction surgery should be considered to excise the pathological section of lung and this may significantly improve symptoms.

Further reading

Tscherno EM, Gruber EM, Jaksch P et al 1998 Ventilatory mechanics and gas exchange during exercise before and after lung volume reduction surgery. *American Journal of Respiratory & Critical Care Medicine* 158: 1424–1431.

Answer 6.5

a. This is an AP supine CXR. The obvious abnormality is the malposition of the nasogastric tube (NGT) which has been placed in the right main bronchus. There is also a left-sided long line which may be placed too long and may be in the right atrium.
b. The patient was a difficult intubation and therefore placement of the NGT under direct vision may also have been

difficult. However, if stomach contents were not aspirated, air should have been injected and the epigastrium auscultated. A CXR should always be taken to confirm position before enteral feeding is commenced.

Answer 6.6

a. This is an AP CXR. The obvious abnormality is an area of opacification in the apex of the right lung field. This represents collapse/consolidation of the right upper lobe. There is also a right internal jugular line in situ in good position.
b. This occurs because of obstruction of the right upper lobe bronchus, usually by sputum plugging or right-sided endobronchial intubation. In this case it is likely to be sputum plugging or aspirated secretions since she was admitted not protecting her airway. Treatment consists of physiotherapy, humidification and bronchoscopy if it does not clear.
c. This often occurs in infants due to the higher position of the right upper lobe bronchus, which may even come off the trachea.

Answer 6.7

a. This is an AP CXR. The obvious abnormality is deviation of the mediastinum to the left-hand side and loss of lung markings on the right lung field. The diagnosis is a tension pneumothorax. This has occurred as a result of barotrauma due to the high inflation pressures required after intubation. Spontaneous pneumothoraces may occur in asthmatics and, if present before intubation, will often result in a tension pneumothorax with positive pressure ventilation.
b. This is an emergency. A needle thoracocentesis should be immediately performed via the second intercostal space in the midclavicular line. Once this has been performed, a chest drain should be inserted.

c. A tension pneumothorax is a clinical diagnosis and this X-ray should never have been taken. Clinical examination will reveal decreased air entry and hyperresonance on the right side, and deviation of the trachea to the left. High pressure on the great vessels in the chest decreases venous return, which leads to a decrease in cardiac output and may lead to an electromechanical cardiac arrest if left untreated.

Further reading
Chest trauma In: *Advanced Paediatric Life Support*. Advanced Life Support Group 1995. BMJ Publishing, London.

Answer 6.8

a. Her GCS is 10 (E3, V2, M5).
b. The predominant picture is one of metabolic acidosis (BE, −10.9) with evidence of a respiratory alkalosis (low P_aCO_2 and bicarbonate), which may or may not be compensatory.
c. The anion gap is +27 [(143 + 2.9) − (101 + 18)]. She has a markedly elevated anion gap which implies the presence of lactic acid (shock, hepatic failure), exogenous acids (salicylic acid, ethylene glycol), ketoacids (diabetes mellitus, alcohol). She is not shocked or jaundiced, her random blood glucose is normal. The diagnosis is therefore likely to be an aspirin overdose as a cause of exogenous acid. This would also contribute to the respiratory alkalosis.
d. In overdose, aspirin initially produces a respiratory alkalosis by direct stimulation of the medullary respiratory centres. This is followed by a metabolic acidosis predominantly secondary to the build-up of ketoacids, but salicylates, dehydration, uraemia and shock contribute. Presenting symptoms involve confusion, tinnitus, abdominal pain, pyrexia and nausea and vomiting. Complications include cerebral and pulmonary oedema, hypotension, dehydration, convulsions and hepatorenal failure. The metabolic effects of aspirin are complex. Oxidative

phosphorylation is uncoupled, leading to accumulation of pyruvic and lactic acids. In addition, gluconeogenesis is stimulated, leading to ketoacidosis in the absence of hyperglycaemia. The accumulation of these acids contributes to the acidosis.

Evidence of other drug overdose should be sought, in particular a paracetamol level should be checked. In addition to general supportive measures, gastric aspiration should be performed, together with the administration of activated charcoal. Since salicylates are acids, in the presence of an acidosis, more free drug will diffuse to body tissues. Therefore any acidosis should be corrected with intravenous bicarbonate, which also increases urinary excretion. Alkalinisation of urine should be considered with plasma concentrations > 500 mg/L. However, forced alkaline diuresis is contraindicated due to potential problems of fluid overload. Despite normoglycaemia, glucose levels may be low in the central nervous system and glucose-containing fluids should be given. Serum clotting and calcium should be monitored and treated. In severe cases (serum level > 700 mg/L) haemofiltration should be considered.

Further reading

Harper NC, Collee GC 1997 Poisoning, overdose and toxic exposure. In Goldhill DR, Withington PS, eds. *Textbook of Intensive Care*. Chapman & Hall Medical, London, pp. 691–692.

Answer 6.9

a. There is air clearly demonstrated under both diaphragms, consistent with bowel perforation. In addition, there is a hiatus hernia with the stomach in the chest (well visualised on the lateral film). In this case, there was a perforated gastric ulcer.

b. Prolonged starvation is the most likely cause; this is also seen in anorexia nervosa. Alcohol, insulin and oral hypoglycaemic medication, e.g.

sulphinylureas, are drug causes to be considered. Acute liver failure, acute and chronic pancreatitis, cardiac failure and sepsis are severe life-threatening conditions associated with hypoglycaemia. Symptoms of agitation, tremor, irritability and faintness start to present at levels of 3 mmol/L or below.

c. 50 mL of 50% glucose intravenously usually works in 5 min, and the patient often wakes up. In systemic illness and drug overdose, e.g. insulin, a glucose infusion 10–20% will be needed for several days. If this is a suicide attempt with insulin, it is worth ultrasounding the injection site and considering surgical incision. It is impossible to administer sufficient intravenous glucose sometimes and other sources of delivery, such as the enteral route, should be utilised.

Further reading

Noone RB, Mythen MG 1999 Hypoglycaemia. In: Webb AR, Shapiro MJ, Singer M, Suter PM, eds. *Oxford Textbook of Critical Care*, Oxford University Press, Oxford, ch. 8.6.

Answer 6.10

a. The head of the pancreas is swollen and enhanced, suggesting a necrotic collection. The tail of the pancreas has formed a pseudocyst.

b. Severe localised pancreatitis is associated with multiple systemic complications, notably respiratory and renal failure and infection. These should be closely monitored and these patients should be managed in a critical care facility. The mortality may be as high as 30%. The patient may require radiologically guided drainage of the pseudocyst, and repeat ultrasound or CT scans will determine when surgical intervention for necrosectomy should be timed. The patient may require weeks in critical care and months in hospital undergoing repeated procedures. Nasojejunal feeding is usually easily established and may help to decrease pancreatic secretions in comparison to nasogastric feeding and avoids the complications of parenteral nutrition. DVT prophylaxis is essential.

c. Hypophosphataemia is a common feature of excessive losses from the gut. It may also be a consequence of diuretic therapy. It may lead to difficulty in weaning from mechanical ventilation. Patients may be profoundly weak and may also fit. A low phosphate also impairs the immune system.

Further reading

Glazer G, Mann DV 1998 United Kingdom guidelines for the management of acute pancreatitis. *Gut* 42(supplement 2).

Answer 6.11

a. This man is mildly jaundiced with raised hepatocellular enzymes indicating severe hepatic damage; bile excretion is unaffected. He is obviously anaemic from acute blood loss; however, there is also a background of chronic liver disease, suggested by the hypoalbuminaemia, macrocytic anaemia, clotting abnormalities and thrombocytopenia. This presentation suggests chronic alcoholic liver disease with the advent of varices. Renal disease should be assessed by serum urea and creatinine measurement; a gamma-glutamyl transferase is a guide to progressive alcoholic liver disease. A viral hepatitis screen should be performed.

b. The CXR is an AP film. The most obvious abnormality is the presence of an opaque tube situated in the midline, likely to be a Sengstaken–Blakemore tube. This has two distinct balloons. The upper thin balloon used to control oesophageal bleeding by direct tamponade is inflated to above venous pressure, usually 20–25 cmH$_2$O (the normal portal venous pressure is 10–12 cmH$_2$O, but may be markedly raised in portal hypertension). The lower, larger gastric balloon is inflated to retain it in the stomach with 400 mL of air. They remain in situ only for a day or so as there is a danger of pressure

necrosis from the oesophageal balloon and this should be deflated for 5 min every hour.

c. Management consists of immediate resuscitation from acute haemorrhage, followed by the management of the presumed varices. Massive gastrointestinal blood loss requires quick intervention. Place the patient on the side, head down, until the airway can be secured with an endotracheal tube; provide high-flow oxygen. Establish at least two large-bore i.v. lines. Cross-match blood but give fluid rapidly while waiting. Ice-cold saline via a nasogastric tube is widely recommended. Central venous access and a urinary catheter are required once control of the patient is established. Once stabilised, octreotide and vasopressin may be used to lower portal pressures.

The blood glucose is commonly low and requires a glucose infusion and should be regularly checked. If conscious, β-blockers are sometimes used to control the tremor and induce calm. Absence of dietary vitamins leads to damage of the nervous system and nutritional diseases, e.g. pellagra. Such patients need a good intake of vitamins and trace elements, particularly thiamine.

The patient may be given lactulose and neomycin to prevent hepatic encephalopathy. Sclerotherapy or ligation may be undertaken via endoscopy once bleeding has stopped. Oesophageal varices tend to re-bleed. Continued bleeding or longer-term management may require portal vein pressure reduction by transjugular intrahepatic portosystemic shunting. Transplantation will be considered in the case of alcoholism if the patient has been abstinent for 6 months.

d. The prognosis from an acute variceal bleed is often quoted as being as high as 50%. The Maddey discrimination score exceeding 32 (serum bilirubin + 4.6 × the prolongation of prothrombin time) has a 1-year mortality of about 60%.

Further reading

Crotty B 1998 Haematemesis and melaena. *Medicine* 26: 16–21.

Day C 1998 Alcohol and the liver. *Medicine* 26: 19–22.

Answer 6.12

a. The catheter can continuously monitor PAPs, CVP, core temperature, cardiac output and S_vO_2. It can intermittently measure PCWP. Catheters that can pace the heart are also available.

b. Normal pulmonary artery occlusion pressure is 6–12 mmHg. Although higher when undergoing positive pressure ventilation, 18 mmHg is likely to represent adequate left ventricular filling. The patient has raised pulmonary pressures suggesting right-sided strain. The cardiac index is very low. The patient is compromised by a poor myocardium and is likely to develop signs of left ventricular failure (pulmonary oedema) and poor tissue perfusion (myocardial ischaemia, acute renal failure, liver damage, compromised peripheral circulation).

c. The high filling pressure and low cardiac output state indicate the patient would benefit from off-loading of the heart plus an inotrope. A dobutamine infusion would be appropriate. This involves greater oxygen consumption, and optimisation of oxygen delivery is a prerequisite for success. There is a likelihood that the patient has suffered a perioperative myocardial infarct due to the blood loss, hypoxia and shock. A postoperative troponin T (replacing the CK-MB level) is indicated. Even in elective aortic aneurysm repair, myocardial infarction is common (up to 20% of cases) and is even higher in emergency cases. It should always be looked for. Serial ECGs also will give some clue as to myocardial damage.

Further reading

Lollgren H 1997 Current choices of inotropes in the intensive care unit. In: Ryan DW, ed. *Current Practice in Critical Illness*, vol II. Chapman & Hall, London.

Answer 6.13

a. This patient probably has severe sepsis which is defined as systemic inflammatory response syndrome (SIRS) + documented infection and associated with cardiovascular compromise or organ dysfunction. SIRS is characterised by:

- core temperature $> 38°C$ or $< 36°C$
- WBC $> 12\,000$ or $< 4000 \times 10^9$/L (or $> 10\%$ immature neutrophils)
- respiratory rate > 20 beats/min; P_aCO_2 < 4.3 kPa
- heart rate > 90 beats/min.

Severe sepsis carries a mortality rate of up to 50%. Establish i.v. access, provide supplemental oxygen if required, and administer 'best guess' antibiotics depending on clinical symptoms. Exclude a diabetic state. Paracetamol and tepid sponging is helpful in controlling the pyrexia.

b. Clinical history and examination may give the clue to the source of infection. The patient should have sputum, urine and blood sent for culture; a vaginal swab should be considered in the female. A lumbar puncture may be indicated. A CXR should be performed. Ear, sinus, scrotal and leg ulcer infections tend to get overlooked. If this fails to reveal the source, the chest and abdomen remain the two most likely sources. Ultrasound scanning, echocardiography and a CT scan need consideration.

c. Consider invasive cardiovascular monitoring, optimise fluid filling and consider inotropes, commonly dobutamine and noradrenaline (norepinephrine). The patient should be moved to a critical care facility. Failure to respond may necessitate mechanical ventilation, a pulmonary artery catheter and renal support. Septic shock has a mortality of over 50%.

Further reading

American College of Chest Physicians/Society of Critical Care Medicine 1992 Definitions for sepsis and organ failure and guidelines for the use of innovative therapies in sepsis. *Critical Care Medicine* 20: 864–876.

Ryan DW 1999 Septicaemia and shock. *European Urology* 2: 1–9.

Vincent JL 1997 Sepsis. In: Goldhill DR, Withington PS, eds. *Textbook of Intensive Care.* Chapman & Hall Medical, London.

Answer 6.14

a. This girl is presenting with diabetic ketoacidosis. She is also dehydrated, hyponatraemic and her blood gases show a severe metabolic acidosis with partial respiratory compensation from hyperventilation.

b. The anion gap is raised at 23 [(125 + 6.6) − (100 + 8)]. This implies the presence of exogenous acid in metabolic acidosis, in this case from ketoacids. There is a spectrum in presentation but mortality depends on delay between onset of ketoacidosis and diagnosis. Mortality is normally 2–5%.

c. The diagnosis is usually straightforward: hyperglycaemia, an acidosis pH < 7.3, a serum bicarbonate < 16 mmol/L, an anion gap exceeding 16, and ketones in the urine and blood. Diabetic ketoacidosis is a medical emergency. The patient needs close monitoring and expert resuscitation, which is best initiated in a critical care area.

Intravenous fluid, as normal saline should be given to support the blood pressure and renal function. Central venous pressure monitoring will help to guide fluid resuscitation. The rate of administration of fluid is controversial. Brisk initial resuscitation is required, particularly to correct acidosis and hyperkalaemia; however, if too rapid, acute changes in sodium predispose to cerebral oedema. An insulin infusion at 20 units/h should be commenced to control the rising blood sugar and counteract the ketoacidosis. Glucose administration should be deferred at this stage but will be needed once the acidosis has resolved. Potassium administration should be delayed until renal function is assessed and the serum potassium is < 5 mmol/L. Sodium bicarbonate is infrequently needed but in the case of circulatory collapse with a pH < 7, it may exceptionally be used. Artificial ventilation may be required if cardiorespiratory collapse or cerebral oedema ensues. If ventilation is required, it is essential to maintain a mild respiratory hyperventilation to partially compensate for the severe metabolic acidosis.

Further reading

Bristow P, Hillman K 1999 Management of hyperglycaemic diabetic emergencies. In: Webb AR, Shapiro MJ, Singer M, Suter PM, eds. *Oxford Textbook of Critical Care,* Oxford University Press, Oxford.

Answer 6.15

a. Weight remains the best long-term guide to overall health. A loss of 10% of body mass is serious; when 25% or more is lost the patient is unlikely to survive. Serum albumin has been cited as a useful investigation; however, being a reactive-phase protein it does not have a great role in the short term, and is limited prognostically. The relatively low serum glucose and low creatinine may suggest there is little glycogen and muscle reserve in the body and this is also seen in anorexia nervosa, as is severe hypokalaemia.

Various formulae exist to assess caloric requirements on a daily basis and the influence of activity. The best known of these is the Harris–Benedict equation, but it is not ideal for the critically ill patient. In the critically ill setting, the Weir formula is sometimes favoured when a metabolic cart can accurately measure oxygen utilisation and carbon dioxide production.

The Harris–Benedict equation

Basal energy expenditure (BEE) (males)
= 66.5 + (13.7 × weight) + (5 × height) − (6.8 × years)

BEE (females)
= 655 + (9.6 × weight) + (1.8 × height) − (4.7 × years)

Formula is 'weighted' for temperature every + 1°C × 1.07; × 1.2 for minor injury; × 1.8 for major injury.

The Weir equation

Energy expenditure
$$= 1440 \times [(3.9 \times V_{O_2}) + 1 \times V_{CO_2}]$$

b. This patient has multiple electrolyte abnormalities and is dehydrated. She is also significantly hypomagnesaemic and hypokalaemic, both of which are often forgotten as causes of perioperative muscle weakness and respiratory failure. Skin and pressure area care is of paramount importance. Similarly, such a frail patient will be less mobile, prone to venous thrombosis and contractures.

c. Until recently, the effect of nutritional support upon short-term survival was not clear. However, two studies involving immunonutritional additives (glutamine i.v.; arginine, RNA and ω-3 fatty acids) have resulted in a lower mortality in critically ill patients.

Further reading

Hardy G 1997 Third Oxford Glutamine Workshop. *Symposium Nutrition* 13: 726.
Beale R 1999 Immunonutrition in the ICU. *International Journal of Intensive Care* 6(1): 12–17.
Christman JW, McCain RW 1993 A sensible approach to the nutritional support of mechanically ventilated critically ill patients. *Intensive Care Medicine* 19: 129–136.

Answer 6.16

a. There is a large amount of ascites, seen as dark areas, with the hepatic bed and gall bladder well visualised.

b. Simple aspiration with needle and syringe, guided by ultrasonography if ascites are not marked or are loculated. Fluid should be sent for protein levels, culture and sensitivity and cytology.

c. Respiration will be compromised by the grossly distended abdomen. Lying such a patient flat to insert a central line or to nurse may precipitate cardiorespiratory arrest. Pain will require treatment, and non-respiratory depressant drugs such

as Tramadol may be preferred. Immobility increases risks of pressure sores and DVTs. Spontaneous bacterial peritonitis should be considered. The cause of the ascites will need further investigation, predominantly devoted to liver and cardiac origins.

d. There are numerous causes of ascites, although chronic liver failure with portal hypertension is the most common. The effects of congestive heart failure, constrictive pericarditis and inferior vena cava obstruction can produce a similar effect. Malignancy, acute or chronic infection, e.g. tuberculosis, *Pneumococcus*, malnutrition, severe hypoalbuminaemia and renal failure need to be considered, as does a pancreatic or biliary leak. It is also worth considering iatrogenic causes such as peritoneal dialysis and a urinary catheter inserted through the bladder.

Further reading

Sanchez-Fueyo A, Rodes J 1999 Ascites. *Medicine* 27: 75–76.

Answer 6.17

a. This is a metabolic acidosis, with incomplete respiratory compensation. A metabolic acidosis is due to either the accumulation of acids or the loss of bicarbonate in the body. The patient is also relatively hypoxic. This can lead to tissue and cellular damage as well as hyperventilation and a respiratory alkalosis.

b. A metabolic acidosis can be defined by either an increased or normal anion gap metabolic acidosis. The anion gap is the difference between the measured cations (Na and K) and anions (Cl and HCO_3). This is normally 12 ± 2 mmol/L and is accounted for by unmeasured anions including albumin, inorganic phosphate, lactate and sulphate. Increased anion gap acidosis is caused by the increase in organic acids, such as lactate, and is therefore a common feature in critically ill patients, as in this case. Normal anion gap acidosis is due to bicarbonate loss and chloride gain (also called hyperchloraemic acidosis).

c. Increased anion gap metabolic acidosis is seen in lactic acidosis, ketoacidosis, ingestion of certain poisons, notably ethylene glycol and methanol, aspirin overdose and uraemia. Tissue hypoxia is such a common feature of critical illness that many patients develop tissue hypoxia leading to anaerobic glycolysis by conversion of pyruvate to lactate. It is also worth remembering that the impact of severe illness also compromises renal and liver function, which can also result in derangement of lactate metabolism.

Normal anion gap acidosis is also more common than appreciated in the critically ill patient. Excessive loss of bicarbonate is common in association with diarrhoea and conditions such as pancreatitis and small bowel fistulae. It can also occur with parenteral nutrition and large-volume saline infusions.

Further reading

Forrest DM, Russell JA 1999 Metabolic acidosis. In: Webb AR, Shapiro MJ, Singer M, Suter PM, eds. *Oxford Textbook of Critical Care*. Oxford University Press, Oxford, ch. 8.3.

Answer 6.18

a. He has a severe respiratory acidosis. The high bicarbonate indicates long-standing CO_2 retention and chronic metabolic compensation, but the severity of the P_aCO_2 rise and acidosis indicates an acute relapse.

b. The CXR is a PA film. There is a severe kyphoscoliosis. There are no visible lung markings on the right-hand side and the ribs are collapsed downwards. There are multiple small areas of calcification in the left lung filed. This is consistent with previous TB and an old right-sided thoracoplasty has been carried out for TB. Although effective treatment when performed, thoracoplasty may severely compromise respiratory function, which is not initially noted, but becomes more marked as the patient ages.

c. This patient is in type II respiratory failure. Lung reserve is severely reduced

and, if intubated and ventilated, weaning will be prolonged and difficult. There is increasing evidence that non-invasive positive pressure ventilation (NIPPV) may improve survival. This should be combined with controlled oxygen therapy aiming for a P_aO_2 around 8 kPa, humidification if chest productive, physiotherapy and nebulised β-agonists if wheeze is present. Steroids and antibiotics should be considered.

If he tires despite this treatment then the outlook is poor. Intubation and ventilation should be carried out if that is in accordance with the patient's wishes. Early extubation should be attempted after 24 h and NIPPV tried again. If this fails, early tracheostomy should be considered. A high P_aO_2 during ventilation may help to decrease respiratory drive, but when weaning, P_aO_2 and P_aCO_2 around 7 kPa are acceptable. Attention should be paid to hydration and nutrition as such patients have often been ill for a number of days and cardiovascular collapse on intubation is common. If ventilated, mortality may be as high as 50%.

Further reading

Juniper MC, Hardinge FM 1998 Noninvasive ventilation: A technique with increasing applications. *Care of the Critically Ill* 14: 201–205.
Plant PK, Owen JL, Elliott MW 2000 Early use of non-invasive ventilation for acute exacerbations of chronic obstructive pulmonary disease on general respiratory wards: a multicentre randomised controlled trial. *Lancet* 355:1931–1935.

Answer 6.19

a. As little as 10 tablets of paracetamol can kill. It is one of the common causes of acute hepatic failure in the UK. The patient should be referred to a regional liver unit. A paracetamol level should be checked with a blood glucose level, prothrombin time (which uncorrected is used as a guide to liver deterioration), electrolytes, as renal failure is common (75% of paracetamol overdoses with fulminant hepatic failure), and routine liver function tests. N-acetylcysteine is a proven antidote for paracetamol. It improves survival if given in the first 36 h and may be beneficial when given later than this. Sucralfate is useful in these cases to provide gastric protection. The progress of such patients is inevitably poor and they should be admitted to a critical care facility and invasively monitored. Pancreatitis occurs in 15%.

b. Progressive encephalopathy, a pH of 7.3, a PT of > 50 s, hypoglycaemia and a serum creatinine > 200 µmol/L are all indications for transfer to a specialist centre. Intracranial hypertension is common. Such patients must be moved anaesthetised and paralysed, and intracranial pressure monitoring may be considered. The patient may deteriorate rapidly. Ideally, all venous lines should be placed in the left side of the neck to leave access if transplantation goes ahead for a RIS (rapid infusion system) and pulmonary artery catheter. As long as the patient is not actively bleeding, it is not necessary to correct the coagulopathy with clotting factors. This interferes with assessment of PT, a useful indicator of hepatic function. Insertion of central access lines should therefore be by an experienced doctor. An orogastric tube should be placed. If renal impairment is present, continuous venovenous haemofiltration (CVVH) may be useful to assist in control of intracranial hypertension and regulate the electrolyte and metabolic changes. These patients frequently appear to be 'septic', usually exhibiting hypotension with an increased cardiac output. Noradrenaline (norepinephrine) may be required. This patient's rapid downhill course suggests he will die unless transplanted soon.

c. Medical treatment alone is insufficient in paracetamol-induced fulminant liver failure and is associated with a high mortality. A liver transplant is often the only solution. The criteria for listing for transplantation are a pH < 7.3, a PT >

100 s, a serum creatinine > 300 µmol/L and grade 3–4 encephalopathy. Survival without transplantation is poor (20%) but with transplantation this rises to 60%.

Further reading
Eckhardt K-M 1999 Renal failure in liver disease. *Intensive Care Medicine* 25: 5–14.
Makin AJ, Williams R 1996 Acetaminophen overdose and acute liver failure: modern management. In: Vincent J-L, ed. *Yearbook of Intensive Care and Emergency Medicine*. Springer Verlag, Berlin, pp. 659–671.

Answer 6.20

a. This is an AP erect CXR. There is opacification of the left hemithorax with loss of the diaphragm and an air bronchogram is visible.

b. This is compatible with a bronchopneumonia.

c. This is a community-acquired pneumonia and in the elderly is likely to be secondary to *Streptococcus pneumoniae* or *Haemophilus influenzae*. Other organisms include *Staphylococcus aureus*, particularly during influenza epidemics, *Klebsiella*, *Pseudomonas aeruginosa*, *Mycoplasma tuberculosis* and Gram-negative organisms, particularly following a history of aspiration. Atypical organisms include *Legionella pneumophila*, *Mycoplasma pneumoniae* and *Chlamydia pneumoniae*. These should respond to erythromycin. If he keeps pigeons or parrots then infection with *Chlamydia psittaci* may be causative and require tetracycline.

Treatment is supportive in the first instance, involving oxygen, intravenous fluid resuscitation to correct dehydration, and consideration for invasive or non-invasive ventilation. Physiotherapy should be instituted. Serology should be sent for atypical community-acquired pneumonias. After taking appropriate cultures, intravenous antibiotics should be commenced. Absolute recommendations depend upon local policy and individual clinical circumstances, but in this case, cefuroxime 750–1.5 g i.v. 8 h + erythromycin 500 mg i.v. 6 h, with the addition of flucloxacillin 1 g 6 h if it follows influenza would be appropriate. Antibiotic therapy should be adjusted once sensitivities are known. In atypical or pneumococcal pneumonias, treatment should usually be for 10 days.

If the patient is intubated and ventilated, then enteral feeding should be commenced immediately and early tracheostomy and weaning considered. A bronchoscopy is recommended during the critically ill phase if diagnosis proves difficult or to clear secretions. If not performed at this time, then a fibreoptic bronchoscopy should be performed during recovery to exclude tumour deposit at the left main stem bronchus, predisposing to obstruction.

Answer 6.21

a. The AP erect CXR shows a large cystic mass in the left side of the chest with a fluid level. The mediastinum is shifted to the right. The lateral CXR shows this mass to cover the entire hemithorax and has a suggestion of septal lines at its base.
b. The differential diagnosis is of an abscess cavity ± bronchopleural fistula, massive hiatus hernia or diaphragmatic hernia with bowel herniated into chest. The clinical history suggests the presence of an acutely decompensating lesion rather than a picture of sepsis. The size and characteristic features on the lateral CXR imply stomach herniation through a diaphragmatic defect, and the suggestion of septal lines within the abscess implies the presence of bowel. This can be confirmed by enteral contrast studies and thoracic CT.
c. Deviation of the mediastinum implies that the mass is under high pressure and is pushing the mediastinum to the right. This may severely impair cardiac output similarly to a tension pneumothorax. Immediate treatment involves decompression of the mass. This is clearly massive gastric dilatation

and insertion of a wide-bore nasogastric tube will decompress it and restore cardiac output. If this was a massive abscess cavity then insertion of a left chest drain may be considered.

Further reading
Gardner S, Gedney J 2000 Mediastinal tamponade due to gastric distension. *Anaesthesia* 55: 296–298.

Answer 6.22

a. The CXR is a supine AP film. The trachea is intubated. There is a right subclavian line in a good position. The cardiac outline is increased, there is bilateral hilar enlargement and there is increased opacification in the lower zones bilaterally. There is also a pleural plaque at the right base.
b. The CT scan shows posterior pulmonary collapse and consolidation, with surrounding pleural effusions.
c. Treatment should include prone ventilation. This may improve oxygenation immediately by redistributing blood to uncollapsed, previously non-dependent lung tissue and redistributing gas flow by altering diaphragmatic position. Other beneficial effects over subsequent hours include redistribution of oedema from previously dependent areas, opening up of collapsed lung units and improvement in sputum clearance. Overall ventilation–perfusion matching should be improved.

Answer 6.23

a. He has a hypochloraemic, hypokalaemic metabolic alkalosis with partial respiratory compensation. He is also dehydrated, has impaired renal function and hypoxaemia.
b. This metabolic profile is a result of duodenal obstruction secondary to inflammation adjacent to the oedematous pancreas. The biochemical picture is similar to that of paediatric pyloric stenosis.

Metabolic alkalosis is due to either a gain in alkali or a loss of non-respiratory acid. In this case there has been continued loss of H+ and Cl− by vomiting. Renal compensation in this situation is usually effective, however the bicarbonate generated in hydrochloric acid (HCl) production has exceeded the renal ability to excrete bicarbonate. Chloride and potassium depletion along with decreased effective blood volume exacerbate the condition. Inappropriate fluid replacement has precipitated the current decline. The urinary chloride concentration is low. This type of alkalosis tends to respond to chloride administration.

c. His clinical condition has deteriorated and his airway is compromised, leaving him at risk of aspiration of gastric contents. He requires endotracheal intubation, oxygen and fluid resuscitation. Ongoing saline resuscitation along with a potassium chloride infusion (titrated to biochemical response) is required. Invasive haemodynamic monitoring is helpful to titrate fluid and electrolyte management. Evidence for the use of hydrochloric acid is sparse. Some suggested indications for its use are:

- serious clinical complications (coma, arrhythmias)
- contraindications to, or ineffectiveness of, other treatments
- severe alkalaemia (pH > 7.55)
- respiratory failure with hypercapnia and/or hypoxaemia.

A nasojejunal tube (cautiously sited via endoscopy) and enteral nutritional support should be considered.

Further reading

Brimioulle S et al 1989 Hydrochloric acid infusion for the treatment of metabolic acidosis associated with respiratory acidosis. *Critical Care Medicine* 17: 232–236.

Answer 6.24

a. This patient has a mixed respiratory and metabolic acidaemia. The clinical history suggests that his underlying metabolic acidosis from his chronic renal failure

has been exacerbated by an acute respiratory acidaemia.

b. This is an AP CXR. There is cardiomegaly (even given the AP projection), bilateral perihilar shadowing, increased vascular markings and Kerly B lines.

c. He has developed acute pulmonary oedema secondary to fluid overload. This results in hypoxaemia and an increased work of breathing. Respiratory decompensation leads to a rise in P_aCO_2, which subsequently worsens his acidaemia, further impairing his respiratory and cardiac function.

d. He is currently unconscious and requires immediate attention to his airway. Endotracheal intubation and mechanical ventilation are indicated. He then requires urgent dialysis to correct his acidosis and remove excess fluid. Underlying sepsis, particularly chest infection or urinary tract infection, should be sought. If his level of consciousness improves with oxygen alone then non-invasive ventilation and vasodilator therapy may be considered. Complications of invasive ventilation in this patient group are common and potentially life-threatening (e.g. myocardial decompensation, nosocomial pneumonia).

Answer 6.25

a. This CXR shows an intubated patient with a PAFC in place. He has ECG and external pacing pads in situ, along with a left internal jugular rapid infusion line, right internal jugular central line. There are also nasogastric and nasojejunal tubes in situ. In addition, there is an area of opacification to the left of the mediastinum around the pulmonary notch and at the tip of the PAFC. This represents a pulmonary artery haematoma.

b. The pulmonary artery haematoma may have been due to overinflation of the balloon in a small pulmonary vessel. This haematoma has subsequently bled into his airways, causing the extensive pulmonary haemorrhage.

c. He may require intubation and ventilation if severely hypoxic. His coagulopathy should be corrected with fresh frozen plasma and a platelet transfusion. He should be placed with the bleeding side in a dependent position to minimise contamination of the healthy lung, and selective main stem endobronchial intubation considered. Positive end-expiratory pressure may assist in tamponading bleeding, especially from pulmonary artery lesions. Massive haemoptysis is defined as blood loss that is greater than 600 mL/h or that is life-threatening. In the event of continued bleeding, bronchoscopy and bronchial irrigation with cold saline or adrenaline (epinephrine) may be attempted. Additional intervention with endobronchial balloon tamponade or arterial embolisation is usually successful. Surgical intervention may ultimately be required.

Further reading

Zürcher Zenklusen R, Jolliet P 1999 Haemoptysis. In: Webb AR, Shapiro MJ, Singer M, Suter PM, eds. *Oxford Textbook of Critical Care*. Oxford University Press, Oxford.

Answer 6.26

a. This patient has presented with acute adrenal insufficiency. This is an Addisonian crisis. Hyponatraemia and hyperkalaemia in a shocked patient suggest Addison's disease. They are frequently associated with hypoglycaemia and hypotension. A Na:K ratio < 25:1 is especially suggestive of acute adrenocortical insufficiency. Gradually worsening symptoms of cortisol deficiency may rapidly deteriorate to a life-threatening shock state, when patients encounter stress such as trauma or infection.

b. Early symptoms may be minimal and vague. Physical signs may include hyperpigmentation occurring on skin exposed to light, skinfolds, gums, tongue, scars, areolae and genitals. This pigmentation is due to raised circulating melanocyte-stimulating hormone and other hormones. Postural hypotension may be present, progressing to shock in severe cases.

c. Investigations helpful in the positive diagnosis of an Addisonian crisis include electrolyte estimation and plasma pituitary and adrenal hormones. Initial random, plasma cortisol levels in a stress situation should be greater than 500 nmol/L. A short synacthen (tetracosactrin 250 mg) test should stimulate a significant rise in cortisol production at 30 and 60 min post-injection. Plasma adrenocorticotrophic hormone (ACTH) will be elevated in primary adrenocortical insufficiency (reduced adrenal function), and low or normal in secondary adrenocortical insufficiency (inadequate secretion of ACTH from the pituitary).

d. Management should involve immediate attention to airway maintenance, breathing and circulation. Corticosteroids should be given as soon as possible. Dexamethasone 10 mg i.v. is given as the first random cortisol level is taken. It does not interfere with the further stages of the synacthen test. Normal saline fluid resuscitation is commenced and titrated to response. This may require invasive monitoring; however, several litres of fluid are frequently required during the first 12 h. Dextrose should simultaneously be infused to prevent hypoglycaemia. Maintenance corticosteroid therapy should then be provided with hydrocortisone. A thorough search for any precipitating pathology (e.g. sepsis) should be initiated. Further investigations will then be required following resuscitation and stabilisation.

Answer 6.27

a. This patient has a high-output, low-resistance shocked state and is hypotensive. She has a low MAP and is particularly at risk of cerebral and renal hypoperfusion. These patients frequently develop cerebral oedema and hence may require an augmented MAP to ensure adequate cerebral perfusion. She has a low left-sided filling pressure.

b. She needs fluid loading to optimise her filling pressure. However, to achieve adequate organ perfusion, her SVR should be increased with a vasoconstrictor, e.g. noradrenaline (norepinephrine). Particular attention to glycaemic and electrolyte control is essential. Her acid–base status is likely to deteriorate and renal replacement therapy may be required. Correction of her underlying coagulopathy should be considered, as the decision to transplant has already been made and her PT is no longer required as a marker of disease severity.

Answer 6.28

a. This patient has a hyperosmolar non-ketotic (HONK) coma. She is profoundly hyperglycaemic, but bicarbonate is 19 mmol/L, suggesting that she is not severely acidotic.

b. The osmolarity can be easily estimated by adding 2 × Na + urea + glucose. In this case, this is 358. The normal range is 280–300.

c. HONK occurs in uncontrolled diabetes mellitus. It is less common than diabetic ketoacidosis (DKA). The syndrome is classically described when the plasma osmolarity is greater than 350 mOsm/L, there is a markedly raised plasma glucose level and minimal or no ketones detectable. Its onset is more insidious than DKA and many of the patients have no previous history of diabetes. Patients are frequently elderly or institutionalised and may be unable to correct their dehydration themselves. The pre-hospital osmotic diuresis is prolonged, leading to life-threatening dehydration on presentation. In contrast to DKA, acidosis is usually mild or absent and insulin deficiency is less severe. Many patients do, however, have ketosis but this is usually only mild. The degree of mental impairment

correlates with the severity of hyperosmolarity. Approximately 50% of patients have a clear diabetic stressor event (such as infection or myocardial infarction).

d. These patients should be managed in a critical care facility. Therapy aims to correct the hyperosmolarity and restore the circulating intravascular volume whilst preventing further complications and seeking a precipitating cause. Glucose levels will correct substantially with saline resuscitation alone and insulin requirements are significantly less than in DKA. Blood glucose measurements should be performed at least hourly and frequent electrolyte (including magnesium and phosphate levels) and arterial gas analyses should be performed. The use of hypotonic solutions is controversial.

Answer 6.29

a. The CXR is an AP film. The most obvious abnormality is a hazy opacification of both lung fields. The cardiac outline is normal. The patient is intubated, has a left internal jugular line in place and a PAFC in a satisfactory position. Sternal wires are seen.

The CT scan of the chest shows the typical appearances of solid areas of consolidated lung, dependent areas of atelectasis and an overall ground-glass appearance. The patchy nature of the disease process is obvious as is the predominance of the congested oedematous lung in dependent areas.

b. The patient has acute respiratory distress syndrome (ARDS). This is characterised by tachypnoea, severe hypoxaemia and the presence of diffuse bilateral pulmonary infiltrates in the absence of signs of left ventricular failure. In left ventricular failure or acute volume overload, the pulmonary artery occlusion pressure (PAOP) should be 18 mmHg or greater. The degree of hypoxaemia distinguishes acute lung injury (ALI), $P_aO_2/F_iO_2 < 40$ kPa, from ARDS, where $P_aO_2/F_iO_2 < 27$ kPa. There

6

A

should also be a recognised precipitating cause to make the diagnosis.

c. Initiating insults may be either direct or indirect pulmonary insults. Inhalation of gastric contents or noxious substances (fumes etc.) along with near drowning and pulmonary emboli directly affect the lungs. Extrapulmonary causes include severe shock (ischaemia and reperfusion injuries), massive transfusion, pancreatitis, infections (systemic and pulmonary), toxins, extracorporeal circulation, trauma and burns.

d. There is no specific treatment for ARDS, and management is essentially supportive. Prevention of further complications is essential, and improved outcomes have been demonstrated using lung protective ventilatory strategies. These minimise peak airway pressures and tidal volumes, whilst maintaining adequate oxygenation. This usually results in a significant rise in P_aCO_2. Additional management strategies have involved changes in patient positioning (prone ventilation, although this may be contraindicated after a recent sternotomy), inhaled nitric oxide and extracorporeal oxygenation. The use of steroids during the fibroproliferative phase of the illness may improve outcome.

Further reading

Acute Respiratory Distress Syndrome Network 2000 Ventilation with lower tidal volumes as compared with traditional tidal volumes for acute lung injury and the acute respiratory distress syndrome. *New England Journal of Medicine* 342: 1301–1308.

Deby-Dupont G, Lamy M 1999 Pathophysiology of acute respiratory distress syndrome and acute lung injury. In: Webb AR, Shapiro MJ, Singer M, Suter PM, eds. *Oxford Textbook of Critical Care*. Oxford University Press, Oxford.

Gattinoni L et al 1991 Body position changes redistribute lung computed tomographic density in patients with acute respiratory failure. *Anesthesiology* 74:15–23.

Meduri GU et al 1998 Effect of prolonged methylprednisolone therapy in unresolving acute respiratory distress syndrome – a randomized controlled trial. *Journal of the American Medical Association* 280: 159–165.

Answer 6.30

a. This is a slightly overpenetrated CXR. The lung fields are hyperinflated with flattening of the right diaphragm. Multiple cavitating lesions are seen in the lung fields, particularly at both bases and both apices. The cardiac outline is normal.

b. The diagnosis is a cavitating bronchopneumonia. The association of a high temperature, rigors and a cavitating pneumonia is strongly suggestive of *Staphylococcus aureus*. Other causes of cavitating pneumonias include *Klebsiella*, histoplasmosis, tuberculosis, hydatid disease and fungi.

c. Staphylococcal pneumonias often spread to the lungs from haematogenous spread or aspiration. This young man is an injecting drug user with a systolic murmur and it is likely that he has staphylococcal endocarditis, probably on his tricuspid valve. He needs repeat blood cultures and echocardiography.

7

OBSTETRIC ANAESTHESIA

Pregnancy is a time of major physiological change in the mother. As a result, the normal ranges for many clinical data are altered. Failure to recognise this may result in misinterpretation of data. In particular, laboratory 'normal' ranges, often printed alongside blood results, may not apply in pregnancy.

PHYSIOLOGICAL CHANGES IN PREGNANCY

Haematological changes (Table 7.1)
Total blood volume increases during pregnancy, due to an increase in both red cell mass and plasma volume. The percentage increase in plasma volume is greater than that of red cell mass, leading to a fall in haematocrit and haemoglobin concentration. This fall occurs even if iron and folate supplements are given. The mean cell haemoglobin concentration (MCHC) is unchanged whilst the mean cell volume (MCV) increases slightly.

Platelet count is unchanged in normal pregnancy. White cell count (WCC) may increase to 9.0×10^9/l by the end of the final trimester due to an increase in neutrophils. There may be a further marked rise in WCC during labour to around 40×10^9/l.

Plasma protein concentration is reduced, mainly due to a fall in albumin concentration of about 10 g/l to around 35 g/l, and plasma globulins increase slightly. As a result of these changes, plasma colloid osmotic pressure falls by around 2 mmHg. Plasma cholinesterase levels fall by around 25%.

Pregnant women are hypercoagulable. Fibrinogen levels rise to around 5.5 g/l from the non-pregnant level of 3 g/l. Clotting factors 7, 8, 9 and 10 are all increased. Fibrinolytic activity is reduced.

Respiratory changes (Table 7.2)
Minute ventilation increases in the second and third trimesters. This is principally due

Table 7.1 Haematological changes during pregnancy

	Non-pregnant	Pregnant
Plasma volume (l)	3	4.2 by 32 weeks
Red cell mass (ml)	1400	1640
Haematocrit	0.4–0.5	0.31–0.35
Haemoglobin g/dl	12.0	11
White cell count ($\times 10^9$)	5–10	9.0
Fibrinogen g/l	2.5–4.0	3.5–6.0

Table 7.2 Respiratory changes during pregnancy

	Non-pregnant	Pregnant
Respiratory rate (per min)	15	15
Tidal volume (ml/min)	500	700
Expiratory reserve volume (ml)	1300	1100
Residual volume (ml)	1500	1200
Oxygen consumption (ml/min)	200	250

to an increase in tidal volume of around 40%. Total lung volume, forced vital capacity, forced expiratory volume and respiratory rate remain unchanged. Functional residual capacity falls as both the expiratory reserve volume and residual capacity are reduced. Typical arterial blood gases in late pregnancy are as follows:

- pH, 7.45
- P_aO_2, 13.5 kPa
- P_aCO_2, 4.0 kPa
- standard HCO_3, 22 mmol/l
- base excess (BE), −3 mmol/l.

Note that:

- Increase in minute volume causes a decrease in arterial CO_2 below non-pregnant levels, which improves the ability of the fetus to excrete CO_2 via a concentration gradient.
- A mild compensatory metabolic acidosis develops, although this is insufficient to compensate for the respiratory alkalosis completely.
- P_aO_2 changes little.

Cardiovascular changes (Table 7.3)
These may be summarised as follows:

- Cardiac output increases by around 40% from the first trimester.

- This is a result of both increased heart rate (15 beats/min) and increased stroke volume.
- Systemic vascular resistance falls.
- Systolic and diastolic blood pressure fall in early pregnancy, returning to pre-pregnant levels towards term.
- Central venous pressure (CVP) is unchanged, although rises occur in labour during contractions and marked rises may occur during maternal expulsive efforts.
- Pulmonary capillary wedge pressure (PCWP) rises slightly. The combination of this and the fall in colloid osmotic pressure predisposes the pregnant woman to pulmonary oedema if there is any further rise in left ventricular pre-load.

Assessment of renal function (Table 7.4)
- Glomerular filtration rate increases by 50% above non-pregnant levels, resulting in increased urea and creatinine clearance. The normal upper level of these substances in plasma is therefore reduced to 4.5 mmol/L and 75 µmol/L, respectively.
- Serum urate levels are reduced in early pregnancy, but rise slightly above non-pregnant levels by term (270 µmol/L). Uric acid levels are raised in pre-

Table 7.3 Cardiovascular changes during pregnancy

	Non-pregnant	First trimester	Third trimester
Cardiac output (l/min)	4.5	6.0	6.0
Heart rate (beats/min)	70	85	85
Stroke volume (ml/beat)	64	71	71
Systolic blood pressure		Unchanged or slight decrease	Unchanged or slight decrease
Diastolic blood pressure		↓ 10–15 mmHg	Return to pre-pregnant level by 32 weeks
CVP (cmH_2O)	2.0–4.5	No change	No change

Table 7.4 Changes in renal function

	Non-pregnant	Pregnant
Urea (mmol/l)	2.5–7.0	2.0–4.5
Glomerular filtration rate (ml/min)	100	170
Serum creatinine (µmol/l)	50–120	25–75
Creatinine clearance (ml/min)	100	120–160
Serum urate (µmol/l)	250	100–270

eclampsia and closely correlate to the severity of the disease and perinatal morbidity and mortality.

- Serum sodium, potassium and chloride levels are unchanged, while serum osmolality declines by approximately 10 mmol/l to 280 mmol/l.
- Glycosuria is common in pregnancy, probably because renal tubular absorption of glucose is impaired.

Liver function tests (Table 7.5)
- Serum alkaline phosphatase (AP) increases two to four times the normal pre-pregnancy level, as a result of rises in both placental and bone isoenzymes. Liver AP does not change significantly.
- Serum gamma glutamyl transferase (γGT) levels do not change significantly.
- The upper limit of normal for aspartate transaminase (AST) and alanine transaminase (ALT) are lower than non-pregnant levels at 30 IU/l.
- Bilirubin levels remain within normal limits.

THE CARDIOTOCOGRAM (CTG)

Cardiotocography was introduced in the 1970s, without prior scrutiny by randomised controlled trials, to identify fetuses at risk of cerebral damage or perinatal death from the consequences of fetal asphyxia, permitting judicious timing and route of delivery. The promised reduction in adverse perinatal events such as cerebral palsy (and subsequent litigation costs) has failed to materialise. The incidence of cerebral palsy has changed little over the last 25 years and is known to be unrelated to intrapartum

events in 90% of cases and therefore little influenced by the introduction of fetal monitoring.

The most commonly used method for monitoring the fetal heart is external Doppler, or ultrasound, with a transducer placed on the maternal abdomen and connected to a CTG machine. A scalp electrode can be attached to the fetal head or buttock after rupture of the membranes, but is only used when external monitoring fails to give a trace of adequate quality.

The use of CTG has many disadvantages, particularly in low-risk women. Mobility in labour is restricted, increasing the need for analgesia and other obstetric interventions, such as augmentation. CTGs, if reassuring, have a high predictive value of a good outcome. However, a non-reassuring CTG has a low predictive value of a bad outcome. The resulting high number of false-positive CTGs dramatically increases both the caesarean section and operative vaginal delivery rate, unless used in conjunction with a fetal scalp pH measurement. 'Fetal distress' cannot, therefore, be diagnosed from a CTG in isolation, the only exception being a prolonged, profound bradycardia. The term 'non-reassuring fetal heart rate' has been introduced into obstetric practice in preference to the more inflammatory term 'fetal distress'.

The second major drawback of CTGs is their use in litigation, with many cases of litigation involving 'misinterpretation', inappropriate response to an abnormal CTG or lack of appropriate monitoring as major parts of the claim. This is compounded by the possibility of interobserver variation in interpretation,

Table 7.5 Changes in liver function

	Non-pregnant	Pregnant
Alkaline phosphatase (AP) (IU/l)	30–160	130–400
Bilirubin (μmol/l)	0–17	0–17
Albumin (IU/l)	35–50	↓ by 40%
Aspartate aminotransferase (AST) (IU/l)	< 40	< 30
Alanine aminotransferase (ALT) (IU/l)	< 40	< 30
Gamma-glutamyl transferase (γGT) (IU/l)	11–50	3–41

resulting in various 'experts' expressing widely differing opinions. CTGs are unhelpful in the successful defence of the majority of these claims.

Fetal monitoring is of most clinical benefit when it is related to the clinical risks of both the mother and fetus, the progress of labour and also combined with the prudent use of fetal blood sampling to identify fetuses likely to suffer the consequences of hypoxia, without unnecessarily increasing operative delivery rates.

Interpretation of a CTG

Interpretation of a CTG should be systematic, and must include assessment of:

- the maternal and fetal risks
- quality of the tracing
- uterine activity
- baseline heart rate
- baseline variability
- accelerations
- decelerations.

Maternal and fetal risks

The CTG provides information on both the fetal heart rate pattern and uterine activity. Antenatal monitors can also demonstrate the presence of fetal movements. The fetal heart rate should not be assessed in isolation as the presence of pre-existing fetal and/or maternal risks will influence the final conclusion (Table 7.6). The presence of particulate meconium, a growth-restricted fetus or maternal diabetes mellitus will influence the weight given to changes in the CTG. For example, in the presence of particulate meconium, one abnormality in the CTG, such as an uncomplicated fetal tachycardia, should

prompt further evaluation of the fetal status; whereas in the presence of clear liquor with no other risk factors, two CTG abnormalities, e.g. tachycardia with reduced variability, would normally be required to prompt further action.

Uterine activity

Similarly, uterine activity should be assessed for the presence or absence of contractions, their frequency and duration, to allow accurate interpretation of decelerations from the baseline. CTGs performed antenatally show the fetal response to Braxton–Hicks contractions or to fetal movement. Overuse of oxytocin in labour will produce hypertonic uterine activity that adversely affects fetal oxygenation leading to CTG changes. During normal labour the fetus will compensate for the temporary reduction in oxygen supply produced by uterine contractions. This mechanism begins to fail when the contractions are too frequent with little or no rest period to allow fetal recovery. The fetus will become hypoxic and develop a metabolic acidosis if this process is not reversed, for instance by switching off the oxytocin infusion.

Fetal heart rate pattern

The fetal heart rate pattern has four identifiable features:

- baseline rate
- baseline variability
- accelerations from the baseline
- decelerations from the baseline.

Baseline rate. The gestation needs to be known before interpreting a CTG, as the fetal heart slows with increasing

Table 7.6 Indications for fetal monitoring in labour

Maternal risks	Fetal risks	Risks in labour
Proteinuric hypertension	Growth restriction	Induced labour
Diabetes mellitus	Oligohydramnios	Augmented labour
Maternal infection	Particulate meconium	Epidural analgesia
Cardiac disease	Breech presentation	Previous caesarean delivery
Renal disease	Prematurity	Prolonged labour
Severe anaemia	Multiple pregnancy	Vaginal bleeding in labour

gestational age due to maturation of the fetal parasympathetic nervous system. The normal range is 110–150 beats/min at term. A change in the baseline rate is said to occur if it persists for more than 10 min and may be a bradycardia or tachycardia. A slow rise in the baseline over time is often missed and may indicate developing fetal hypoxia. Always inspect the full length of the CTG tracing.

Bradycardia. A mild bradycardia, 100–109 beats/min only, indicates hypoxia if associated with other suspicious CTG features, such as loss of variability or decelerations. Rates less than 100 beats/min may be associated with fetal congenital heart block. Prolonged, profound bradycardias with rates < 80 beats/min are often associated with severe hypoxia and should prompt urgent action to exclude reversible causes, such as maternal hypotension.

Tachycardia. A fetal heart rate of >150 and < 180 beats/min in the presence of an otherwise normal trace is rarely associated with hypoxia and does not require a scalp pH in labour unless another adverse factor exists, e.g. particulate meconium. More likely causes are maternal anxiety, tachycardia, dehydration, the use of beta-adrenergic agents (ritodrine) or fetal prematurity. However, a gradually increasing baseline with decreasing variability and/or decelerations is often associated with hypoxia.

Baseline variability. This relates to the fluctuations in the fetal heart rate around the baseline over a short period of time, usually 1 min. Variability may be normal at 10–25 beats/min, reduced at 5–10, or absent. The presence of normal variability reflects central nervous system activity and normal cardiac conductivity and, along with the presence of accelerations, is a positive indicator of fetal well-being.

Reduced variability is seen in healthy fetuses during the sleep–rest cycle which usually lasts for 20–40 min. Reduced variability may be caused by analgesia and anaesthesia, barbiturates and magnesium sulphate as well as steroid therapy to improve fetal lung maturation. Loss of

variability, particularly if associated with an increasing baseline rate or decelerations, suggests the presence of fetal hypoxia and is therefore a non-reassuring heart rate pattern.

Accelerations. These are increases in the baseline of at least 15 beats/min, which last for at least 15 s and are found in association with fetal movements or contractions. Their presence, almost always in a trace with normal variability, suggests fetal well-being. Hypoxia may develop gradually during labour with loss of accelerations as the first indication, followed by a rise in the baseline rate and loss of variability.

Decelerations. Decreases in the fetal heart rate from the baseline may be described by their relationship to the uterine contractions as early, late, variable or prolonged.

Early decelerations. These are mirror images of the contractions, the peak of the contraction corresponding to the nadir of the deceleration, and are not usually associated with fetal hypoxia. Early decelerations rarely go below 100 beats/min and are thought to be a vagal response to head compression, seen usually in the late first stage of labour.

Late decelerations. These begin after the contraction starts and return towards the baseline after the finish of the contraction. They may suggest the presence of fetal hypoxia due to uteroplacental insufficiency, particularly when persistent and associated with increasing frequency and depth or loss of variability.

In the initial stages of hypoxia, the increasing depth of the deceleration and prolonged recovery time reflect the increasing degrees of hypoxia. However, as hypoxia further increases in severity, the decelerations become shallower as a result of myocardial rather than CNS depression.

Occasional late decelerations are common in labour, often due to overstimulation with oxytocin. Epidural analgesia may also precipitate late decelerations, although this can largely be avoided by preventing maternal hypotension.

The simplest method to determine the type of deceleration present is to line a ruler, or piece of paper, vertically across the CTG paper, with its edge on the peak of a contraction. The nadir of an early deceleration will line up with the peak of the contraction, whereas a late deceleration has its nadir beyond the edge of the ruler.

Variable decelerations. These vary in their shape and onset in relation to the contraction, with a rapid descent and recovery. They occur frequently in the second stage of labour, due to cord compression. Normal variability (return to a normal baseline after the deceleration with accelerations immediately prior to and after the deceleration) is a reassuring feature. Features that change the CTG to a non-reassuring trace are loss of variability, increasing or decreasing baseline, loss of accelerations and slow recovery.

Prolonged decelerations. Decelerations lasting more than 60 seconds may occur in response to vaginal examination, cord prolapse or rapid descent of the fetal presenting part. A reversible cause should be sought immediately, turning the patient on her side, switching off the oxytocin infusion and excluding a cord prolapse. Lack of improvement in the CTG trace despite these measures should prompt delivery.

The speed with which delivery should occur depends on the urgency of the fetal situation and relates to:

- the gestation – premature babies have low tolerance levels for hypoxia
- the fetal heart rate – the lower the rate, the more urgent is the delivery
- loss of variability
- no evidence of recovery towards the baseline.

ASSESSING THE NEED FOR INTERVENTION

The CTG findings should be interpreted after consideration of the complete clinical picture. The CTG may then be described as:

- *Reassuring* – when there is no evidence of fetal compromise and all that is required is continued observation.
- *Non-reassuring* – the CTG contains abnormalities suggestive of fetal compromise, particularly if combined with adverse clinical features. Further action is required to reverse the underlying cause. If this fails to bring about improvement, fetal scalp sampling should be performed. Failure to obtain a fetal blood sample should prompt urgent delivery.
- *Pathological* – a prolonged, profound deceleration unresponsive to simple interventions. The fetus requires urgent delivery.

FURTHER READING

American College of Obstetricians and Gynecologists 1994 *Fetal Distress and Birth Asphyxia*. ACOG Committee Opinion. American College of Obstetricians and Gynecologists, Washington DC.

Balen AH, Smith JH 1992 *The CTG in Practice*. Churchill Livingstone, Edinburgh.

Blair E, Stanley FJ 1988 Intrapartum asphyxia: a rare cause of cerebral palsy. *Journal of Pediatrics* 112: 515–519.

Blair E, Stanley FJ 1993 When can cerebral palsy be prevented? The generation of causal hypothesis by multivariate analysis of a case control study. *Paediatrics & Perinatal Epidemiology* 7: 272–301.

Donker DK, van Geijin HP, Hasman A 1993 Interobserver variation in the assessment of fetal heart rate recordings. *European Journal of Obstetrics, Gynaecology & Reproductive Biology* 52: 21–28.

Ramsey MM, et al 2000 *Normal Values in Pregnancy*. WB Saunders, London.

Redman CWG, Beilin LJ, Bonnar J, Wilkinson RH 1976 Plasma urate measurements in predicting fetal death in hypertensive pregnancy. *Lancet* i: 1370–1373.

Rooth G, Huch A, Huch R 1987 Guidelines for the use of fetal monitoring. *International Journal of Obstetrics & Gynaecology* 25: 159–167.

Williams DJ 1997 Renal disease in pregnancy. *Current Opinion in Obstetrics & Gynaecology* 7: 156–162.

Yudkin PL, Johnson A, Clover LM, Murphy KW 1995 Assessing the contribution of birth asphyxia to cerebral palsy in term singletons. *Paediatrics & Perinatal Epidemiology* 9: 156–170.

QUESTIONS

Fetal heart rate (FHR)

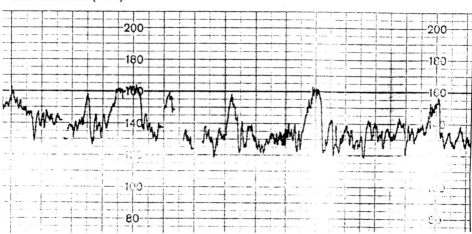

Uterine activity (UA)

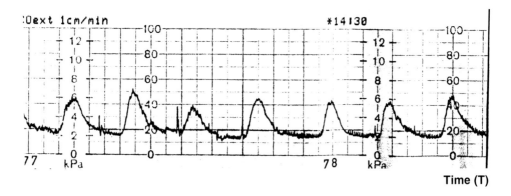

Time (T)

Question 7.1

A 21-year-old primigravida at term, with a normally grown fetus, is admitted in spontaneous labour. She is normotensive, the liquor is clear and the cervix is 2 cm dilated with a cephalic presentation at the spines. Her admission CTG is shown.

a. What clinical risks are present?
b. Describe the CTG findings.
c. What is the anaesthetic plan of action?
d. What obstetric actions should now be taken?

7

Q

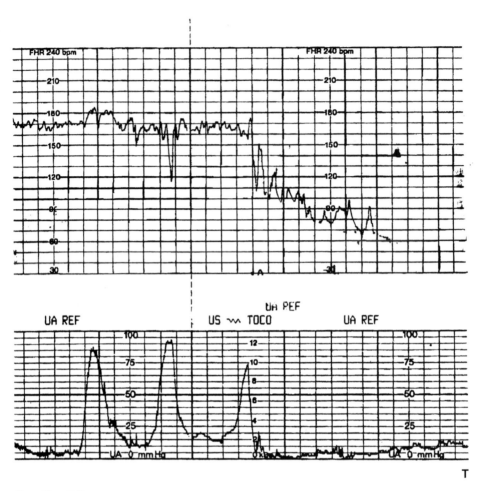

T

Question 7.2

The intrapartum CTG from a 40-year-old multiparous patient with a history of a previous caesarean section is shown. She is being induced at term because of proteinuric hypertension. She has not been seen by an anaesthetist at present.

a. What clinical risk factors are present?
b. Describe the CTG findings.
c. What should happen now?
d. Describe your anaesthetic plan.

FHR

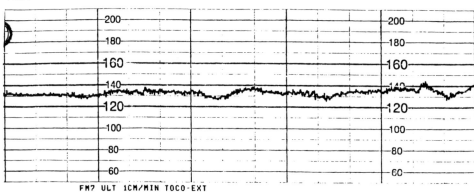

FM? ULT 1CM/MIN TOCO-EXT

UA

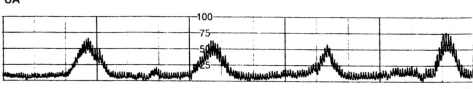

T

Question 7.3

This is an antenatal CTG from a 28-year-old primigravida seen in clinic at 37 weeks because of suspected fetal growth restriction. She gives a history of vague abdominal tightenings for 6 h, during which time she felt no fetal movements. The fundal height measures 28 cm. A scan shows oligohydramnios with the fetal abdominal circumference and biparietal diameter below the fifth centile. The cervix is very unfavourable on vaginal examination.

a. What clinical risks are present?
b. Describe the CTG findings.
c. What should be done now?
d. What is your anaesthetic management?

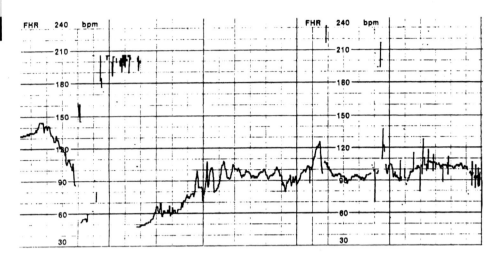

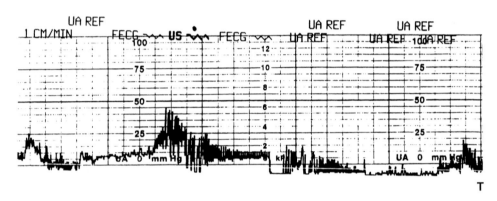

Question 7.4

This is the CTG from a 16-year-old unbooked primigravida admitted fully dilated at 39 weeks after a vaginal bleed. The mother is clammy and pale and very anxious. Her blood pressure is 120/70 mmHg with a heart rate of 100 beats/min. The presentation of the fetus is cephalic with 0/5 palpable per abdomen.

a. What clinical risks are present?
b. Describe the CTG findings.
c. What clinical conditions would give rise to these features?
d. Outline further management.

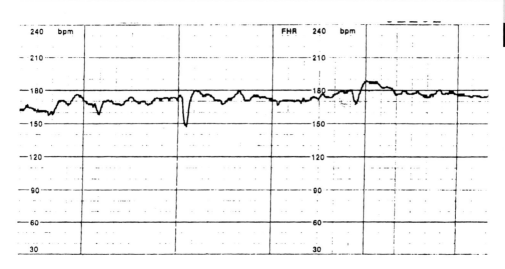

22:20

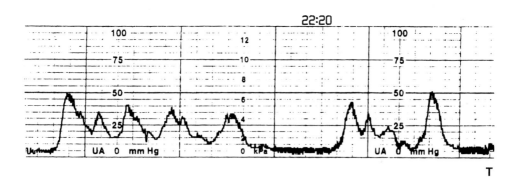

T

Question 7.5

This is the CTG of a 28-year-old woman, para 3, in spontaneous labour at 38 weeks. The fetus is normally grown. The cervix is 5 cm dilated with a cephalic presentation at the spines. Fresh, particulate meconium is obtained at artificial rupture of the membranes (ARM).

a. What clinical risks are present?
b. Describe the CTG findings.
c. What obstetric interventions are required?
d. What anaesthetic interventions are likely to be required?

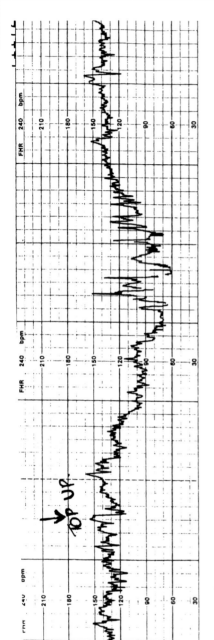

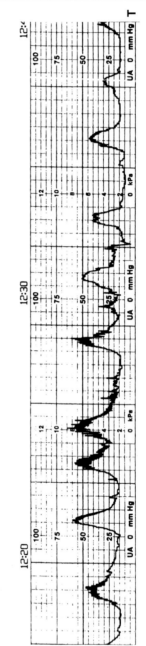

Question 7.6

This is the CTG from a 25-year-old woman, in her first pregnancy, at 41 weeks' gestation in spontaneous labour. She has an epidural in situ for analgesia and has just received a top-up with 10 mL of 0.25% bupivacaine. She complains of feeling nauseated and light-headed and her recorded blood pressure is now 90/50 mmHg, from a previous pressure of 120/70 mmHg.

a. What are the clinical risks?
b. Describe the CTG findings.
c. What is an appropriate management plan?

Question 7.7

A 30-year-old gravida 2, para 1, with a previous normal delivery at term, presented at 39 weeks' gestation in spontaneous labour. She was contracting 1 in 10, the presentation was cephalic, three-fifths palpable abdominally and the fetal heart was 140 beats/min and regular. A vaginal examination revealed a cervix 3 cm dilated with the head 2 cm above the ischial spines. The membranes were left intact.

Two hours later she had a spontaneous rupture of the membranes and a vaginal examination was performed to exclude cord prolapse. The cervix was 8 cm dilated with the head at 0–1 above the ischial spines. The fetal heart rate fell to 80 beats/min after the vaginal examination and she became sweaty and disorientated. She was immediately transferred to theatre for a caesarean section were she was found to be fully dilated and delivered by forceps of a stillborn male.

She had a massive postpartum haemorrhage (PPH) after delivery of the placenta and became hypotensive with a BP of 60/40 mmHg and a pulse of 140 beats/min. An examination under anaesthetic (EUA) was planned to exclude surgical causes of bleeding. On arrival in theatre she was noted to be cyanosed (oxygen saturation 60%). The patient was pre-oxygenated, anaesthetised and ventilated. No traumatic cause for the bleeding was found, although she was bleeding from vaginal grazes. Her full blood count and clotting results taken after the collapse are as follows: prothrombin time (PT), 44 s; activated partial thromboplastin time (APTT), 73 s; fibrinogen, < 0.5 g/l; D-dimer, > 32 000, < 64 000; haemoglobin, 10.6 g/dl; platelets, 90×10^9/l.

a. What are the differential diagnoses?
b. What do the blood results show?
c. Discuss the immediate management.

Question 7.8

A 25-year-old primigravida at 36 weeks' gestation presents with a 2-day history of upper abdominal pain, nausea, vomiting and stabbing pain between shoulder blades and passing dark urine. On examination she is jaundiced and afebrile with a blood pressure of 140/90 mmHg. Her chest is clear. The fundal height measures 33 cm, with a cephalic presentation, three-fifths palpable abdominally. The fetal heart cannot be heard and the diagnosis of an intrauterine death is confirmed on scan. Her blood results are as follows:

Na, 133 mmol/l	amylase, 64 IU/l	Hb, 12.6 g/dl
K, 3.9 mmol/l	bilirubin, 171 μmol/l	WCC, 19.6×10^9/l
urea, 9.8 mmol/l	ALT, 455 IU/l	platelets, 172×10^9/l
creatinine, 184 μmol/l	AST, 412 IU/L	PT, 24 s
HCO_3^-, 21 mmol/l	alkaline phosphatase, 598 IU/l	KCCT, 84 s
glucose, 6.2 mmol/l	albumin, 28.2 g/l	fibrinogen, 0.94 g/l
urine osmolarity, 533 mOsm		FDPs, > 80, < 160
plasma osmolarity, 277 mOsm.		

a. Describe the biochemical abnormalities.
b. Discuss the differential diagnoses and the most likely diagnosis.
c. Discuss the acute management of this patient.

7

Q

Question 7.9

A 27-year-old multigravida presents at term with a blood pressure of 170/115 mmHg, with ++proteinuria on dipstick. She is asymptomatic and the fetus appears to be normally grown. The following blood results are obtained: Hb, 11.0 g/dl; WCC, 10×10^9/l; platelet count, 110×10^9/l; urea, 5.6 mmol/l; urate, 500 mmol/l; creatinine, 100 µmol/l.

a. Describe the abnormal blood results.
b. What is the likely diagnosis?
c. Outline the management of this patient.

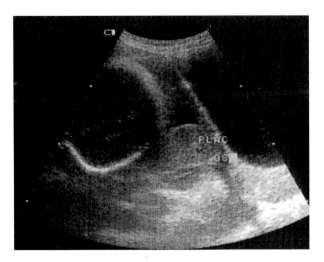

Question 7.10

A 35-year-old multiparous woman at 37 weeks' gestation presents with a history of slight vaginal bleeding. The estimated blood loss is 50 ml, the uterus is non-tender with a non-engaged fetal head presenting. The woman's blood pressure is 120/70 mmHg, pulse 80 beats/min, and the fetal heart is regular at 140 beats/min with a reassuring CTG. The ultrasound scan performed at 35 weeks is shown.

a. What does the scan show?
b. What is the likely obstetric plan?
c. Discuss her anaesthetic management.

ANSWERS

Answer 7.1

a. This woman has no obvious clinical risks.

b. There is uterine activity demonstrated with contractions occurring regularly, with five contractions every 10 min. The baseline rate is 130–135 beats/min with normal variability. Accelerations are present with no decelerations. Overall assessment: reassuring CTG from a low-risk labour.

c. This is a normal labour progressing satisfactorily. The provision of analgesia could safely be raised now, if it has not been discussed earlier, and placing of the epidural catheter, if requested, could be performed. Discussion with the mother and midwife followed by prescription of an appropriate regimen for labour and delivery is appropriate.

d. If epidural analgesia is not required, the CTG should be discontinued. The use of electronic monitoring will restrict the woman's mobility, increase her analgesic requirements and potentially lengthen her labour.

Answer 7.2

a. This woman has five risk factors: her age; multiparity; induction of labour; history of a previous caesarean section; proteinuric hypertension. Administering syntocinon to a multiparous woman exposes her to an increased risk of uterine hypertonicity and rupture. Multiparity is not a contraindication to the use of syntocinon, although great care must be employed and senior obstetric involvement in decision-making is advised.

b. There is uterine activity with powerful contractions followed by the apparent loss of uterine action. The fetal heart trace shows a tachycardia of 170 beats/min with reduced variability. There are no accelerations and a prolonged, sustained deceleration to 60 beats/min, the onset of which corresponds to the loss of uterine activity. The overall assessment is of a pathological CTG demonstrating the effects of uterine rupture on the fetal heart.

c. Immediate abdominal delivery is the only option. Both fetal and maternal mortality and morbidity are increased in the presence of a uterine rupture.

d. This is an obstetric emergency, and urgent delivery by caesarean section is necessary. Measures to reduce gastric pH – intravenous ranitidine and oral sodium citrate – are needed. The urgency of delivery probably precludes the option of regional anaesthesia and this should be discussed with the mother. Rapid-sequence induction of anaesthesia will be required, and measures taken to reduce the hypertensive response to intubation. This might include the use of alfentanil or i.v. magnesium. The presence of proteinuric hypertension requires very close perioperative monitoring and control of hypertension and fluid balance. Postnatal monitoring in an HDU environment for 24–48 h after delivery is appropriate.

Answer 7.3

a. Clinical risks: the fetus is growth-restricted; oligohydramnios.

b. There is uterine activity with contractions occurring every 4 min. The baseline rate is 135 beats/min with almost absent variability. There are no accelerations, but two shallow, late decelerations are seen, which are easily missed without close inspection. Overall assessment: non-reassuring CTG.

c. The clinical picture and CTG suggest a fetus requiring urgent delivery. Scalp pH sampling is not an option as the woman is not in labour.

d. This is an obstetric emergency in a patient from the antenatal clinic. Urgent delivery is essential to try to rescue the fetus but the risks of a full stomach and poor preoperative preparation are key factors in management. Immediate operation is not necessary, so there is some time to review the mother before surgery. Antacid prophylaxis and blood

7

A

cross-matching can be achieved whilst theatre is being organised. Regional anaesthesia is the safest option for the mother. Maternal hypotension must be avoided at all costs because of the already compromised fetus. Neonatal resuscitation must be available at delivery, and the baby may require to be transferred to the special care baby unit.

Answer 7.4

a. Clinical risks: no antenatal care; intrapartum bleeding.

b. The contraction trace is of poor quality and is therefore unhelpful. The baseline rate initially is 130 beats/min and falls rapidly to 90 beats/min with a sustained bradycardia. There are no accelerations present and the variability is reduced. Overall assessment: pathological CTG.

c. The history of blood loss in a woman who is clammy with a mild tachycardia could suggest that a significant degree of hypovolaemia is present, even though the blood pressure is normal. Common causes of significant bleeding in late pregnancy include both placenta praevia and placental abruption. In this case, placenta praevia is unlikely as the head is deeply engaged. Ultrasound can be used to exclude placenta praevia, but the urgent need for delivery precludes its use in this case.

d. The assessment of blood loss may be difficult, and you should be suspicious that she has a compensated hypovolaemia. Intravenous access with a large-bore cannula is essential, even if there is going to be an attempt at vaginal delivery. Blood should be taken for full blood count, clotting screen and cross-matching. This fetus requires urgent delivery in theatre, vaginally, if this would be a technically easy procedure; otherwise deliver by caesarean section.

If caesarean section is required, the urgency of delivery, likelihood of hypovolaemia, and possibility of clotting abnormalities associated with abruption all make general anaesthesia the preferable option. Neonatal support should be available at delivery.

Answer 7.5

a. Clinical risks: particulate meconium at ARM.

b. There is irregular uterine activity with contractions every 3–5 min. The baseline rate increases throughout the tracing from 160 to 180. The variability is reduced, with no acceleration and one late deceleration to 150 beats/min. Overall assessment: a non-reassuring CTG.

c. Fresh meconium increases the likelihood of acidosis in the presence of CTG abnormalities. As a general rule, one CTG abnormality in the presence of fresh meconium should prompt consideration of fetal blood sampling. Obstetric intervention will be on the basis of the pH result.

d. Although an epidural obstetric intervention will be on the basis of the pH result. Although an epidural would ensure comfort for the woman during the scalp sampling, the clinical situation would not allow time to establish epidural analgesia. It would certainly be appropriate to meet the mother at this stage and obtain an anaesthetic history since progression to caesarean section is likely.

Answer 7.6

a. Clinical risks: epidural analgesia; recent top-up.

b. The CTG shows regular uterine activity with four contractions every 10 min. The baseline rate is 130 beats/min initially with a prolonged bradycardia to 60 beats/min, the fetal heart recovering to a normal baseline thereafter. Accelerations are present prior to the deceleration with normal variability. The overall assessment is of a non-reassuring CTG due to a hypotension secondary to the epidural top-up. CTG becomes reassuring after treatment of hypotension.

c. Initial management should include

placing the mother in the full lateral position, increasing the rate of fluid administration and administration of a vasopressor (ephedrine). The value of fluid 'preloading' in preventing hypotension in this situation has frequently been questioned. Examination of the mother must exclude excessively high nerve blockade. Subsequently the mother should be discouraged from lying in an unwedged supine position.

Answer 7.7

a. Salient features are: sudden-onset fetal distress following rupture of the membranes; onset of hypotension, tachycardia and hypoxia in the mother. There are many causes of sudden-onset fetal bradycardia. However, if this follows recent rupture of the membranes, the possibility of an amniotic fluid embolus (AFE) should be considered. The mother exhibits typical features of AFE, which often starts with sweating, confusion and coughing, followed by cardiovascular collapse and hypoxia. Other differential diagnoses would include:

- Haemorrhagic shock from uterine rupture or placental abruption – although hypoxia is not normally a feature. Massive haemorrhage can obviously result in a coagulopathy, although this is not usually present immediately.
- Pulmonary thromboembolism – does not normally cause a coagulopathy.

b. The blood results show a coagulopathy with an elevated PT and APTT. Platelet count and fibrinogen levels are low, suggesting the presence of a disseminated intravascular coagulopathy. This supports a diagnosis of AFE.

c. The management of AFE is largely supportive. Tracheal intubation and IPPV with 100% O_2 should be instituted, and invasive cardiovascular monitoring used to guide fluid therapy and inotropic support. Correction of clotting abnormalities is likely to require fresh

frozen plasma (FFP) and platelet or cryoprecipitate infusions, as guided by laboratory results and expert haematological advice. Mortality has been quoted as high as 86%, although this must depend on the accuracy with which the diagnosis is made, minor cases often being missed.

Further reading
Noble W, St-Amand J 1993 Amniotic fluid embolus. *Canadian Journal of Anaesthesia* 40: 971–980.

Answer 7.8

a. Liver function tests show evidence of an acute hepatitic process, with raised transaminase levels, elevated bilirubin levels, deranged clotting and reduced fibrinogen levels. Renal function is also impaired with elevated plasma urea and creatinine. Plasma osmolarity is within the normal range for pregnancy (normally 10 mOsm below non-pregnant levels). The WCC is elevated, with normal haemoglobin and platelet counts.

b. The biochemistry suggests that this is an acute hepatitis which, in pregnancy, may result from:

- infection, particularly viral causes, e.g. hepatitis A, B or C or glandular fever
- chemical poisons and drugs
- pregnancy-induced causes including intrahepatic cholestasis of pregnancy, HELLP syndrome (haemolysis, elevated liver enzymes, low platelets) and acute fatty liver of pregnancy.

In the absence of evidence of infection or chemically induced hepatitis, the likely diagnosis in this case is acute fatty liver of pregnancy. Normal platelet count and haemoglobin effectively exclude a diagnosis of HELLP syndrome, although the management in both cases may, in practice, be similar.

Intrahepatic cholestasis of pregnancy classically presents in the third trimester of pregnancy with pruritus caused by a marked rise in serum bile acids. Jaundice is often absent and liver transaminases only moderately raised. This condition resolves after delivery and the prognosis for the mother is good. The condition does pose risks for the fetus, however, with increased risk of pre-term delivery and intrauterine death.

c. The diagnosis of acute fatty liver of pregnancy is usually made from the clinical picture and exclusion of other causes such as viral hepatitis. Liver biopsy shows fatty infiltration of hepatocytes, which is most prominent in the pericentral region, although in practice this is often not performed because of clotting derangement. Clinically the patient usually presents in the third trimester with anorexia, malaise, vomiting and abdominal pain. Jaundice may not be present initially. Signs of pre-eclampsia often coexist, with increased blood pressure, and raised serum urea and uric acid. AFL probably represents one end of the spectrum of this disease.

Coagulopathy is common, as a result of both a decreased production of clotting factors and a coexisting consumptive coagulopathy. Hypoglycaemia is also common. Left untreated, the patient may proceed to fulminant hepatic failure, with hepatic coma, renal failure and hypoglycaemia.

Treatment first consists of urgent delivery of the fetus, after which the condition usually resolves. If caesarean section is required, clotting abnormalities are likely to preclude regional anaesthesia. Other treatment is largely supportive, including careful fluid management, treatment of hypoglycaemia, renal support where necessary, and protein restriction and oral lactulose for the treatment of hepatic encephalopathy.

Further reading

Nelson-Piercy C 1997 Liver disease in pregnancy. Current Obstetrics and Gynaecology 7: 36–42.

suggesting impaired renal function.

b. The combination of the abnormal blood results and the presence of a raised BP and proteinuria is highly suggestive of pre-eclampsia.

c. The management of this patient should include the following:

- Carry out further investigations, including LFTs and clotting screen.
- Monitor blood pressure and treat if persistently > 160/90 mmHg. Labetalol and hydralazine are the most commonly used agents in the UK.
- Assess fetal well-being, usually by ultrasound and CTG.
- Delivery is indicated in the presence of significant proteinuric hypertension at term. Vaginal delivery would be anticipated following induction of labour in a multiparous woman.
- Monitor fluid balance and consider CVP monitoring, particularly if urine output is poor.
- Epidural analgesia in labour should be suggested as this is an aid to blood pressure control.
- The role of magnesium sulphate in the management of severe proteinuric hypertension is unclear although widely used in the USA. Its role, in this condition, is currently the subject of a multicentre trial (Magpie Trial).

Further reading

Anumba DOC, Robson SC 1999 Management of pre-eclampsia, elevated liver enzymes, and low platelets syndrome. Current Opinion in Obstetrics and Gynaecology 11: 149–156.

Linton DM, Anthony J 1997 Critical care management of severe pre-eclampsia. Intensive Care Medicine 23: 248–255.

Mushambi MC, Halligan AW, Williamson K 1996 Recent developments in the pathophysiology and management of pre-eclampsia. British Journal of Anaesthesia 76: 133–148.

Williams DJ, de Swiet M 1997 The pathophysiology of pre-eclampsia. Intensive Care Medicine 3: 620–629.

Answer 7.9

a. The platelet count is normal. Urea, creatinine and urate are all raised

Answer 7.10

a. The scan shows a posterior placenta praevia covering the cervical os. The

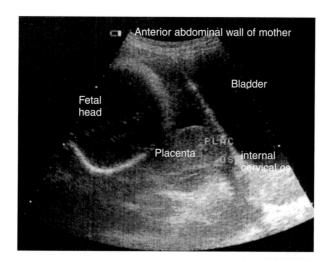

Labels on the scan: Anterior abdominal wall of mother; Bladder; Fetal head; Placenta; internal cervical os

illustration above identifies the main features of the scan.

b. This woman is at term with a posterior placenta praevia and a history of vaginal bleeding. Delivery by caesarean section is indicated.

c. Anaesthetic management of placenta praevia is controversial. Traditional advice has often been that the likelihood of increased blood loss associated with placenta praevia means that general anaesthesia is the technique of choice. However, surveys have indicated that many experienced obstetric anaesthetists are willing to perform regional anaesthesia in women with this condition. Regional anaesthesia obviously avoids the well-known risks of general anaesthesia in the pregnant woman. In a retrospective survey of 350 cases of placenta praevia, regional anaesthesia was used in 60% of cases.

Control of blood pressure in the presence of major haemorrhage did not appear to be a problem, and regional anaesthesia was associated with a significantly reduced estimated blood loss.

Whatever technique of anaesthesia is used, the possibility of major blood loss should always be anticipated. A senior anaesthetist and obstetrician should always be immediately available, as should cross-matched blood.

Further reading

Bonner SM, Hayes SR, Ryall DM 1995 The anaesthetic management of caesarean section for placenta praevia; a questionnaire survey. *Anaesthesia* 50: 992–994.

Parekh N, Husaini SWU, Russell IF 2000 Caesarean section for placenta praevia: a retrospective study of anaesthetic management. *British Journal of Anaesthesia* 84: 725–730.

8

PAEDIATRIC ANAESTHESIA

INTRODUCTION

Children are not little adults. They are physiologically different, with some values that are normal for an adult being abnormal in a small child. They have a wide range of clinical presentations, with congenital abnormalities forming a significant proportion of the underlying conditions. Some age-related aspects of normal data are discussed, and then data are presented to illustrate these fundamental differences.

HAEMATOLOGY

Haemoglobin at birth is often higher than in an adult but it is extremely variable, being dependent on birth weight as well as maternal factors. Neonates have a high proportion of fetal haemoglobin, resulting in left shift of the oxygen dissociation curve, which is necessary to increase the ability of the fetus to pick up oxygen in utero. After birth, haemoglobin falls, largely due to a decrease in fetal haemoglobin, and reaches a nadir at 2–3 months of age. However 2,3-DPG levels rise so that, with a Hb of 10 g/dL, oxygen delivery is the same as that for an adult with a Hb of 13 g/dL. Blood volume is higher for the first year of life, around 80–85 mL/kg, falling to a normal value of 60–65 mL/kg by 3 years of age. Figure 8.1 shows the investigation of anaemia in childhood.

The white cell count (WCC) is generally higher at birth, falling to normal levels by the age of 12 years. The platelet count is similar to that in adults, as are tests of clotting.

BIOCHEMISTRY

The reference ranges for standard electrolytes are shown in Table 8.1.

Urea is the main nitrogen-containing metabolite of protein catabolism. It is synthesised in the liver and 90% is excreted via the kidneys. Because of tubular reabsorption, urea is not an accurate reflection of glomerular filtration rate (GFR). Plasma urea is increased in babies who are fed excessive protein or insufficient water and in states of dehydration and renal insufficiency. Reference ranges for urea are as follows:

- Newborn, 2–10 mmol/L
- 1–2 years, 1.8–5.4 mmol/L
- 2–16 years, 2.9–7.1 mmol/L.

Creatinine is an endogenous product of muscle metabolism. The rate of production is proportional to muscle mass. Clinically, creatinine is excreted primarily through glomerular filtration with little tubular reabsorption or secretion. It therefore approximates to glomerular filtration rate (GFR). Small children have reduced muscle mass and, therefore, a lower creatinine level. From the age of 2 years upwards, normal GFR is 110–125 mls/min/1.73 m². Figure 8.1 allows the estimation of GFR knowing the child's age, creatinine and weight centile. For example, an 11-year-old on the 50th centile for weight, with a creatinine of 120 µmol/l, has a GFR of half normal.

THE ELECTROCARDIOGRAM

The difficulty in interpreting the electrocardiogram (ECG) in childhood is

Table 8.1 Reference ranges for standard electrolytes

	Term infant	Child
Na	132–142	135–143
K	4.5–6.5	3.5–4.5
Ca (total)	1.8–3.0	2.25–2.74
Ca (ion)	1.1–1.5	1.14–1.29
Mg	1.5–2.3	1.4–1.9

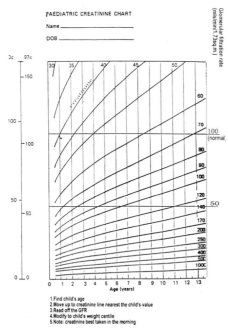

PAEDIATRIC CREATININE CHART

Name

DOB

1. Find child's age
2. Move up to creatinine line nearest the child's value
3. Read off the GFR
4. Modify to child's weight centile
5. Note: creatinine best taken in the morning

Fig. 8.1 Paediatric creatinine chart.
(Reproduced with kind permission of Dr
M Coulthard, Royal Victoria Infirmary, Newcastle
upon Tyne.)

Table 8.2 Age-specific ECG changes in children

Heart rate	
Newborn	110–150 beats/min
2 years	85–125 beats/min
4 years	75–115 beats/min
6 years	65–100 beats/min
> 6 years	60–100 beats/min

PR interval (lower limits of normal)	
< 3 years	0.08 s
3–16 years	0.10 s
> 16 years	0.12 s

QRS axis	Mean	Range
Newborn	125°	180–30°
1 month	90°	130–10°
3 years	60°	120–20°
Adult	50°	110–30°

QRS duration	
Premature	0.04 s
Term	0.05 s
1–3 years	0.06 s
> 3 years	0.07 s
Adult	0.08 s

the natural variation with age. Even the resting heart rate varies substantially, meaning that adult definitions of tachycardia and bradycardia do not apply. It is therefore important to have access to age-specific values when approaching the paediatric ECG (see Table 8.2).

The QT interval is the time for ventricular depolarisation followed by repolarisation. It varies with heart rate but not with age except in infancy. As yet there are no normal values for preterm babies, however the QT interval must be corrected (QTc) for heart rate, which tends to be higher in younger age groups. Use Bazett's formula to correct the QT, which should be less than 0.44 s, except in infants when it should be less than 0.49 s.

$$\text{Bazett's Formula } QTc = \frac{QT \text{ measured}}{\sqrt{(RR \text{ interval})}}$$

THE CHEST X-RAY (CXR)

The CXR in neonates, infants and small children varies considerably from that in adults, both in terms of projection and in terms of the existence of specific paediatric pathology. Infant chest radiographs are usually obtained with the child supine and therefore are in an anteroposterior projection, producing apparent enlargement of the cardiac shadow and mediastinum.

The chest in an infant is more cylindrical in shape than in an adult, and small degrees of rotation will cause quite marked distortion of the mediastinum, which should not be mistaken for pathology. The degree of rotation can be assessed by looking at the relationship of the inner ends of the clavicles to the vertebral bodies at the same level. The inner ends of the clavicles should be equidistant from the midpoint of the adjacent vertebral body.

It can be difficult to obtain a chest radiograph in full inspiration on a child. If the film has been taken in the expiratory phase, the mediastinum can appear to be enlarged, and the pulmonary vasculature becomes very prominent, giving a false impression of pulmonary pathology. Count the anterior ends of the ribs – at least five should be visible above the diaphragm if the lungs are to be adequately assessed.

THE CERVICAL SPINE

A number of principles underlie assessment of lateral X-rays of the cervical spine, equally applicable in both adults and children. Most importantly, the radiological investigations must be considered in the light of clinical findings and never considered in isolation. A neck may only be considered normal if both radiology and clinical examination are normal and this is particularly true in children, in whom ligamentous injury is more common. The stability of the neck is due to soft tissues (ligaments and facet joint capsules) as well as bones. Indirect evidence of cervical trauma not involving fractures of bony structures must be looked for.

Examination of the cervical spine is discussed in detail in Chapter 4, but there are several points of particular note in the examination of the paediatric cervical spine film.

- It is vital to have adequate films, which should include the C7–T1 junction; this may be more problematic to obtain in children than in adults.
- The prevertebral soft tissue may be expanded by haematoma or swelling following a major neck injury. However, this may be difficult to assess in children since this may also appear widened by adenoidal enlargement or in children who are crying vigorously. Above C4, soft tissue width should be less than one-third the width of the vertebral body at that level; and below C4, soft tissue width should be less than the width of the whole vertebral body at that level.
- The atlantoaxial distance (distance between posterior aspect of the atlas and front of the odontoid peg) should be less than 5 mm.
- Never be reassured with normal radiology in a child with a painful neck.

FURTHER READING

Park MK, Guntheroth WG. *How to Read Paediatric ECGs*, 3rd edn. Mosby, London.
Soldim SJ, Rifai N, Hicks JMB 1995 *Biochemical Basis of Paediatric Disease*. American Association for Clinical Chemistry Washington, DC.

QUESTIONS

Question 8.1

A 4-month-old baby boy, born at 25 weeks' gestation with a birth weight of 760 g, is admitted for repair of bilateral inguinal hernias. His current weight is 3 kg and he is oxygen-dependent at home requiring 200 mL/min via nasal cannulae to keep his saturations above 94%. He is bottle-fed and just starting to wean. On examination, he has mild subcostal and intercostal recession with a hyperinflated chest. Auscultation reveals good air entry with only transmitted upper respiratory tract noises. The heart rate is 110/min with full pulses. His full blood count and a capillary blood gas are available for your preoperative visit, as follows: *FBC*: Hb, 9.8 g/dl; WCC, 10.9 × 10^9/l; platelets, 243 × 10^9/l. *Capillary blood gases*: pH, 7.33; P_aCO_2, 8.8 kPa; P_aO_2, 6.4 kPa; HCO_3, 28 mmol/l; base excess (BE), +4.6 mmol/l.

a. Comment upon the blood results.
b. Comment upon the blood gases.

Question 8.2

A 7-year-old Afro-Caribbean boy presents with swelling, pain and redness of his right ankle. The surgeons are concerned that this is an osteomyelitis, which they wish to drain. The following blood results are obtained: Hb, 7.1 g/dl; WCC, 20 × 10^9/l; platelets, 470 × 10^9/l; MCV, 76 fl; reticulocyte count, 12%; bilirubin, 70 µmol/l.

a. What do these results show?
b. Define anaemia and its classification?
c. What further haematological investigation would be helpful.
d. Based on the ethnic background, what is the most likely diagnosis and what confirmatory tests are helpful?
e. What is the genetics of this condition?

Question 8.3

An 18-month-old Bangladeshi child presents with a previously undiagnosed congenital dislocation of the hip. An open reduction is planned. The routine preoperative full blood count is as follows: Hb, 9.5 g/dl; WCC, 8 × 10^9/l; platelets, 200 × 10^9/l; MCV, 67 fl; mean corpuscular haemoglobin (MCH), 22 pg; reticulocytes, 1%.

a. What does the full blood count show?
b. What is the differential diagnosis, and what further haematological investigations help in the differential diagnosis?
c. Assuming normal elemental dietary intake and absorption, and noting the ethnic origin, what is the likely diagnosis and underlying genetics of this condition.

Question 8.4

A 7-year-old boy undergoes routine adenotonsillectomy for recurrent tonsillitis. In the first 12 h postoperatively, he oozes from both tonsillar beds requiring return to theatre. The following results are obtained: Hb, 8.1 g/dl; MCV, 85 fl; WCC, 11 × 10^9/l; platelets, 430 × 10^9/l; prothrombin time (PT), 12 s (normal for lab); activated partial thromboplastin time (APTT), 42 s (upper limit of normal for lab = 38 s); fibrinogen, 6.5 g/l.

a. Comment on these investigations.
b. What is the differential diagnosis and what further haematological investigations would you request?
c. Based on the new information supplied in the answer to 'b', what is the diagnosis and how would you treat it preoperatively?

Question 8.5

A 4-year-old boy is admitted with anorexia, nausea, vomiting and abdominal pain for the previous 15 h. The pain was central and has now moved to the right iliac fossa. He is referred to the surgeons who diagnose appendicitis and he is scheduled for surgery. On examination he has a temperature of 37.9°C and is slightly flushed. His sclera are slightly yellow. He has pain, especially localised to the right iliac fossa, with generalised tenderness and guarding. The following investigations are available: Hb, 12.4 g/dl; WCC, 18.9×10^9/l; platelets, 380×10^9/l; MCV, 80 fl; Na, 132 mmol/l; K, 4.3 mmol/l; Cl, 101 mmol/l; Ca, 2.32 mmol/l; urea, 5.8 mmol/l; creatinine, 40 μmol/l; bilirubin, 120 μmol/l; alkaline phosphatase, 170 IU/l; GGT, 35 IU/l; ALT, 10 IU/l; AST, 11 IU/l.

a. What further investigations would you request?
b. Apart from appendicitis, what are the differential diagnoses?
c. What precautions should be taken after surgery?

Question 8.6

A 2-year-old boy presented as an emergency with a traumatic laceration of his palate requiring repair. A standard rapid-sequence induction is undertaken. At the end of a 1 h procedure he fails to breathe and is taken to ITU. The following blood results are subsequently obtained: serum cholinesterase, 663 U/l (ref. range 650–1450); fluoride no., 17; Dibucaine no., 16.

a. Please explain what these tests indicate.
b. What is the diagnosis and likely underlying genotype?

Question 8.7

A 5-week-old male infant presents with a 3-day history of projectile vomiting. Following a test feed, a diagnosis of pyloric stenosis is made. The following serum electrolytes are obtained: Na, 128 mmol/l; K, 2.9 mmol/l; bicarbonate, 35 mmol/l; Cl, 2.8 mmol/l; pH, 7.63; BE, +10 mmol/l.

a. Describe the electrolyte abnormalities.
b. How do these arise in this case?
c. How would you correct these abnormalities prior to surgery?
d. What levels would you consider acceptable before surgery?

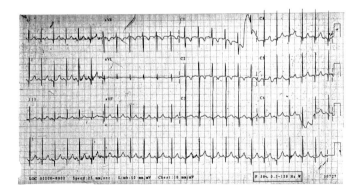

Question 8.8

A neonate presents for operation with antenatally diagnosed exomphalos. Ectopic beats were noted on the antenatal scans and an ECG is performed, as shown above.

a. Describe this ECG. What does it show?

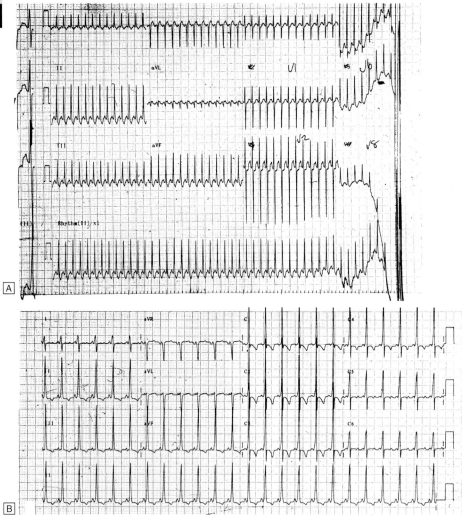

Question 8.9

A 6-month-old baby presents for surgical repair of a right inguinal hernia. Preoperative assessment is completely normal. At induction the heart rhythm changes, with an ECG trace as shown in (A).

a. What is the diagnosis?
b. What is the treatment of choice?
c. The rhythm reverts with treatment and a postoperative ECG is performed (B). What is the likely diagnosis?
d. What is the appropriate action in an otherwise asymptomatic child?

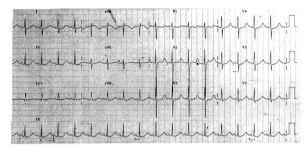

Question 8.10

Preoperative assessment of an 11-year-old girl reveals a history of fainting associated with exercise. The patient's brother died suddenly aged 8. Until that time he had been a normal child but was thought to have mild aortic stenosis. A bicuspid aortic valve was found at postmortem and the family were told that he had a brain abnormality, which may have contributed to his death.

Examination of the girl reveals no abnormalities, with a clear chest, regular pulse and normal heart sounds. Her blood pressure whilst supine is 105/55 mmHg in the right arm which rises to 110/60 on standing. An ECG is performed, as shown.

a. What other history would you want?
b. What is the diagnosis?
c. What is the treatment?

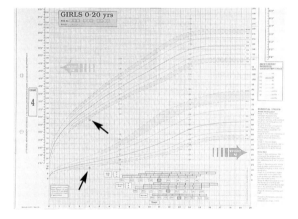

Question 8.11

A child with Turner's syndrome (XO), aged 4 years, is admitted for insertion of grommets, having had a long history of secretory otitis media and a hearing deficit which may have caused speech delay. The child has the following findings on examination: weight, 11 kg; height, 89 cm; growth chart marked as shown; no lymph nodes, jaundice, anaemia, clubbing; webbing of neck. *ENT*: slight nasal discharge; fluid behind both tympanic membranes; throat: fleshy tonsils. *Chest*: slightly nasal breathing; respiratory rate, 20/min; no recession; clear air entry, no added sounds. *Cardiovascular*: heart rate, 95/min; pulse, good volume; praecordium, normal; heart sounds I and II, normal with no added murmurs; blood pressure, 130/75 mmHg. *Abdomen*: soft non-tender; no masses palpable; normal genitalia.

a. What relevance is the weight and height?
b. What part of the examination would you repeat?
c. What further examination would you perform?
d. What investigations would you request?

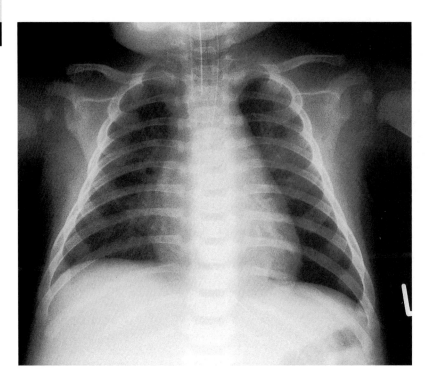

Question 8.12

An infant of 5 weeks has a 2-day history of increasing shortness of breath in a peripheral hospital. The baby has been unable to feed because of dyspnoea and has been hydrated intravenously. Increasing respiratory distress and apnoea require ventilation and the baby is transferred to the regional PICU. The admission CXR is shown. The following results are also available:

Arterial blood gas		Full blood count		Biochemistry	
pH	7.28	Hb	13.2 g/dL	Na	126 mmol/l
P_aCO_2	8.9 kPa	WCC	5.6×10^9/L	K	3.9 mmol/l
P_aO_2	9.5 kPa	Platelets	236×10^9/L	U	2.4 mmol/l
				Cr	35 µmol/l
				Bil	17 µmol/l

a. What features does the X-ray show?
b. What is the likely diagnosis?
c. What is the next likely course of action?
d. What further test would you perform?
e. Comment upon the biochemistry?

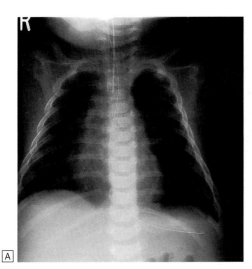

A

Question 8.13

The child from Question 8.12 is pressure-ventilated on 24/4, F_iO_2 0.75, inspiratory time 0.5 s at a rate of 40/min. The CXR 1 h later is shown in (A) and the flow trace from the pulmonary graphics is shown in (B). The blood gas 1 h after pressure ventilation is as follows: pH, 7.23; P_aCO_2, 10.8 kPa; P_aO_2, 13.9 kPa.

a. What has happened?
b. What needs to be done to improve the blood gases?

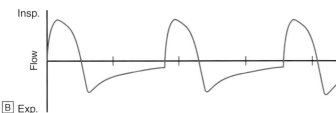

Insp.

Flow

B Exp.

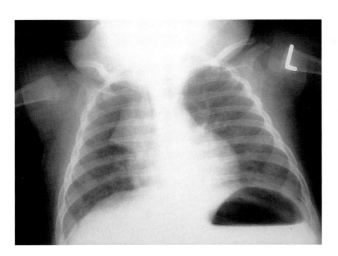

L

Question 8.14

This 5-month-old infant presents with recurrent, nocturnal cough and possible asthma. A chest film is obtained, as shown.

a. What does this film show?
b. What should be done about this?

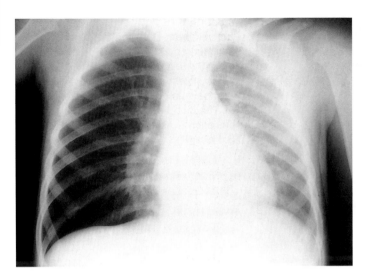

Question 8.15

A 9-year-old boy presents as an emergency with a sudden onset of repeated coughing. This followed eating some small round sweets, which he had been throwing up into the air and trying to catch in his mouth. On examination, expiratory wheeze is present throughout the right side of the chest. The following radiograph is obtained.

a. What does this film show?
b. What is the likely cause of these findings?
c. How may this problem present in children?
d. What needs to be done and what are the anaesthetic considerations?

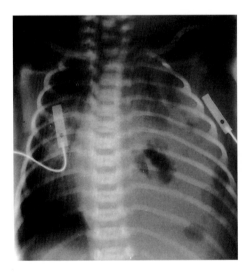

Question 8.16

This 6-year-old term infant presents with increasing respiratory rate, cyanosis and tachycardia. Examination shows a scaphoid abdomen. This CXR is obtained.

a. What does the X-ray show?
b. What is the differential diagnosis?
c. What is the likely diagnosis in view of the clinical history?
d. Describe the management of this case.

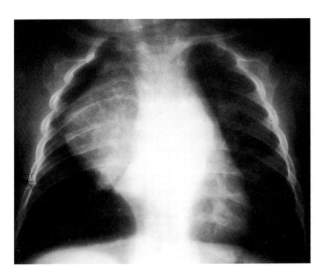

Question 8.17

A child presents with a four-week history of being off colour, fever and bruising easily. Initial investigations have shown anaemia and pancytopenia. The following chest X-ray has been obtained.

a. Describe the abnormality shown in this film.
b. How is the mediastinum divided into compartments?
c. What are the major causes of masses in each compartment in children?
d. Where exactly does the abnormality lie and thus what is the differential diagnosis?
e. Why may you be asked to anaesthetise this child?

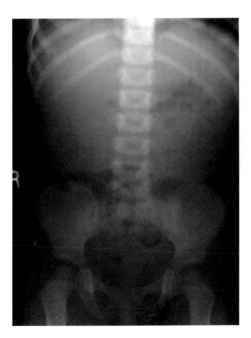

Question 8.18

A previously well, 3-month-old male infant presents with a 24-h history of screaming attacks, becoming pale and drawing his knees up. The episodes, which last 3–4 min, have occurred several times per hour and been associated with vomiting. Only a small amount of loose stool has been passed. This plain abdominal X-ray was obtained. .

a. What is the main abnormal feature and diagnosis?
b. How is the diagnosis most commonly obtained?
c. How is it treated?

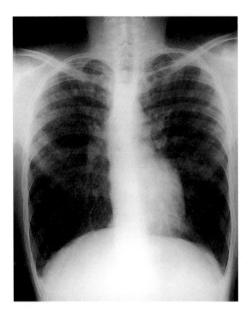

Question 8.19

An 8-year-old boy presents on a planned ENT list with nasal obstruction due to polyps. He has a long history of persistent cough, recurrent chest infections and failure to thrive. A CXR is available, as shown.

a. What does this X-ray demonstrate?

b. What is the likely diagnosis and how is this confirmed?

c. Why are these X-ray changes encountered?

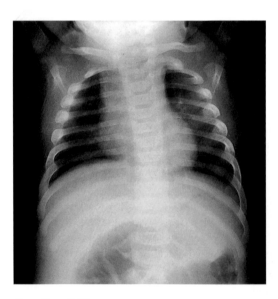

Question 8.20

This 6-month-old infant presents for repair of a torn frenulum. This is reported to have occurred due to a fall from a high chair. There is widespread bruising across the chest. A CXR is obtained, as shown.

a. What are the important features?

b. What diagnosis must be considered?

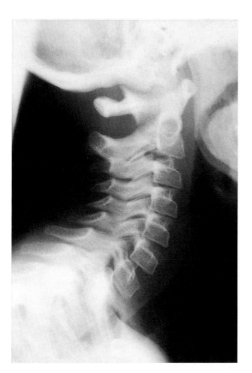

Question 8.21

An 8-year-old girl presents to A&E after being struck by a car whilst running across a road. The X-ray shown is one of a series of primary X-rays taken soon after presentation.

a. Describe your approach to interpretation of a lateral X-ray of the neck
b. Describe the findings on this film.
c. Can the stiff collar be removed?

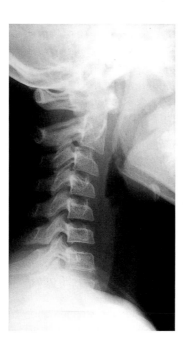

Question 8.22

This 7-year-old child was thrown forward from her pony. She was wearing a hard hat and has a bruise on her right cheek. She is fully alert and orientated, and has no neurological abnormality on examination. She has no neck pain or limitation of movement. Her lateral neck film is shown.

a. Please comment on the film.
b. What other variants exist on paediatric as opposed to adult neck films?
c. At what levels do neck injuries in children commonly occur?

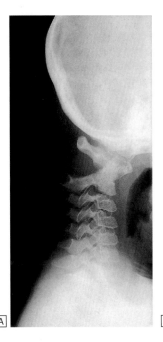
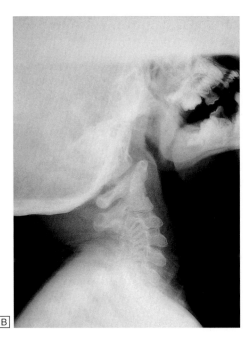

A | B

Question 8.23

An 8-year-old boy with Down's syndrome presents for planned adenotonsillectomy. Lateral neck X-rays have recently been taken and are shown (A, B).

a. What do these films show?
b. Should all children with Down's syndrome have a preoperative lateral neck X-ray?

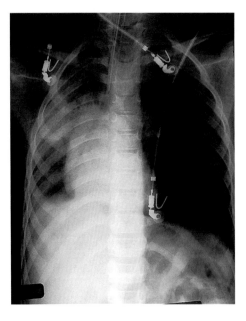

Question 8.24

A 6-year-old girl presents with a fractured wrist for manipulation under anaesthesia. She is starved for 6 h preoperatively. She undergoes intravenous induction of anaesthesia and a facemask is held with the patient spontaneously breathing under inhalational anaesthesia. However, on manipulation of her wrist, she coughs and desaturates, necessitating intubation and controlled ventilation. Her F_iO_2 is 1.0, oxygen saturation is 94% and a CXR is performed, as shown.

a. Describe this CXR. Which lobe is most affected?
b. What has happened and why?
c. What is the immediate treatment?
d. What is the mortality and the long-term complications?

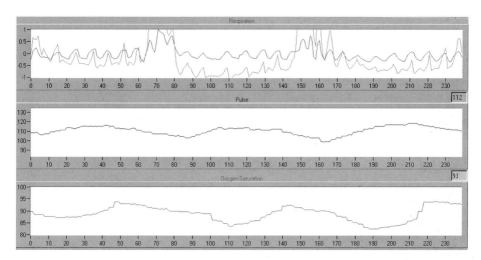

Question 8.25

A 6-month-old boy is listed on your ophthalmic list for an 'Examination under Anaesthesia' (EUA). He appears to have a repaired cleft palate and a relatively small jaw. His parents have noticed that he snores at night and appears very restless. You find this printout of a sleep study in his notes.

a. What does the tracing display?
b. What sequence is he most likely to be displaying?
c. What is the commonest syndrome to cause this?
d. What other abnormalities may be present?
e. What are the anaesthetic implications of this case?

ANSWERS

Answer 8.1

a. The haemoglobin, WCC and platelets are within the normal ranges for a child of this age and with this birth weight. The normal blood count values according to age are shown in Table A8.1.

b. The capillary blood gas demonstrates a compensated respiratory acidosis consistent with bronchopulmonary dysplasia. This is secondary to extremely preterm delivery and ventilation. Care will be needed to avoid overventilation, causing alkalosis. Care will also be required to enable extubation at the end of the procedure.

   Capillary gases are more commonly performed in children and infants than in adults. They can be very useful but require care in interpretation. In a well perfused child (such as one with chronic $P_aCO_2 = 8.8$ kPa) the pH and P_aCO_2 will be similar to arterial values. The P_aO_2 may be significantly lower. In poorly perfused patients, the capillary blood gas becomes less useful as values may be very different from arterial samples.

Further reading

Hinchliffe RF 2000 In: Lilleyman J, Hann I, Blanchette V, eds. *Paediatric Haematology*, 2nd edn. Churchill Livingstone, London, pp. 1–20.

Answer 8.2

a. A normocytic anaemia (low Hb, normal MCV).

b. Anaemia is a decrease in the concentration of haemoglobin in the blood below the reference range for a specific age. Anaemia may be classified according to the underlying mechanism or morphological appearance. Mechanisms of anaemia include:

- increased blood loss
- impaired red cell function
- decreased red cell life span
- A combination of the above.

   The mean cell volume (MCV) divides anaemias morphologically into micro, normo and macrocytic anaemias (see fig below). Causes of a normocytic anaemia, as in this case, include:

- acute blood loss
- haemolysis
- bone marrow failure
- chronic disease states (malignancy, renal failure).

c. The raised blood bilirubin concentration (unconjugated) and high reticulocyte count in this case suggests excessive red cell destruction with some compensatory increase in marrow activity. The shortened red cell life indicates the diagnosis to be a haemolytic anaemia.

Table A8.1 Normal full blood count values according to age

Age	Hb (g/dL) (by birth weight)			MCV(fL)
	1000–1500 g	1501–2000 g	> 2000 g	
Birth			14.9–23.7	100–125
2 weeks	11.7–18.4	11.8–19.6	13.4–19.8	88–110
2 months	7.1–11.5	8.0–11.4	9.4–13.0	84–98
3 months	9.1–13.1	9.3–11.8		
6 months	9.4–13.8	10.7–12.6	10.0–13.0	73–84
1 year			10.1–13.0	70–82
2–6 years			11.0–13.8	72–87
6–12 years			11.1–14.7	76–90
Platelets	150–450 × 10⁹/L			
WCC	10–26 × 10⁹/L at birth, falling to 4.5–14.5 × 10⁹/L at 12 years			

d. Causes of haemolytic anaemia in childhood may be congenital or acquired. Congenital causes are:

- red cell membrane abnormalities (e.g. hereditary spherocytosis)
- red cell enzyme defects (e.g. glucose-6-phosphate dehydrogenase deficiency)
- haemoglobin abnormalities (e.g. sickle cell disease, β-thalassaemia major, haemoglobin H disease).

Acquired causes outside the neonatal period are uncommon, but include:

- immune causes (e.g. autoimmune haemolytic anaemia)
- red cell destruction (e.g. haemolytic uraemic syndrome)
- infections (e.g. malaria)
- miscellaneous (e.g. drugs).

Investigations helping in the differential diagnosis include a blood film. Certain abnormal red cell forms or inclusions in a film suggest specific causes of haemolysis, e.g. spherocytes in hereditary spherocytosis and autoimmune haemolytic anaemias, elliptocytes in hereditary elliptocytosis, sickle cells in sickle cell anaemia, and Heinz bodies in red cells in glucose-6-phosphate deficiency.

The Afro-Caribbean background makes sickle cell anaemia a high probability. If not confirmed on the film, a screening sickle solubility test (e.g. Sickledex Test) will confirm the diagnosis in minutes. This involves adding a reducing agent, such as sodium metabisulphite, which sickles the abnormal sickle haemoglobin, allowing it to polymerise and thus form a precipitate. It does not differentiate sickle cell anaemia from sickle cell trait.

Haemoglobin electrophoresis and high-pressure liquid chromatography (HPLC) take substantially longer but give further information regarding the type and concentration of many different haemoglobin variants. Values of 98% haemoglobin S, 2% haemoglobin F would suggest sickle cell anaemia, with approximately 35% haemoglobin S and 60% haemoglobin A (normal adult haemoglobin) suggesting sickle cell trait. HPLC has the advantage of being faster and allowing easy discrimination of many different haemoglobin variants, whereas electrophoresis is much more

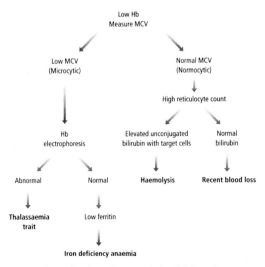

Investigation of anaemia in childhood.

demanding but involves considerably less expensive equipment.

e. Sickle cell anaemia results from two abnormal genes (the homozygous state) on chromosome 11. Almost all the haemoglobin formed is the abnormal haemoglobin S, which has a single amino acid substitution in the β-globin chain. Heterozygotes (sickle cell trait) have one normal and one abnormal gene, producing about 60% normal haemoglobin (Hb A) and 40% abnormal Hb S. Sickling only occurs at oxygen saturations less than 40%, rarely reached in venous blood.

Further reading

Weatherall DJ 1998 The hereditary anaemias. In: Provan D, Henson A, eds. *ABC of Clinical Haematology*. BMJ Publishing, London.

Answer 8.3

a. A low Hb, a low MCV and a reduced MCH (normal range at 6 months to 6 years is 24–30 pg). This is a hypochromic microcytic anaemia.

b. The differential diagnosis is: iron deficiency anaemia; thalassaemia minor; lead poisoning; anaemia of chronic disease. Any test assessing body iron stores is helpful. A low serum ferritin would suggest iron deficiency. Ferritin is an iron storage protein present in many tissues and in low levels in serum. It usually directly reflects the amount of iron stored in the bone marrow. A serum lead excludes lead poisoning. Diagnosis of anaemia of chronic disease is difficult and involves exclusion of the other causes in combination with evidence of an underlying disease process.

c. α- or β-thalassaemia trait. Both are asymptomatic, presenting as a minor hypochromic, microcytic anaemia on routine testing. They can be differentiated from iron deficiency by a normal serum iron and ferritin level. The inheritance is complex. In β-thalassaemia, mutation of the genes for β-globin chain formation results in reduced or absent β-chain production.

A single abnormal gene results in the asymptomatic β-thalassaemia trait. Two abnormal genes (homozygote) cause severe anaemia (which is in part haemolytic) due to precipitation of the excess α-chains within red cells.

Four genes in total are responsible for α-globin chain production (two close together on each chromosome 16). Impaired α-chain production leads to an excess of β- or γ-chains, forming unstable tetramers. The severity of reduction in α-chain reduction varies with the number of abnormal genes present. There are two varieties of abnormal chromosome. In the first, one of the two genes on the chromosome may be deleted. In the second, both genes are deleted – this genotype is restricted to Far Eastern ethnicity. Deletion of a total of one or two genes is essentially asymptomatic (α-thalassaemia trait). Deletion of three genes gives very low rates of α-chain production, a marked excess of β-chains, and clinically moderately severe haemolytic anaemia (Hb H disease). Four abnormal genes result in stillbirth.

Further reading

Hoffbrand AV, Pettit JE 1993 *Essential Haematology*. Blackwell Science, Oxford.

Answer 8.4

a. The patient is anaemic. The platelet count is raised, in keeping with recent blood loss. PT measures the extrinsic and common pathways, whilst APPT measures the intrinsic and common pathways. There is a defect in the intrinsic pathway.

b. The likely diagnoses include: haemophilia A (reduced factor VIII); haemophilia B (reduced factor IX); von Willebrand's disease (reduced or abnormal von Willebrand factor [vWF]). Therefore levels of factor VIII, factor IX and vWF will establish the clotting abnormality. The following results are obtained: factor VIII C level, 22%; vWF, 19%; factor IX level, 98%.

c. The child has von Willebrand's disease; vWF is low. This is the most common inherited bleeding disorder, occurring in about 1 in 1000 individuals. As well as facilitating platelet adhesion, vWF also serves as a carrier for factor VIIIC. Reduced levels of vWF result in a reduced half-life for factor VIIIC and thus its reduced blood levels. DDAVP (0.3 µg/kg) mobilises vWF stores and therefore can raise vWF blood levels. It is generally effective in mild or moderate von Willebrand disease and might well provide adequate haemostasis in this instance. If ineffective in controlling bleeding, alternatives are intermediate-purity factor VIII, vWF concentrate or cryoprecipitate.

Further reading
Howard MR, Hamilton PH 1999 Von Willebrand's disease and other inherited coagulation disorders. In: Haematology: an illustrated colour text. Churchill Livingston, Edinburgh.

Answer 8.5

a. The full blood count presents a normal picture with a slightly raised WCC. The biochemical profile shows a low sodium which may be due to vomiting or a degree of water retention. The urea at the high end of normal makes the former more likely. The urea may also be higher because of starvation and catabolism. However, it is the high bilirubin that should excite comment. This suggests a liver problem but the other liver enzymes remain in the normal range. In this situation it would be appropriate to request clotting profile, a differentiation between conjugated and unconjugated bilirubin, urobilinogen and further history.
b. The differential depends upon the type of jaundice:

• Unconjugated bilirubin may be elevated in the absence of a raised conjugated bilirubin in marked haemolysis, haematoma formation, physiological jaundice in the newborn, and rare metabolic disorders. It may also be raised in liver disease.

• Elevated conjugated bilirubin is an insensitive but specific indicator of hepatobiliary disease.
• Urobilinogen increases in haemolytic states. There is no evidence of haemolysis or other evidence of liver disease in this case. Further history should be sought for previous jaundice, prolonged jaundice postnatally or a family history of jaundice. This is most likely to be a metabolic disorder with the increase secondary to the appendicitis.

Metabolic disorders giving hyperbilirubinaemia include:

• *Unconjugated*: Crigler–Najjar syndrome type I and II; Gilbert's syndrome.
• *Conjugated*: Dubin–Johnson syndrome; rotor disease.

c. This child needs an appendicectomy. However, further advice should be taken. The hyperbilirudinaemia is unconjugated and family history reveals similar episodes of jaundice in other family members. This child has type II Criglar–Najjar syndrome. This is an autosomal dominant condition which usually presents in infancy but may present later in childhood prompted by intercurrent infection. There is a small but real risk of kernicterus and therefore bilirubin levels must be monitored carefully postoperatively as some children will require haemofiltration.

Answer 8.6

a. The amount of cholinesterase in serum is the lower end of normal. However, this is measured using test substrates such as acetylcholine or benzoylcholine, not suxamethonium. In 1957, Kalow reported that the plasma of healthy individuals who had experienced a prolonged response to suxamethonium contained an abnormal (atypical) enzyme. This atypical enzyme has a reduced ability to hydrolyse test substances but is totally unable to

8

A

hydrolyse suxamethonium. He went on to demonstrate that the local anaesthetic cinchocaine (Dibucaine) inhibits the hydrolysis of benzoylcholine by the normal enzyme by 70% or more, whereas it inhibits the hydrolysis by the abnormal variant by only 30% or less. The degree of inhibition of hydrolysis by Dibucaine (the Dibucaine number) allows one to differentiate between patients with normal and atypical cholinesterase enzyme.

The type of cholinesterase in an individual's plasma is determined genetically by two allelic, autosomal, co-dominant genes. Two genes for the normal enzyme (E^u, E^u) result in normal enzyme activity and a Dibucaine number of 70 or more; 1 in 2500 individuals has two abnormal genes (E^a, E^a) resulting in markedly reduced enzyme activity and a Dibucaine number of 30 or less; 1 in 25 has one normal and one atypical gene (E^u, E^a) and has plasma containing both types of enzyme, very mild prolongation of action of suxamethonium, and a Dibucaine number of between 40 and 70.

Subsequently, sodium fluoride has also been shown to be a differential inhibitor of the normal and atypical variants of plasma cholinesterase. However, a number of patients were found to have moderately prolonged paralysis with suxamethonium, a small change in inhibition to hydrolysis with Dibucaine (Dibucaine number = 20, like atypical variant) but marked inhibition with sodium fluoride (fluoride number = 70, unlike atypical variant). There is thus a second abnormal allele (E^f), which occurs in a homozygous state in 1 in 300 000 of the population. A further rare, silent gene (E^s) also exists.

b. The subject has low normal cholinesterase levels with little inhibition of hydrolysis by Dibucaine or fluoride. The cholinesterase genotype is homozygous for the atypical gene (E^a, E^a), and the patient will be markedly sensitive to suxamethonium.

Further reading

Pantuck EJ 1993 Plasma cholinesterase: gene and variations. *Anesthesia & Analgesia* 77: 380–386.

Answer 8.7

a. The infant has a hypochloraemic, hypokalaemic alkalosis.

b. The obstruction is between stomach and duodenum. Losses are essentially gastric secretions of hydrogen ions and chloride ions. Initially the body attempts to correct the resulting acid–base disturbance by losing bicarbonate ions in the urine and hypoventilation (compensatory respiratory acidosis). As the obstruction continues, absorbed oral intake falls, the infant becomes hypovolaemic, and maintenance of circulating volume takes precedence over the acid–base status. Sodium ions are reabsorbed in the kidney to maintain extracellular fluid volume in exchange for potassium and hydrogen ions. This results in the paradox of an acid urine being secreted in the presence of a systemic metabolic alkalosis.

c. If the infant is significantly dehydrated, a bolus of 10–20 mL/kg of 0.9% saline will partially restore circulating volume. Electrolyte changes should be corrected gradually over at least 24 h, with regular blood sampling. It is easiest to use 0.45% saline in 5% dextrose at 4–6 mL/h (adding 10–20 mmol potassium to each 500 mL bag).

d. Acceptable thresholds before undertaking surgery include a chloride above 90 mmol/L, potassium above 3 mmol/L and bicarbonate of 30 mmol/L.

Answer 8.8

a. This is an ECG from an infant, the rhythm is sinus, the rate is 140 beats/min. The PR interval is normal at 0.1 s, the axis is +60° and the QT interval is 0.26 s. This represents a normal ECG for a neonate.

Answer 8.9

a. This ECG shows a fast ventricular rate approaching 300 beats/min, with no visible P waves. This is a paroxysmal supraventricular tachycardia, which represents the most common arrhythmia in childhood and infancy; 70–80% of children presenting with paroxysmal supraventricular tachycardia have normal hearts, but it is also associated with atrial septal defects, Ebstein's anomaly, mitral valve prolapse, corrected transposition and disease of the cardiac muscle.

b. Treatment depends upon the state of the child. If there is time, and it is safe, an ECG taken in tachycardia (even a rhythm strip assists in diagnosis). In the anaesthetised patient who is stable (as most will be), the tachycardia can be terminated by use of adenosine. Treatment should be according to the Advanced Paediatric Life Support algorithm as shown below.

c. The ECG demonstrates sinus rhythm but with a PR interval of 0.06 s. A short PR interval may be found in Wolf–Parkinson–White syndrome (WPW); Lown–Ganong–Levine syndrome, and glycogen storage disease. This is WPW syndrome and a clear delta wave is demonstrated, seen most clearly as an upstroke in the anterior chest leads. Inhalational

anaesthesia may cause supraventricular tachycardia in susceptible children with accessory pathways.

d. It is appropriate to refer the child to a paediatrician or paediatric cardiologist according to the local referral pattern. Any long-term drug therapy should be discussed with a paediatric cardiologist before implementation.

Further reading
Jordan SC, Scott D 1995 *Heart Disease in Paediatrics*, 3rd edn. Butterworth, London.
Advanced Life Support Group 2001 *Advanced Paediatric Life Support*, 3rd edn. BMJ Publishing, London.

Answer 8.10

a. More family history is required. Is there any history of sudden death, especially in children but also young adults? Any history of dizziness or loss of consciousness? A family history of deafness should be sought. Obviously, is there any history of family members having problems with anaesthesia?

b. The diagnosis is one of long QT syndrome. The QT interval is measured from the earliest portion of the QRS complex to the end of the T wave. It is affected by both heart rate and age, with the normal range being 0.2 s at birth and 0.4 s in adolescence. It may be increased in hypothermia, hypothyroidism, myocarditis and hypocalcaemia, but it may also be familial, sometimes associated with deafness (Lange–Nielsen syndrome). If it is familial, it is an autosomal dominant with variable penetrance. It is children who are most at risk of life-threatening ventricular arrhythmias. These are thought to occur during episodes of tachycardia when T and P waves coincide.

    The corrected QT should be less than 0.44 s, except in infants when it should be less than 0.49 s. In this case it is more than 0.61 s when corrected. It can be calculated by using:

```
                Shock present?
            No                  Yes

Vagal manoeuvres    Synchronous DC shock
                         0.5 J/kg
     Adenosine
     50 µg/kg       Synchronous DC shock
                         1.0 J/kg
     Adenosine
     100 µg/kg      Synchronous DC shock
                         2.0 J/kg
     Adenosine
     250 µg/kg

     Consider:      Consider antiarrhythmics
     DC shock
     Antiarrythmics
```

8

A

Bazett's formula: $QTc = \dfrac{QT \text{ measured}}{RR \text{ interval}}$

$= \dfrac{0.48}{\sqrt{0.6}} = 0.61$

c. Treatment in children is usually by β-blockade to limit rapid sinus tachycardia. This treatment is usually continued throughout life, but should be commenced by a paediatric cardiologist once a firm diagnosis has been made.

Answer 8.11

a. The child is small and short for her age, which is in keeping with a diagnosis of Turner's syndrome. Later in life, at around the age of 11 years, she may be commenced on growth hormone to improve her overall height at the end of puberty. Children with Turner's syndrome are likely to be of smaller than expected stature.

b. Particular attention should be directed at the cardiovascular examination, and the blood pressure should be repeated as it is beyond the 95th centile for her age. Particular care should be taken in . listening for murmurs, especially at the back. A rough estimate of expected systolic blood pressure can be obtained from the following formula: 80 + (age × 2) = expected systolic blood pressure (mmHg), i.e. 88 for a 4-year-old. However, values for systolic and diastolic 90th centiles by age are as shown in Table A8.2.

c. Pulses should be felt and any sign of radiofemoral delay detected. If the blood pressure is high then it should be obtained from a lower limb to detect a fall caused by a coarctation.

d. If the blood pressure is as high as this, then it requires further investigation. An ECG and a referral to a paediatric cardiologist will be appropriate. Ultimately, with this history, the child will have an echocardiogram. However, other causes of hypertension should not be forgotten and blood urea and electrolytes should be checked. Children with Turner's are more likely to have renal problems, the most common of which is a horseshoe kidney.

In this case, the diagnosis is coarctation of the aorta. About 20% of children with Turner's syndrome have heart disease, of which 75% have coarctation of the aorta, which is more common in children with webbing of the neck. Thus, overall, 15% of children born with XO chromosomes will have coarctation.

Further reading

Second Task Force on Blood Pressure Control in Children 1987 Report. *Pediatrics* 79: 1–25.

Child Growth Foundation 1996 *Girls Four in One Growth Charts (Birth–20 yrs)*. Child Growth Foundation, London.

Answer 8.12

a. The chest radiograph shows: markedly hyperinflated lungs (low flat diaphragms, narrow mediastinum); coarse perihilar lung infiltrate with bronchial wall thickening; patchy atelectasis.

b. The diagnosis is bronchiolitis. Acute bronchiolitis is a form of viral respiratory tract infection. It is usually seen in infants, and about 10% of infants will have had it by their first birthday. Very young infants, as in this case, or those with underlying cardiorespiratory problems, are most at risk. Respiratory syncytial virus is the most common cause, but influenza virus, rhinovirus and adenovirus can

Table A8.2 Values for systolic and diastolic 90th centiles by age.

Age	1	2	3	4	5	6	7	8	9	10	11	12	13
Systolic	105	106	107	108	109	111	112	114	115	117	119	121	124
Diastolic	69	68	68	69	69	70	71	73	74	75	76	77	79

cause similar symptoms. The illness starts with rhinorrhoea and a low-grade fever, progressing to a harsh, dry, cough and wheeze. Children with severe disease become increasingly tachypnoeic. Young infants may experience apnoea, which may be the presenting symptom. Fewer than 1 in 50 need hospitalisation, with only a small proportion requiring ventilation.

The major differential diagnosis would be asthma, but this is unlikely due to patient age and the predominance of fine crepitations. The bronchioles develop oedema and necrosis. Secretions and bronchial wall swelling can lead to partial bronchial obstruction, giving a ball valve effect (hyperinflation). More complete obstruction gives patchy areas of atelectasis.

c. In a small child who is clinically exhausted or getting apnoeic episodes, intubation and controlled ventilation are required.

d. The diagnosis is based on the clinical picture and presentation and is confirmed by identifying the virus on nasopharyngeal aspirate.

e. This biochemical profile shows a low serum sodium. This would normally be due to fluid retention in this situation. It is not unusual for infants requiring ventilation for bronchiolitis to exhibit a degree of inappropriate secretion of antidiuretic hormone. In this case a urine and serum osmolality should confirm the diagnosis. Fluid restriction is all that is usually required and no infant ventilated for bronchiolitis should be receiving more than 100 mL/kg per day in intravenous fluids, even though its normal oral intake may be 150 mL/kg per day.

Further reading

Landau LI 1997 Bronchiolitis. In: David TJ (ed) *Recent Advances in Paediatrics* vol. 15.

Answer 8.13

a. The oxygenation has improved but the carbon dioxide retention has got worse. The flow waveform shows that there is gas trapping. The picture is one of obstructive airways disease. There is insufficient exhalation time before the ventilator delivers the next breath. The CXR now appears better aerated but is overdistended because of the gas trapping.

b. The rate needs to be slowed to give adequate exhalation time. Ventilated infants with bronchiolitis may need to be ventilated at very slow rates for their age. This may require careful sedation, or at times even paralysis, to coordinate the slow rates required. A slower rate permits adequate expiratory time. With sufficient minute ventilation the p_aCO_2 will move towards normal limits. The flow trace below shows a slower respiratory rate allowing expiration to fully occur, before the next breath.

Answer 8.14

a. This film shows a typical thymic shadow, which is normal in an infant. The thymus gland is relatively large in infants. It occupies the anterior and superior mediastinum, extending inferiorly adjacent to the heart. The thymus gland can also have a characteristic shape; in this case the lateral and inferior borders on the right form a very clearly defined 'sail' shape.

Being a soft organ, the thymus may also mould to the shape of the thoracic

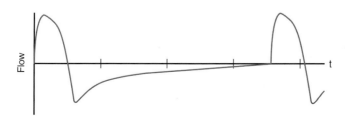

cage. This commonly leads to indentations on the gland from the overlying ribs, giving a 'wavy' appearance, especially on the left (see film below).

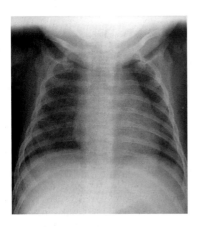

b. This is normal and nothing should be done. The thymus is particularly prominent from birth to the age of 4 and becomes relatively smaller as the child grows. It should not be confused with a pathological mediastinal mass.

Answer 8.15

a. This film is taken in expiration. It shows hyperexpansion of the right lung due to air trapping. There is shift of the mediastinum into the left hemithorax.

b. The most likely diagnosis, given this history, is of a foreign body in the right main bronchus. Partial airway obstruction leads to a ball valve effect impeding expiration of that lung. The lung distal to the obstruction becomes overdistended due to air trapping. If marked, this leads to a low hemidiaphragm and widening of the rib spaces on the affected side with shift of the mediastinum contralaterally. These features are much more obvious on an expiratory film. More complete obstruction will lead to complete collapse of the segment distal to the obstruction.

c. The diagnosis may be easy, as in this case with a clear history of eating round sweets, or classically peanuts, followed

by coughing or stridor. However, infants may present with no clear history but simply with respiratory difficulty and signs relating to both the upper and lower airway. Although air trapping, as in this case, is classically described, the child may just present with lobar collapse or consolidation. An inhaled foreign body should always be considered in such cases. It is important to remember that in the small child, the narrowest part of the airway is at the level of the cricoid. Airway resistance increases 16-fold for a decrease of 50% in airway diameter and critical obstruction at this level may be life-threatening, particularly since children require a large oxygen consumption.

d. At this stage, the child is unlikely to cough this out, and rigid bronchoscopy under general anaesthesia is invariably required. With high obstruction (trachea/larynx), spontaneous respiration should be maintained with inhalational anaesthesia. For obstruction lower in the airway, debate exists as to whether ventilation should be spontaneous or controlled. A deep plane of anaesthesia should be established before airway manipulations. The problems of a shared airway in a small, potentially hypoxic child mean that these cases should be undertaken by experienced anaesthetists.

Further reading
Badgewell JM 1997 *Clinical Paediatric Anesthesia* Lippincott, Raven, Philadelphia.

Answer 8.16
a. There is shift of the mediastinum into the right hemithorax, with a mixed density 'mass' in the left hemithorax.

b. The differential diagnosis includes diaphragmatic hernia, cystic adenomatoid malformation (a congenital lung abnormality) and multiple pneumatoceles following staphylococcal pneumonia.

c. The likely diagnosis is a congenital diaphragmatic hernia. This occurs in 1 in 2500 live births. It is more common on the left. Initially the hemithorax may be opaque due to fluid-filled bowel loops. As the child swallows air after birth, radiolucencies begin to appear in the hemithorax.

d. These children represent a high-risk group and often have associated cardiac disease, gut malrotation and a hypoplastic lung. They may present in severe respiratory distress and acidosis, requiring immediate artificial ventilation. The lungs will be of low compliance, but airway pressures should be minimised to decrease the significant risk of pneumothorax. A nasogastric tube should be inserted to deflate the stomach of gas.

The child should be stabilised for laparotomy to remove the gut contents from the chest and close the diaphragmatic defect. The main problems faced in the perioperative period include pulmonary hypertension and lung hypoplasia.

Further reading
Lui LMP, Paig LM 2001 Neonatal surgical emergencies. In: Hamid RKA (ed) Anesthesiology Clinics of North America. Vol 19:2. WB Saunders, Philadelphia.

Answer 8.17

a. This film shows a large mass superiorly within the upper part of the mediastinum, mainly right-sided.

b. The mediastinum is bound anteriorly by the sternum and posteriorly by the vertebral bodies, paravertebral gutters and ribs. The superior and inferior borders are the thoracic inlet and diaphragm. A simple approach is to divide the mediastinum into three compartments: (i) anterior to the pericardial sac = anterior mediastinum; (ii) the pericardial sac and its contents = middle mediastinum; (iii) behind the pericardial sac = posterior mediastinum.

c. Mediastinal masses in children are commonly neoplastic (primary or

secondary), infective or cystic. In a review of 429 mediastinal masses reported by Filler et al, 40% of masses were in the posterior mediastinum, and were predominately neurogenic tumours, approximately 15% in the middle mediastinum (lymphomas, bronchogenic cysts etc.); 45% of masses lay in the anterior mediastinum, being predominately thymic or lymphomatous in origin.

d. The posterior aspects of the ribs adjacent to the mass on the right are eroded and splayed, indicating that this mass is within the posterior mediastinum. In a child, the differential diagnosis includes neurogenic tumours (neuroblastoma, ganglioneuroblastoma, ganglioneuroma), neurenteric cyst and oesophageal duplication cyst.

e. This child had a neuroblastoma. These tumours arise from cells of neural crest origin in the adrenal medulla or sympathetic chain; 60% occur in the abdomen but the thorax is the next most common site. The diagnosis is usually confirmed by a bone marrow aspiration and raised 24-h urinary catecholamines. If both these findings are not present, surgical biopsy will be needed to confirm the diagnosis. Beware anaesthesia for children with mediastinal masses (particularly anterior mediastinal masses). Anaesthesia is fraught with problems, mainly due to compression of large airways. This may require the use of rigid ventilating bronchoscopes and should only be performed by experienced paediatric anaesthetists in specialist centres.

Further reading
Cheung SLW, Lerman J 1998 Mediastinal masses and anaesthesia in children. *Anesthesiology Clinics of North America* 16(4): 893–910. WB Saunders, Philadelphia.
Filler RM, Simpson JS, Ein SH 1979 Mediastinal masses in infants and children. *Pediatric Clinics of North America* 26: 677–691. WB Saunders, Philadelphia.

8

A

Answer 8.18

a. The supine abdominal film shows a soft tissue density mass in the right upper quadrant of the abdomen. There is no evidence of small bowel dilatation or perforation. This appearance is typical of intussusception. In infants, intussusception is usually idiopathic, possibly related to inflammation of Peyer's patches in association with viral illnesses. In older children and adults, there is usually a predisposing abnormality giving rise to the lead point. These include Meckel's diverticulum, polyp, lymphoma and inspissated faeces in children with cystic fibrosis.

b. The diagnosis is now often made on ultrasound in which the intussusception has a characteristic 'pseudokidney' appearance (see below).

c. Uncomplicated cases can usually be reduced radiologically using contrast medium or air under general anaesthesia. If this fails, then a laparotomy will be required. These infants are often extremely dehydrated since large amounts of fluid are sequestered in the bowel and this needs to be carefully considered in their preoperative assessment – 40 mL/kg of intravenous fluid resuscitation is often required perioperatively.

Further reading

Paes RA, Hyde L, Griffith DM 1988 The management of intussusception. *British Journal of Radiology* 67: 187–189.

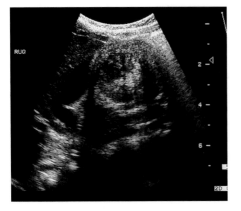

Answer 8.19

a. This film shows marked hyperinflation of the lungs (low flat diaphragms, narrow mediastinum), bronchial wall thickening, ring shadows and small mottled opacities. These changes are often maximal in the mid and upper zones. The diaphragm is low due to airflow obstruction. These features are typical of cystic fibrosis.

b. The diagnosis is cystic fibrosis. A sweat test is the most commonly used test in the diagnosis of cystic fibrosis. It usually measures the chloride, sodium and osmolality of sweat. Some antibiotics may cause false-positive results and the test should therefore be delayed until after a treatment course is finished. Gene probes are increasingly being used. They can detect up to 95% of the commonly occurring mutations resulting in cystic fibrosis.

c. In this condition, the lungs appear normal at birth but abnormal mucociliary clearance soon leads to obstruction of small airways causing hyperinflation of the lungs due to air trapping. Infection supervenes leading to microabscesses, which appear as small peripheral opacities on the chest radiograph. Inflammatory infiltrates in the bronchial walls lead to an accentuation of the bronchial wall pattern; this is seen as parallel lines or ring shadows. Eventually, there is evidence of bronchiectasis.

   Infection can cause segmental consolidation. Areas of segmental collapse can also be seen if a mucous plug occludes a larger airway. In some cases, the hila are enlarged. This can be due either to lymph node enlargement as a response to infection, or, in advanced cases, to pulmonary hypertension leading to enlargement of the proximal pulmonary arteries.

Further reading

Walsh TS, Young CH 1995 Anaesthesia and Cystic Fibrosis. *Anaesthesia* 50: 614–622.

Answer 8.20

a. This film shows healing fractures of the second to fifth ribs on the right and the third to fifth ribs on the left. There is apparent widening of the ribs due to callus formation. Rib fractures in infants and small children are very unusual due to the springiness of children's bones.

b. The presenting injury and X-ray findings should always arouse suspicion of non-accidental injury (NAI). In NAI, fractures typically occur in the posterior and lateral aspects of the ribs. They are due to extreme compressive forces when the child is held around the thorax and tightly squeezed. This may also explain the presentation of this child. This child will need to be treated sensitively in the perioperative period.

Answer 8.21

a. • Check patient details.
   • Is the film adequate?
   • Anterior soft tissue.
   • Spinal lines – the cervical spine bony elements should form a relatively smooth curve. Four lines may be constructed (as in the figure below):

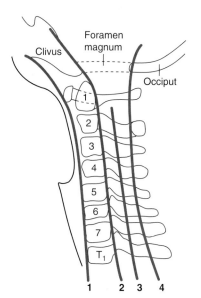

Reproduced with permission from *Advanced Paediatric Life Support* manual.

(1) the anterior spinal line follows the anterior spinal ligament; (2) the posterior spinal line follows the posterior spinal ligament; (3) the spinolaminar line follows the laminae; (4) a final line should link the tips of the spinal processes.
   • Disc spaces should be equal.
   • Spinous processes.
   • Facet joints – these should be parallel with equal joint spaces.
   • The atlantoaxial distance.

b. This is a normal lateral cervical neck X-ray.

c. Little clinical information has been made available to you, and radiological information must not be considered in isolation. If the child is complaining of cervical pain, is tender to palpation, has muscle spasm or restricted movements or is unconscious, the collar should stay in place, and senior assessment and further investigations undertaken. In a recent series, 44% of children with spinal cord injuries had normal lateral neck X-ray plain films (SCIWORA – **s**pinal **c**ord **i**njury **w**ithout **r**adiographic **a**bnormality).

Further reading

Baker C, Kadish H, Schunk JE 1999 Evaluation of pediatric cervical spine injuries. *American Journal of Emergency Medicine* 17: 230–234.
Interpreting trauma X-rays. In: Advanced Life Support Group. 2001 Advanced Paediatric Life Support; the practical approach. 3rd ed. BMJ Publishing, London.

Answer 8.22

a. The posterior spinal line at C2/3 is broken with an obvious step present. This is a normal variant, present in up to 40% of children under the age of 8 years. In the child's neck, the fulcrum for flexion and extension is roughly at C2/3 or C3/4 (as opposed to C5/6 in adults). This, in combination with generalised laxity of ligaments and a film taken somewhat flexed, gives the appearance of cervical subluxation, called 'cervical pseudosubluxation'. The clue that this is pysiological rather than traumatic is due to the lack of assoicated soft tissue swelling. As with many paediatric radiographs, this requires an experienced radiological opinion.

b. Multiple other variants from adult appearances occur in children, due to developing growth plates, the development of a cervical lordosis with increasing age etc. This makes interpretation of paediatric neck X-rays difficult. Important ones to be aware of include:

- The odontoid peg does not fuse with the body of the axis until 3–6 years of age. This synchondrosis may be misinterpreted as a fracture.
- Anterosuperior edges of vertebral bodies are commonly wedged.
- An increased distance of anterior aspect of the odontoid peg and posterior aspect of the anterior arch of the atlas (the atlanto-dens interval) – up to 4.5 mm is acceptable.
- The presence of vertebral body growth plates.

c. Fortunately, cervical spine injuries in children are uncommon (0.2% of all fractures and dislocations). In infants and children under the age of 8 years, fractures most commonly occur at the level of the atlas, axis and dens. In older children the pattern of injury is similar to adults and is centred on the lower cervical vertebrae.

Further reading
Glasgow JFT, Kerr GH 1997 *Management of Injuries in Children*. BMJ Publishing, London.

Answer 8.23

a. The atlanto-dens interval is 5 mm during flexion, representing atlantoaxial subluxation.

b. Although there are case reports of subluxation and cord injury after intubation, the majority of anaesthetists would probably not obtain radiographs preoperatively in asymptomatic children. X-ray criteria are not felt to be predictive of a tendency to dislocate. In addition,

signs and symptoms typically precede dislocations.

Further reading
Davidson RG 1988 Atlanto-axial instability in Down's syndrome: a fresh look at the evidence. *Pediatrics* 81: 857–865.
Mitchell V, Howard R, Facer E 1995 Down's syndrome and anaesthesia. *Paediatric Anaesthesia* 5: 379–384.

Answer 8.24

a. This is an AP CXR of a 6-year-old child. It is well centred and penetrated. The mediastinum is shifted to the right with opacification throughout the right lung field. An air bronchogram is shown involving the right main bronchus. The diaphragm is visible on the right and is elevated, suggesting pulmonary collapse. The opacification is greatest above the horizontal fissure; therefore the right upper lobe is predominantly affected. This is consistent with aspiration of gastric contents leading to pulmonary collapse.

b. The diagnosis is aspiration pneumonia. She has regurgitated and aspirated gastric contents on manipulation of her wrist. Gastric emptying ceases after trauma and therefore routine fasting times should be viewed with caution, particularly in children and particularly if anxious or in pain.

c. Pulmonary aspiration is a significant cause of morbidity and mortality from anaesthesia. Indeed, the first anaesthetic death, that of Hannah Greener in 1848, is thought to have occurred secondary to gastric aspiration during chloroform anaesthesia. The current incidence of aspiration has been estimated at 4.7 cases per 100 000 anaesthetics. Gastric contents of more than 25 mL (in an adult) and with a pH < 2.5 are especially damaging to the lung and associated with a high mortality. Problems may be divided into immediate airway obstruction requiring bronchoscopy and lung damage secondary to pneumonitis. There is a spectrum of presentation from mild soiling requiring suction, physiotherapy and oxygen, to one of severe bronchospasm and hypoxia requiring mechanical ventilation, inotropes and bronchodilators. Ventilating in the lateral or prone position may help to clear pulmonary secretions. Steroids are not beneficial except as a bronchodilator. Antibiotics are indicated when infection is evident.

d. Repeated aspiration is a feature in the elderly and intubated patients in ITU. Bacterial infection is a problem in about 40% of cases and this may lead to long-term complications, including empyema and abscess formation and fibrosis. The patient may develop acute respiratory distress syndrome (ARDS). The immediate mortality is 10% but can rise in intractable cases to 50%.

Further reading

Cooper DJ 1997 Aspiration syndromes. In: Oh TE, ed. *Intensive Care Manual*, 4th edn. Butterworth Heinemann, Oxford.

Olsson GL, Hallen B, Hambraeus-Jonzon K 1986 Aspiration during anaesthesia: a computer-aided study of 185,358 anaesthetics. *Acta Anaesthesiologica Scandanavica* 30: 84–92.

Answer 8.25

a. These are sleep study tracings. Airflow measurement was absent, since it was tolerated by the child. Periods of oxygen desaturation are demonstrated, associated with a rise in heart rate and vigorous respiratory effort. the respitrace shows regular arousals, confirmed on video footage. This is a typical picture of obstructive sleep apnoea.

b. This is a classical description of the Pierre–Robin sequence (mandibular hypoplasia and glossoptosis). A sequence is where a constellation of factors or abnormalities occur together to form a characteristic clinical pattern.

By itself, a sequence does not describe the underlying genetic cause of the clinical picture.

c. The commonest genetic cause for Pierre–Robin sequence is the Stickler syndrome. (This has been blamed for Abraham Lincoln's appearance, amongst others.) Stickler is most commonly an autosomal dominant mutation of the type II collagen (COL2a., {120140.0005) gene.

d. The associated abnormalities are due to the collagen defects; there are facial abnormalities, with a flat face, depressed nasal bridge, cleft palate and tooth abnormalities. The visual aspects include retinal detachment, glaucoma, occasional cataracts and progressive myopia. There is often sensorineural hearing loss. Cardiovascular problems relate to mitral valve prolapse. Skeletal problems are due to joint laxity and these may lead to scoliosis, kyphosis, arachnodactyly, arthropathy and irregular femoral epiphyses.

e. Anaesthetic considerations include:

- An airway that may be extremely difficult to maintain and to intubate. This is especially true in this case that has demonstrated severe sleep apnoea. It is likely to be associated with right heart failure and this should be investigated preoperatively.
- The mitral valve disease will require consideration of prophylactic antibiotics, and ideally a Doppler visualisation of the heart should be available.
- Positioning problems. The joint laxity may lead to pressure of direct nerve injury.

Further reading

Stickler syndrome. In: Baum VC, O'Flaherty JE, 1999. *Anaesthesia for Genetic, Metabolic and Dysmorphic Syndromes of Children*. Lippincott, Williams & Wilkins.

9

PAIN MANAGEMENT

Injections and practical procedures obviously play only a small part in the whole range of biopsychosocial methods in pain management. Historically, the involvement of anaesthetists in pain management arose largely from their familiarity with techniques of neural blockade. In recent years, there has been a swing away from a solely invasive approach to a multidisciplinary and broad-based physical, pharmacological and behavioural approach. Injections are only a small part of the overall armamentarium of the pain clinician, and a considerable range in the degree of invasiveness of approach exists between individual clinicians.

Despite this, a range of invasive procedures remains useful in pain management and knowledge of details of these is important. In anaesthetic examinations, images of X-ray appearances during procedures may be used as foci for questioning and this is the format adopted in this section: the procedures are a selection of those in common clinical use, and of which knowledge might be expected of a trainee sitting the Anaesthetic Fellowship examination. For all the procedures discussed below, it is of course essential that fully informed consent is obtained, that there is immediate availability of resuscitation drugs and equipment and that contraindications to the procedures are excluded. It must be stressed that though there is no single correct method of performance of these procedures, the brief descriptions here are of methods that work and are distilled from various sources as well as experience in practicing and teaching them. The detailed techniques are not described, but these may be sought from the authoritative texts described below. A detailed knowledge of relative anatomy is crucial.

FURTHER READING

Adriaensen H et al 1998 The place of nerve blocks and invasive methods in pain therapy: evidence-based results in chronic pain relief. In: Zenz M, ed. *Baillière's Clinical Anaesthesiology* 12(1): 69–87.

Cousins MJ, Bridenbaugh PO (eds) 1998 *Neural Blockade in Clinical Anesthesia and Management of Pain*, 3rd edn. JB Lippincott Company, Philadelphia.

Diamond AW, Coniam SW 1997 *The Management of Chronic Pain*, 2nd edn, Oxford University Press, Oxford.

Dolin S, Padfield N, Pateman J (eds) 1996 *Pain Clinic Manual*. Butterworth-Heinemann, Oxford.

Wedley JR, Gauci CA 1994 *Handbook of Clinical Techniques in the Management of Chronic Pain*. Harwood Academic Publishers, Reading.

9
Q

QUESTIONS

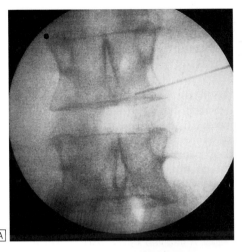

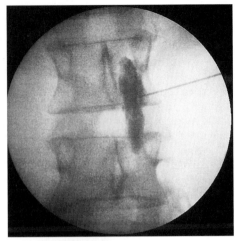

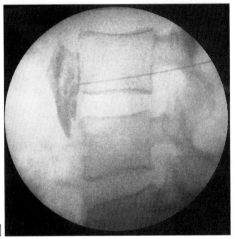

Question 9.1

The vascular surgical team refer a 68-year-old man complaining of rest pain and a non-healing superficial ulcer on his left ankle to you. Amongst other findings, their investigations showed an ankle brachial pressure index (ABPI) of 0.7 and the angiographic appearances confirmed that this patient was unsuitable for surgery. They requested assistance in improving skin blood flow in the affected lower extremity and pain relief.

As a result, a procedure was carried out under radiological guidance, and (A)–(C) are a series of images generated during the procedure. They have been reproduced from the image intensifier for storage in the medical records of this patient.

a. What is this procedure?
b. Describe the relevant anatomy.
c. What side-effects and complications might be encountered?

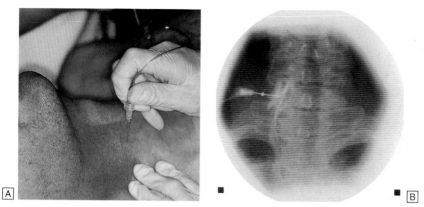

Question 9.2

A 40-year-old man presents following referral from the orthopaedic surgeon with a history of an injury to his right wrist. He subsequently developed a complex regional pain syndrome (CRPS) type 1 with marked colour change and sweating. As part of his management, the procedure illustrated was performed (A, B).

a. What is this procedure?
b. What might be the indications for its performance?
c. What are the anatomical considerations and describe a technique for performing this block.
d. What effects would you look for?
e. What are the possible side-effects of this procedure?

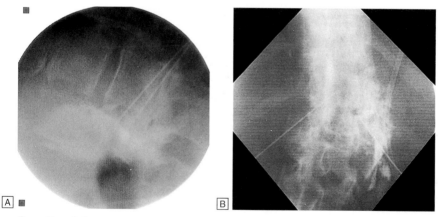

Question 9.3

A 63-year-old woman with a long previous history of back pain presents with pain from a recurrence of carcinoma of the pancreas demonstrated on CT scanning 9 months after a Whipple's operation. After initial attempts to manage her pain non-invasively, she undergoes the procedure whose radiographic appearance is shown here (A, B), with excellent relief of her symptoms.

a. What procedure is shown here, and what other indications are there for its performance?
b. Describe the relevant anatomy.
c. What side-effects and complications may be encountered?
d. What initial methods might be used to manage her pain?

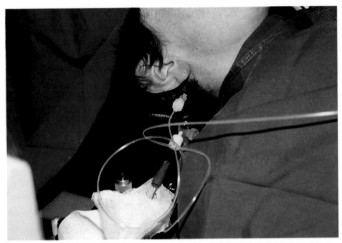

A

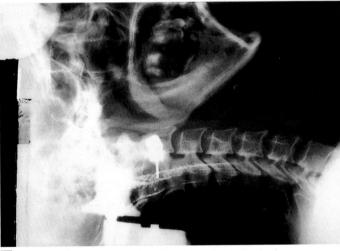

B

Question 9.4

A 36-year-old woman with secondary spread of cervical carcinoma develops tumour invasion of the femoral nerve, with very severe unremitting pain unresponsive to non-invasive methods. After consideration of further options and discussion with the patient, the procedure depicted is performed (A, B), with good relief of her symptoms.

a. Briefly outline the initial management methods that might be used for this neurogenic pain.
b. What is the procedure shown?
c. What might be the indications for it?
d. What complications may be encountered?

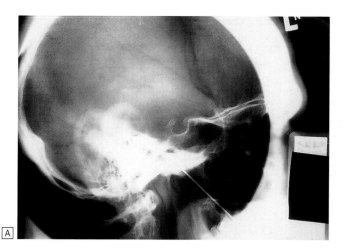

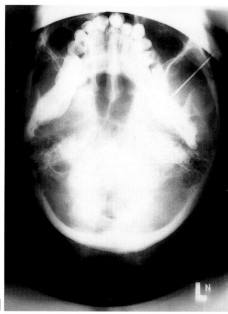

Question 9.5

A 56-year-old woman is referred from her general dental practitioner with a history of severe attacks of left-sided facial pain in the distribution of the mandibular division of the trigeminal nerve. The pain is episodic and is described by the patient as being like a severe electric shock. She gives a history of previous episodes when she had experienced the pain, with periods of remission in between. Previously the pain had responded to oral medication, but on this occasion it is ineffective. Clinical examination reveals no neurological abnormality, although she has two discrete areas where light touch could precipitate her pain.

a. What procedure is shown in (A) and (B) and what is the likely diagnosis?
b. Describe the clinical presentation and pathogenesis of this condition.
c. What is the differential diagnosis?
d. What is the usual initial medical treatment?
e. What other approaches are there for the treatment of this condition?

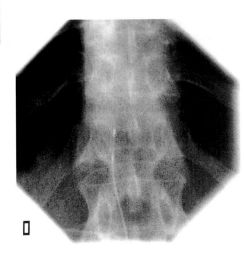

Question 9.6

A 39-year-old woman developed severe neurogenic pain in her left lower leg after knee surgery, refractory to extensive treatment. Eventually she proceeded to undergo the procedure during which this radiograph was taken, with resulting good relief of her pain.

a. What is this procedure?

b. What are the indications for this procedure?

c. Briefly outline what you know about the technique.

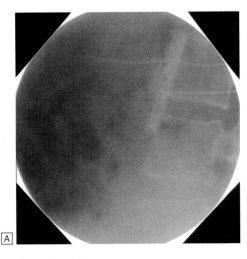

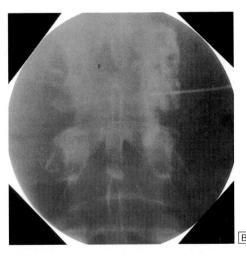

A

B

Question 9.7

A 67-year-old man with intractable lower limb pain from ischaemia has been seen by the pain team and has failed to improve on drug therapy alone. A trial block with local anaesthetic was performed which resulted in a marked improvement in his symptoms. A more permanent neurolytic block is performed during which these images (A, B) are taken from the image intensifier.

a. What block has been performed?

b. Describe a suitable and safe technique for this procedure.

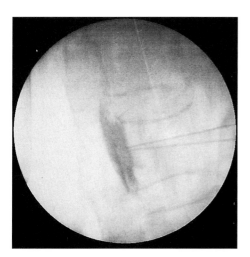

Question 9.8

A 74-year-old patient presents with lower limb pain in both legs. After unsuccessful medical treatment, he presents for the treatment shown.

a. What procedure has been performed?
b. What complications could arise from this?
c. What are the technical problems associated with performing such blocks?

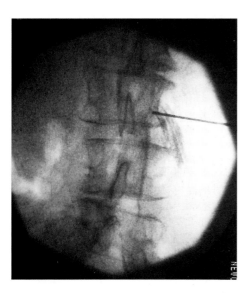

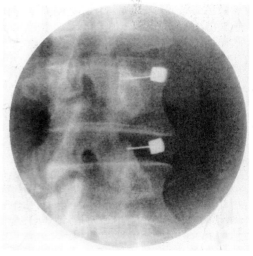

Question 9.9

A 78-year-old man undergoes a lumbar sympathetic block. During the procedure this image is taken on injection of contrast medium.

a. Describe the image.
b. What has happened?
c. What are the potential complications of this?

Question 9.10

A 50-year-old man presented with back pain. As part of his management, combined with rehabilitative measures, a procedure with this radiographic appearance was performed.

a. What is this procedure?
b. What clinical scenario might lead to its performance?
c. Discuss the anatomy and briefly outline the procedure used.

ANSWERS

Answer 9.1

a. This is a lumbar sympathetic block. (A) shows the ideal needle position in the position of the sympathetic chain. (B) and (C) are PA and lateral views, respectively, of the ideal spread of contrast medium within the anatomical boundaries occupied by the lumbar sympathetic chain. This patient represents one of the commonest reason for a neurolytic lumbar sympathetic block, with vascular insufficiency and rest pain of the lower extremity.

Local anaesthetic blockade of the sympathetic chain may be used as a diagnostic and prognostic block for proposed neurolytic blockade. Local anaethetic block may also be used as part of treatment for neurogenic pain.

b. The sympathetic outflow from the spinal cord is thoracolumbar from T1 to L2 or L3. At each level the rami communicantes carry fibres from the anterior spinal nerve roots anteriorly to the sympathetic chain. The lumbar sympathetic chain lies on the anterolateral aspect of the vertebral bodies just anterior to the psoas fascia in the paracolic gutter. An important relation is the genitofemoral nerve which runs down the anterior surface of the psoas sheath and which may be affected by lateral spread of neurolytic agent.

c. Side-effects and complications are:

- Local bruising, haematoma formation and discomfort.
- Postural hypotension is unusual after unilateral sympathectomy, and if it occurs it generally settles rapidly.
- Groin pain is relatively common after neurolytic sympathectomy and is usually of short duration. It is frequently burning or aching in nature and often responds to treatment with tricyclics or TENS. The cause for this pain is uncertain, although it has been thought to be genitofemoral neuralgia. It also occurs on occasion after open surgical sympathectomy.
- Ejaculatory incompetence can occur with bilateral high lumbar neurolytic blocks.
- In patients with large vessel occlusion and an ABPI below about 40%, there is a potential for 'steal' from the muscles to the skin after neurolytic sympathectomy. This may worsen claudication, and many reserve sympathectomy for the treatment of rest pain or skin ulceration.

Further reading

Dobrogowski J 1995 Chemical sympathectomy. *The Pain Clinic* 8: 93–97.

Hughes JH 1996 Reflex sympathetic dystrophy – causalgia. In: Dolin S, Padfield N, Pateman J, eds. *Pain Clinic Manual*. Butterworth-Heinemann, Oxford, pp. 17–37.

Wang JK, Erikson RP, Ilstrup DM 1985 Repeated stellate ganglion blocks for upper extremity reflex sympathetic dystrophy. *Regional Anaesthesia* 10: 125.

Answer 9.2

a. (B) is an X-ray image taken during a stellate ganglion block (A).

b. Sympathetic blockade of the upper extremity is used for the following:

- to cause temporary vasodilatation, particularly in acute vascular disorders such as post-traumatic vasospasm, inadvertent intra-arterial irritant injection or cold injury
- for diagnosis and management of neurogenic pain of the arm or head and neck
- it may be of use in the management of angina
- there is some evidence that sympathetic blockade very early in the course of shingles may reduce the incidence of post-herpetic neuralgia.

c. The stellate ganglion is formed by the fusion of the seventh and eighth cervical and first thoracic sympathetic ganglia. It lies anterior to the prevertebral fascia and longus colli muscle over the transverse processes of the C7 and T1 vertebrae, posterior to the carotid sheath and, at its lower end, the dome of the pleura. The surface markings are a point level with the cricoid cartilage, 3 cm above and 2 cm lateral to the suprasternal notch. As with all regional blocks, intravenous access must be established and availability of resuscitation drugs and equipment ensured. Although the procedure is often performed without screening, the availability of x-ray screening makes it far easier and safer, particularly in patients with thick necks.

The patient's neck should be extended, and he should be asked to open his mouth and breathe to discourage swallowing, with resultant needle movement and increased risk of trauma. The transverse process of C6 may occasionally be felt at the point described above, and the carotid sheath may be distracted laterally. After cleaning the skin a small skin bleb of local anaesthetic is injected and then a suitable needle is inserted directly backwards to contact the tubercle of the C6 transverse process or the lateral aspect of its body (some authors advise C7 but that places the needle much nearer the pleura). After touching bone, the needle is withdrawn 2 mm to lie anterior to the prevertebral fascia.

After careful aspiration (an extension tube on the needle, with an experienced assistant manipulating the syringe, can make this much easier), a very small test dose of approximately 0.5 ml is made and then slow injection of up to 10–15 ml of local anaesthetic solution. The patient should be closely observed for a period afterwards in case of side-effects.

d. A Horner's syndrome should be seen. The earliest sign of a Horner's syndrome is dilatation of the ipsilateral conjunctival blood vessels, followed by the appearance of miosis, ptosis and stuffiness of the nose on the affected side. Enophthalmos and ipsilateral anhidrosis are rarely noted clinically.

Increased skin temperature and vasodilatation of the ipsilateral hand and arm should also be noted.

e. Side-effects include:

- local bruising and pain
- systemic toxicity – the stellate ganglion is in a very vascular area
- vertebral artery puncture and intra-arterial LA – this is the main reason for the small test dose and slow injection, since negative aspiration is no absolute guarantee of safe needle placement. If local anaesthetic is inadvertently injected into the vertebral artery, immediate loss of consciousness and convulsion are likely.
- brachial plexus block
- intrathecal block by penetration of a dural nerve root sleeve
- recurrent laryngeal block resulting in a transiently husky voice
- phrenic nerve block
- pneumothorax – the dome of the pleura comes up to the level of C7
- oesophageal perforation and mediastinitis, osteitis of the transverse process.

Further reading
World Health Organisation 1986 *Cancer Pain Relief.* World Health Organisation, Geneva.

Answer 9.3

a. This is the X-ray appearance of a coeliac plexus block. The indications may be either diagnostic or therapeutic: the coeliac plexus carries sympathetic afferent sensation of pain from the pancreas and other upper abdominal viscera, and blockade may allow the differentiation of visceral or somatic sources of pain in this area. Neurolytic blockade of the coeliac plexus is a valuable technique in the relief of pain from malignant disease in the organs innervated through it, particularly pancreatic carcinoma.

In this context, it is being used as an alternative analgesic technique, because her pain is inadequately controlled by the use of oral opioids and adjuvant medications, or in whom the use of these drugs gives unacceptable side-effects.

b. The coeliac plexus is formed by the union of the greater, lesser and least splanchnic nerves with the coeliac branch of the right vagus. The splanchnic nerves penetrate the crura of the diaphragm, pass into the coeliac ganglia anterior to the body of L1 and their post-ganglionic fibres and form the coeliac plexus on the anterior surface of the aorta anterior to the body of L1, carrying sensation from the upper gastrointestinal tract, liver, pancreas, ureters, upper colon and the vessels to the abdominal viscera.

c. Side-effects and complications include:

- initial bruising and discomfort
- diarrhoea, hypotension, bleeding – indeed, some practitioners feel that a drop in blood pressure is an essential indicator of a successful block. This is not, however, a reliable sign. Some degree of postural hypotension is common, although this generally settles in a few days
- failure of ejaculation due to interruption of the central connections of the hypogastric plexus
- haematuria
- groin pain from damage to L1 root
- rare cases of paraplegia, probably from anterior spinal artery syndrome, have been reported, and very occasional transient weakness of the lower extremities can occur.

d. Initially, her pain must be assessed to ensure that the pain is indeed that of pancreatic carcinoma, to check for other sources and types of pain and to establish what analgesia is being used already. The initial pharmacological management should be with analgesics according to the WHO analgesic ladder, and in patients like this it is often necessary to move rapidly to the strong opioid level on this. The initial dose requirement should be titrated with an immediately acting oral morphine preparation given regularly four hourly, with additional immediately acting oral morphine also available for breakthrough analgesia. Once adequate analgesia has been established then the daily dose requirement can be given as a sustained release preparation, maintaining availability of immediate release oral morphine for breakthrough analgesia. It is also worth giving adjuvant medication, such as paracetamol or another non-steroidal drug, and ensuring that laxative cover is given and antiemetic medication, if required, is prescribed.

Further reading

Davies DD 1993 Incidence of major complications of neurolytic coeliac plexus block. *Journal of the Royal Society of Medicine* 86: 264–266.

Eisenberg E, Carr DB, Chalmers TC 1995 Neurolytic celiac plexus block for treatment of cancer pain: a meta-analysis. *Anesthesia & Analgesia* 80: 290–295.

Answer 9.4

a. The nature of the pain should be assessed and, in particular, assessment should be made of its causes. Likely findings, which were present in this case, are weakness of the affected area with sensory abnormalities and loss, allodynia (abnormal painful sensation to light touch, often described as burning and stinging in nature) and hyperpathia (exaggerated and escalating painful response on repetitive stimulation, continuing for a prolonged period after cessation of stimulation).

Neurogenic pain of this sort may frequently be poorly responsive to opioids alone, although a trial of opioids according to the WHO ladder should be considered. In addition, the use of adjuvant medications such as tricyclic antidepressants, anticonvulsants and membrane-stabilising agents should be tried. Other techniques that may be of use include transcutaneous nerve stimulation (TENS), and if oral medications have not been successful then the use of subcutaneous infusions of ketamine, spinally administered analgesics, intrathecal neurolysis or the procedure shown may be considered.

b. (B) is the X-ray appearance of percutaneous cervical cordotomy (A), a technique that involves creating a radiofrequency lesion in the anterolateral spinothalamic tract at the level of the C1–C2 interspace in the neck.

c. The indications for a cervical cordotomy include:

- unilateral pain below C5 unresponsive to simpler methods of treatment
- short life expectancy – although the lesion is permanent, CNS plasticity means that the relief may not last more than 6–18 months and 'de-afferentation pain' may ensue.

The use of percutaneous cordotomy, although still potentially very valuable in the management of cancer pain, has reduced in recent years due to improvements in the use of spinal opioid and other drug administration.

d. Complications include the following:

- bilateral high cervical cordotomy carries a risk of central sleep apnoea ('Ondine's curse') and respiratory compromise
- motor deficit and bladder dysfunction
- headache
- thermo-anaesthesia on the side opposite the lesion
- Horner's syndrome
- infection and meningitis
- sympathetic fibre lesioning.

Answer 9.5

a. These images are taken during Gasserian ganglion radiofrequency neurolysis. The needle tip is passing through the foramen ovale into the trigeminal ganglion. The most likely diagnosis is trigeminal neuralgia.

b. Trigeminal neuralgia is an intensely painful condition. The typical presentation is as described in the question: there is severe episodic pain, the attacks being of brief duration and recurring frequently, with the periods of painful episodes being followed by remissions, although there is often a tendency for the painful periods to become more frequent. It may occur in any of the three divisions of the trigeminal nerve, although it most frequently occurs in the mandibular division. There are often one or more areas where very light stimulation, even talking or air currents over the skin, may precipitate attacks. This may lead to the patient avoiding stimulation of the face, including washing or shaving. Some patients may find, paradoxically, that firm pressure over the face can relieve the pain. Examination should not reveal any sensory or other neurological abnormalities and these, if present, should raise the suspicion of other causes of the pain, such as tumour or demyelinating disease.

In a large number of patients, trigeminal neuralgia may be caused by, or at least associated with, compression of the roots of the trigeminal nerve by an aberrant loop of artery, which may lead to local demyelination and ectopic electrical activity of the nerve. Microvascular decompression may lead to long-term relief of symptoms.

c. Multiple sclerosis, vascular abnormalities or tumours may cause similar symptoms, but these may be associated with more persistent background pain, as well as facial sensory or other neurological abnormalities. Certainly in young patients the diagnosis of multiple sclerosis should always be considered. Other sources of facial pain may include cluster headaches, atypical facial pain and post-herpetic neuralgia, although clinically the latter is very distinct from trigeminal neuralgia. The diagnosis of trigeminal neuralgia is mostly made on the history and the findings on examination of the patient, but MRI and, if equipment and expertise permit, MR angiography, may be used to demonstrate compression and to eliminate other causes such as tumour and demyelinating disease.

d. Initial treatment of the condition should be with oral medication, with carbamazepine remaining the drug of first choice. A good response to the use of carbamazepine makes the diagnosis of trigeminal neuralgia more likely. It used to be held that response of the pain to treatment with carbamazepine was pathognomonic, and that failure of response implied that the diagnosis was not trigeminal neuralgia. This is now known to be false, and indeed only 60–70% of patients do respond to a useful degree. The addition of baclofen or clonazepam may increase the success of treatment. Other anticonvulsant drugs have also been used, including phenytoin, valproate and more recently gabapentin.

e. Other approaches to the treatment of this condition include:

- Peripheral blockade of branches of the trigeminal nerve or even section or avulsion of its branches has been used in trigeminal neuralgia but is less useful than more central approaches.
- Local anaesthetic and steroid blockade at the foramen ovale may be of use in some patients and is often done before radiofrequency or other permanent lesioning to assess effect and to allow patients to assess whether the resulting anaesthesia will be acceptable to them.
- Radiofrequency lesioning of the trigeminal ganglion where it lies in Meckel's cave within the foramen ovale has been extensively used. This procedure carries potential complications of infection, anaesthesia dolorosa (the development of dysaesthetic neurogenic pain in the anaesthetic distribution of the lesioned nerve) and ophthalmic anaesthesia with the potential for corneal ulceration. Herpes zoster activation may follow blockade of the Gasserian ganglion. It is an unpleasant procedure

for the patient and, with the increasing use of microvascular decompression, it is increasingly reserved for patients unfit for this procedure.

- Gasserian ganglion glycerol blockade is an alternative technique and may be associated with less risk of corneal anaesthesia. Blockade with alcohol is less commonly performed nowadays.
- Surgical treatment: microvascular decompression or potentially partial sensory rhizotomy. Surgical treatment has good efficacy and is increasingly considered as the invasive method of first choice, after failed medical treatment, in patients who are fit to undergo this treatment. Success rates in excess of 90% may be achieved.

Further reading
Hakanson S 1984 Tic douleureux treated by the injection of glycerol into the retrogasserian subarachnoid space; long term results. *Acta Neurochirurgica Supplementum* 33: 471–472.

Janetta PJ 1977 Treatment of trigeminal neuralgia by suboccipital and transcranial operations. *Clinical Neurosurgery* 24: 538–549.

Answer 9.6

a. The X-ray shows the electrode of a spinal cord stimulator positioned in the thoracic epidural space.

b. Indications for this procedure include:

- ischaemic pain, particularly angina and peripheral vascular disease – these indications have the most encouraging outcomes for this technique
- phantom limb pain
- arachnoiditis and other neurogenic pains
- other somatic pains resistant to treatment, although opinion varies on this and in particular the results of spinal cord stimulation in patients with failed back surgery may be poor.

c. Electrical stimulation has been used to produce analgesia for centuries; the first recorded use was in Egyptian records, of electric fish being applied to treat painful conditions. After the publication of the gate control theory of pain in 1965, the use of electrical stimulation-produced analgesia expanded and dorsal column stimulation by implanted electrodes has been used in pain management since the late 1960s. This technique can be useful for pain and also for other conditions such as spasticity, bladder control, peripheral vascular disease and angina. The mechanism by which it achieves its results is uncertain.

The procedure involves implantation of electrodes into the epidural space to overlie the dorsal columns, either surgically at laminectomy or percutaneously. Usually multipolar electrodes are used, with testing at insertion to ensure that the stimulation evoked is in the area of the pain. Patient selection for this procedure needs to be very stringent: full psychological assessment needs to be performed and trial stimulation prior to implantation of a permanent system is essential. Generally a trial period of 5–7 days' stimulation is performed before implantation of a permanent stimulator in order to assess the results.

Permanent stimulation may be by an internal or an external power source, the internal one being fully implanted with its own power source and stimulus generator, re-programmable by an external telemetric control, and the external one working via an induction loop implanted under the skin powered by an external loop and stimulus generator. This is bulky, but has the advantage that in the event of the need for battery change or reprogramming, further surgical intervention is avoided. Financial issues also arise – this is an expensive treatment with a high revision rate.

Further reading

Melzack R, Wall P 1965 Pain mechanisms: a new theory. *Science* 150: 971.

Shealy CN 1967 Electrical inhibition of pain by stimulation of the dorsal column. *Anaesthesia & Analgesia* 46: 489–491.

Answer 9.7

a. A lumbar sympathectomy has been performed using a neurolytic agent, commonly phenol.

b. This block may be performed with the patient lying prone or in the lateral position, with the side to be blocked uppermost on an X-ray screening table whilst the entry site is identified. There are various methods for this but a simple one is to take the midpoint between the 12th rib and the iliac crest and drop posteriorly along this line to the lateral edge of the erector spinae muscle. This is usually about 10 cm from the midline, and can be clearly felt by asking the patient to cough. For a patient in the lateral position, the inferior border of L3 is identified via X-ray screening (for a single-needle technique). Local anaesthetic is progressively infiltrated using a 5.25 inch 20G needle with the bevel orientated towards the vertebral body (to avoid digging into the periosteum and to allow it to slide anteriorly along the body). This is advanced onto the vertebral body and then walked anteriorly until it is felt to pass through the psoas sheath. This should be accompanied by a loss of resistance to injection. The needle tip should be level with the anterior border of the vertebral body on the lateral view, and within the line of the shadows of the pedicles (the 'owl's eyes') on the AP view.

A small amount of radio-opaque contrast medium is then injected and should spread up and down the anterior margin of the vertebral bodies on lateral screening (as shown in A and B). On AP screening, the spread of contrast should be along the line of the sympathetic chain, and within the confines of the body of the vertebrae. At the end of the injection, the needle should be cleared of neurolytic agent by injecting a small amount of air to avoid depositing phenol near the somatic nerves during its withdrawal. After the neurolytic block the patient should be kept lying in the lateral position for about 30 min to avoid lateral spread of neurolytic agent onto the genitofemoral nerve.

Needle positioning at the mid-body of the vertebra should be avoided: at this level there are vessels and a fibrous tunnel for the rami communicantes. If this is entered, it may result in posterior spread of the injected drug onto the somatic nerve roots. For this reason, intermittent observation of a lateral X-ray view of the spread of neurolytic agent mixed with contrast medium during the injection is desirable.

Answer 9.8

a. The patient has undergone bilateral lumbar sympathetic block.
b. Bilateral lumbar sympathetic block presents the potential for increased circulatory problems secondary to hypotension as well as care required with the dose of phenol.
c. There are also problems from a technical point of view. As this image shows, it is difficult to identify which side's contrast shadow is which. This may require rocking the patient or the image intensifier tube from side to side.

Answer 9.9

a. This is an AP image intensifier view of a lumbar sympathetic block on injection of contrast medium. The medium can be seen to spread out laterally away from the vertebral column in a distinct space.
b. This represents spread within the psoas sheath. This spread gives a characteristic appearance, with contrast outlining the muscle on the anteroposterior view.
c. Spread within the psoas sheath should be avoided since this may increase the risk of genitofemoral pain following a neurolytic block and will of course also reduce the effectiveness of the lumbar sympathetic block.

Answer 9.10

a. This is the radiographic appearance during injection of the right lumbar facet joints.
b. A typical history would be of a patient complaining of low back pain radiating into the buttocks and thighs in a non-dermatomal pattern, not normally extending below the knees. It is frequently worse on rising in the mornings and after prolonged sitting or standing, and exacerbated by extension and rotation of the back. Palpation over the facet joints is tender. Examination should not reveal any abnormal neurological signs, though straight leg raising may result in back pain.
c. The lumbar facet or zygapophyseal joints are true synovial joints, between the superior and inferior articular processes of adjacent vertebrae. Their capsules are richly innervated. Each joint receives innervation from a medial branch of the dorsal ramus at the same level as the vertebra as well as fibres from the dorsal ramus at the level above.

The procedure is performed with the patient prone under radiographic guidance, and either the patient is rotated slightly laterally or the image intensifier is rotated about 25 degrees from the AP plane to give an image of the facet joints. In this plane the characteristic appearance of 'scotty dogs' may be seen with the facet joint forming the back of the ear of each dog. Under aseptic conditions a needle is advanced into the joint and a small quantity of local anaesthetic with a depot steroid preparation is injected.

Some clinicians, as an alternative, block the medial branch of the posterior ramus and may, after good results from diagnostic injections, perform radiofrequency lesioning of the medial branch to provide longer term pain relief.

TABLE OF NORMAL VALUES

Haematology

Full Blood Count

Haemoglobin	(Hb)	
men		13.5–18 g/dl
women		11.5–16.5 g/dl
White Blood Cell Count		
(WBC)		$4–11 \times 10^9/l$
Platelet count		$150–400 \times 10^9/l$
Reticulocyte count		0–2% of rbcs
Mean corpuscular volume (MCV)		76–96 fl
Mean Corpuscular Haemoglobin Concentration (MCHC)		31–35 g/dl
Mean Corpuscular Haemoglobin (MCH)		27–32 pg

Clotting

Prothrombin time	14–18 s
Activated partial thromboplastin time	35–45 s
Fibrinogen	2–4 g/l
Fibrinogen degradation products	<10 mg/l

Biochemistry

Sodium	132–146 mmol/l
Potassium	3.5–5 mmol/l
Chloride	96–106 mmol/l
Bicarbonate (standard)	22–26 mmol/l
Urea	2.3–6.7 mmol/l
Creatinine	45–110 µmol/l
Random blood glucose	3–7.7 mmol/l
Alanine aminotransferase	<48 IU/l
Albumin	35–49 g/l
Alkaline phosphatase	30–100 IU/l
Aspartate aminotransferase	<45 IU/l
Bilirubin (total)	<17 mmol/l
Calcium (total)	2.25–2.62 mmol/l
Creatinine-phosphokinase	<60 IU/l
γ-glutamyl transferase	9–44 IU/l
Lactate (plasma)	0.63–2.44 mmol/l
Magnesium	0.7–1.1 mmol/l
Phosphate	0.8–1.6 mmol/l

Arterial Blood gases

pH	7.36–7.44
P_aO_2	12–14.7 kPas (90–110 mmHg)
P_aCO_2	4.53–6.13 kPas (34–46 mmHg)
Base excess	+/– 2 mmol/l

(Note: 1 kPa ≈ 7.52 mmHg)

The ECG

P wave	<2.5 mm tall
P-R interval	0.12–0.21 s
QRS width	<0.12 s
QRS height	S in V1 + R in V5 <35 mm
Frontal Axis	−30° to +90° (or 120°)

Pathological Q wave if >25% following R wave and >0.04 s width

Q-T interval	0.35–0.43 s

(Corrected to 60 bpm using Bazett's formula, $Q = QT \ int/\sqrt{R - R}$)

S-T elevation pathological if >1 mm and depression if > 0.5 mm

(Note: The term adrenaline is used interchangeably with epinephrine and noreadrenaline interchangeably with norepinephrine throughout the text)

INDEX

I

I